Color Atlas of Anatomy

A Photographic Study
of the Human Body

Second Edition

Color Atlas of Anatomy

A Photographic Study of the Human Body

Second Edition

JOHANNES W. ROHEN

Professor Dr. med., Dr. med. h. c.
Chairman, Department of Anatomy
University of Erlangen-Nürnberg, Germany

CHIHIRO YOKOCHI

Professor Emeritus, M. D.
Department of Anatomy
Kanagawa Dental College, Yokosuka, Japan

With the collaboration of E. C. B. Hall-Craggs
M. A., M. B., B. Chir., Ph. D., Professor of Anatomy
University of Maryland School of Medicine
Baltimore, Maryland

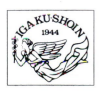

IGAKU-SHOIN New York • Tokyo

Published and distributed by

IGAKU-SHOIN Ltd.,
5-24-3 Hongo, Bunkyo-ku, Tokyo

IGAKU-SHOIN Medical Publishers, Inc.
1140 Avenue of the Americas, New York, N. Y. 10036

Library of Congress Cataloging-In-Publication Dats

Rohen, Johannes W. (Johannes Wilhelm)
  Color atlas of anatomy.

  Includes index.
  1. Anatomy, Human–Atlases, I. Yokochi, Chihiro,
II. Hall-Craggs, E. C. B. [DNLM: 1. Anatomy–atlases.
QS 17 R737c]
QM25.R55 1988   611'.0022'2   87-33906
ISBN 0-89640-141-3

ISBN 0-89640-141-3 (New York)
ISBN 4-260-14141-4 (Tokyo)

Printed in Germany

10 9 8 7 6 5 4 3 2 1

Preface to the Second Edition

The success of our photographic atlas has encouraged us to work intensively on its further improvement. Three years after the first printing, this second edition incorporates a number of photographs taken from newly dissected specimens as well as important CT scan figures and MR images. In addition, new drawings were included to facilitate the repetition of basic anatomical facts needed for an understanding of the macroscopic dissections. To avoid an undesirable increase in the volume size we omitted all figures of minor quality.

Each chapter in the second edition consists of two parts. The first part describes the anatomical structure of the organs in a systematic manner, e.g., in the case of an extremity: bones, joints, ligaments, muscles, blood vessels, and nerves. In the second part, the regional anatomy is depicted, so that the description of the superficial layers is followed by the deeper and deepest layers: thus the student in the lab can find the orientation needed for the dissection of the cadaver. When viewing the macrophotographs, the use of a magnifier is strongly recommended in order to identify more precisely the three-dimensional structure of the tissues and organs depicted.

While preparing this new edition, the authors were reminded of how precisely, beautifully, and admirably the human body is constructed. If this book helps the student or medical doctor to appreciate the overwhelming beauty of the anatomical architecture of tissues and organs in the human, then it greatly fulfills its task. Deep interest and admiration of the anatomical structures may create the "love for man", which alone can be considered of primary importance for daily medical work.

The new specimens were dissected with great skill and knowledge by Dr. M. Takahashi (Tokyo), Dr. G. Lindner-Funk, and Dr. P. Landgraf. Dr. Takahashi worked for two years in the Department of Anatomy in Erlangen and prepared the new specimens of the head, the face, the nasal cavity, the shoulder girdle, and the autonomic nervous system. Dr. Lindner-Funk dissected the new specimens of the cranial nerves, the orbit, the olfactory region, and the heart. Dr. Landgraf dissected those new specimens of the back and shoulder. All other specimens were dissected by the authors themselves.

We would like to express our great gratitude to all coworkers for their skilled work. Without their help the improvement of the atlas would not have been possible. We are indebted to the artists, Mrs. E. Ott-Freiberger, Ch. Wittek, and Mr. A. Atzenhofer, who made the new drawings in such an excellent manner, and particularly to the photographer, Mr. M. Gösswein, who made the very excellent macrophotographs. Thanks also to Dr. Lindner-Funk and all other coworkers, whose untiring and skilled work on this new edition of the atlas sped us to its finish.

We also express our sincere thanks to those at Igaku-Shoin and F. K. Schattauer who always listened to our suggestions and invested again a great deal of their effort into improving this book.

December 1987   J. W. Rohen, Erlangen
                                                   C. Yokochi, Yokosuka

Contents

Chapter I
General Anatomy

General Organization of the Human Body

In contrast to most other mammals the human body is adapted for bipedal locomotion. Three general principles in the architecture of the human organism are recognizable:

1. The principle of **segmentation,** which dominates in the trunk. The vertebral column and the thorax consist of relatively equal, segmentally arranged elements.

2. The principle of **bilateral symmetry.** Both sides of the body are separated by a midsagittal plane and resemble each other like image and mirror-image.

3. The principle of **polarity** between the head at one end of the body and the lower extremities at the other. As the center of the information system the head contains the main sensory organs and the brain. The head has a predominantly spherical form while the extremities consist of radially formed skeletal elements, the number of which increases distally.

A. The **skull** consists of two parts: 1. a **cranial part** containing mainly the brain and the sensory organs and 2. a **facial part** which contains the nasal and oral cavity and the chewing apparatus. The cranial cavity is continuous with the vertebral .canal which contains the spinal cord.

B. The **thorax** contains the respiratory and circulatory organs (lung, heart, etc.) but also some of the abdominal organs which are located underneath the diaphragm.

C. The **abdominal cavity** contains the organs of metabolism such as the liver, the stomach and the intestinal tract as well as the excretory and genital organs (kidney, uterus, urinary bladder, etc.). The latter are located primarily in the **pelvic cavity** (C_2) with the exception of the testes.

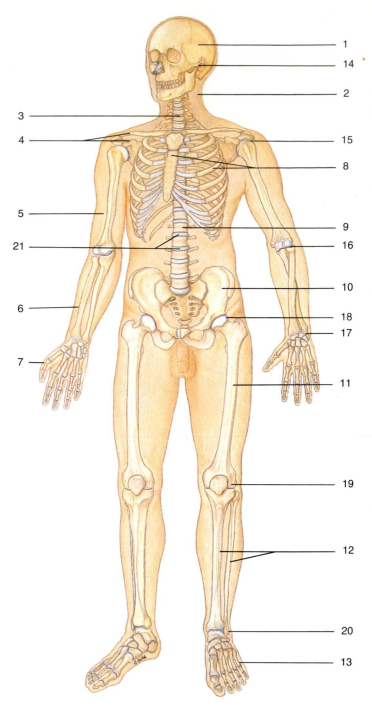

General view of the body and the skeleton.
Blue = joints.

1	Head
2	Neck
3	Vertebral column (cervical part)
4	Shoulder girdle
5	Arm (brachium)
6	Forearm (antebrachium)
7	Hand (manus)
8	Thorax and sternum
9	Vertebral column (lumbar portion)
10	Pelvic bones (pelvis)
11	Femur
12	Tibia and fibula
13	Foot

Joints (articulations)

14	Temporomandibular joint
15	Shoulder joint
16	Elbow joint
17	Radiocarpal joint
18	Hip joint
19	Knee joint
20	Ankle joint
21	Intervertebral discs

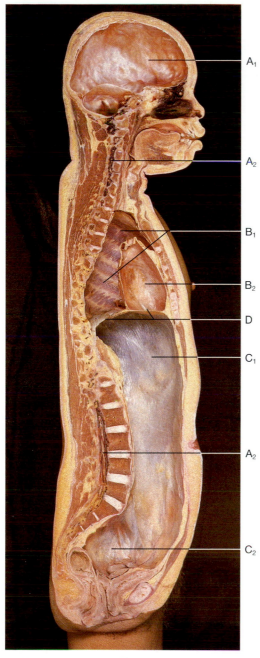

Sagittal section through the human body (female).
Demonstration of the main cavities of the body.
Internal organs are removed.

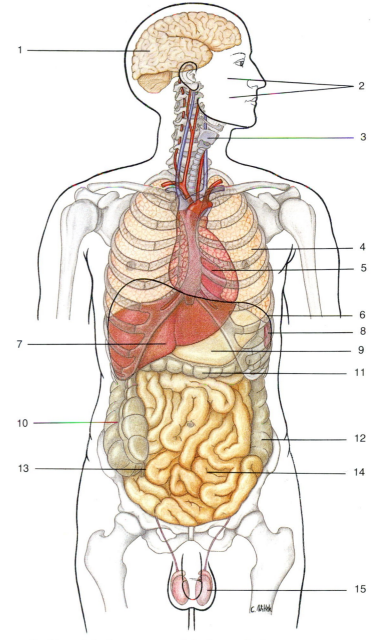

Position of the inner organs of the human body
(anterior aspect).
The three main cavities of the body and their contents.

A₁ Cranial cavity
A₂ Vertebral canal
B₁ Thoracic cavity
B₂ Pericardial cavity
C₁ Abdominal cavity
C₂ Pelvic cavity
D   Diaphragm

1   Head (neurocranium) with the brain
2   Facial bones with oral and nasal cavities
3   Larynx
4   Thorax with the lungs
5   Heart
6   Surface projection of the diaphragm
7   Liver
8   Spleen
9   Stomach
10 Ascending colon
11 Transverse colon
12 Descending colon
13 Appendix
14 Small intestine
15 Testes

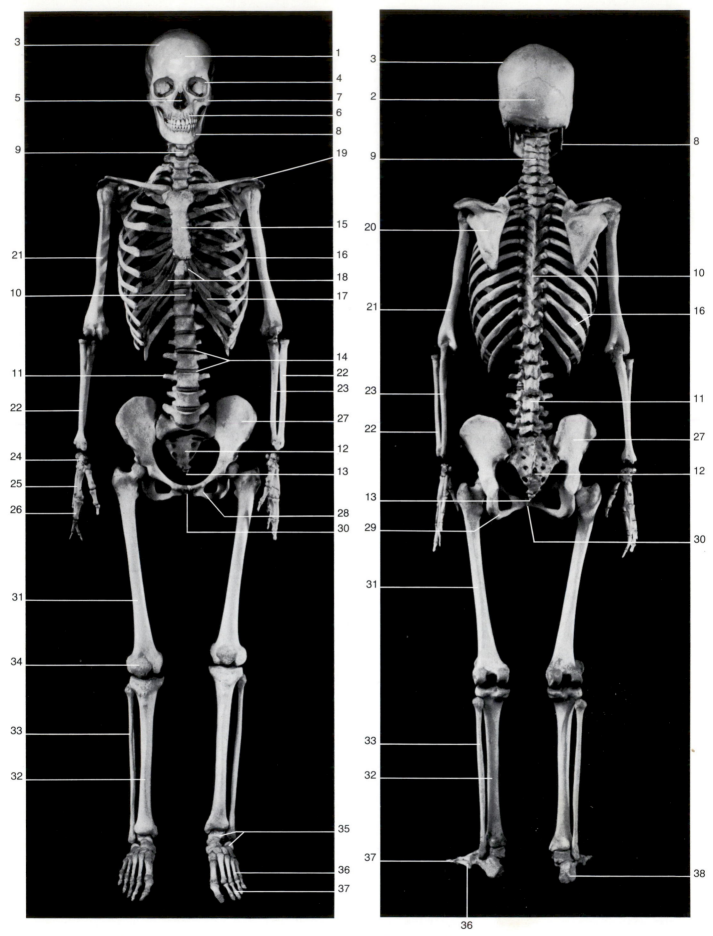

Skeleton of the adult (anterior aspect).

Skeleton of the adult (posterior aspect).

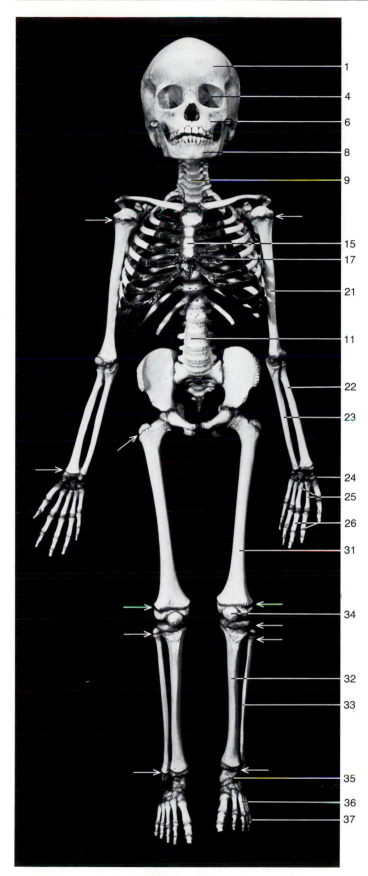

Head
1 Frontal bone
2 Occipital bone
3 Parietal bone
4 Orbit
5 Nasal cavity
6 Maxilla
7 Zygomatic bone
8 Mandible

Trunk and thorax
Vertebral column
9 Cervical vertebrae
10 Thoracic vertebrae
11 Lumbar vertebrae
12 Sacrum
13 Coccyx
14 Intervertebral discs

Thorax
15 Sternum
16 Ribs
17 Costal cartilage
18 Infrasternal angle

Upper limb and shoulder girdle
19 Clavicle
20 Scapula
21 Humerus
22 Radius
23 Ulna
24 Carpal bones
25 Metacarpal bones
26 Phalanges of the hand

Lower limb and pelvis
27 Ilium
28 Pubis
29 Ischium
30 Symphysis pubis
31 Femur
32 Tibia
33 Fibula
34 Patella
35 Tarsal bones
36 Metatarsal bones
37 Phalanges of the foot
38 Calcaneus

Skeleton of a 5-year-old child (anterior aspect).
The zones of the cartilaginous growth plates are seen (arrows).
In contrast to the adult, the ribs show a predominantly
horizontal position.

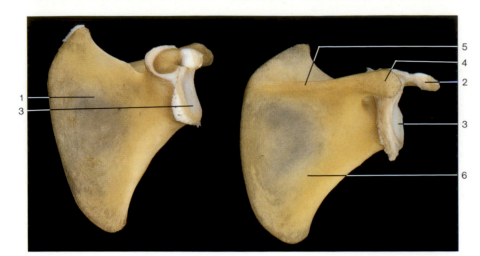

1 Subscapular fossa
2 Coracoid process
3 Glenoid fossa
4 Acromion
5 Spine of scapula
6 Infraspinous fossa

Ossification of the scapula
(left: anterior aspect; right: posterior aspect).

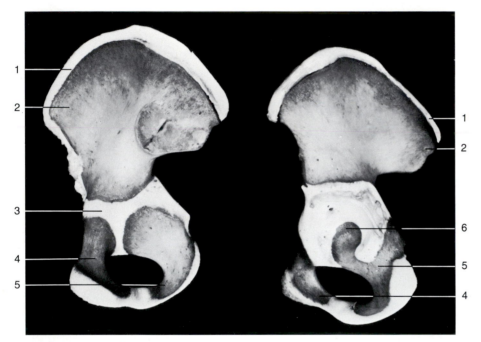

1 Cartilage of the iliac crest
2 Ilium
3 Cartilage
4 Pubis
5 Ischium
6 Acetabulum

Ossification of the hip bone
(left: medial aspect; right: lateral aspect).

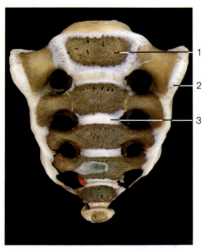

1 Bone tissue
   (vertebral body)
2 Cartilaginous tissue
   (lateral epiphysis)
3 Intervertebral discs

Ossification of the sacrum (anterior aspect).
Note the five vertebral bones which are still separated
from each other.

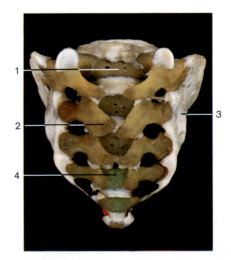

1 Bony tissue
   (center of
   ossification)
2 Vertebral arch
   (not completely
   united)
3 Cartilaginous
   tissue
   (lateral epiphysis)
4 Sacral canal

Ossification of the sacrum
(posterior aspect).

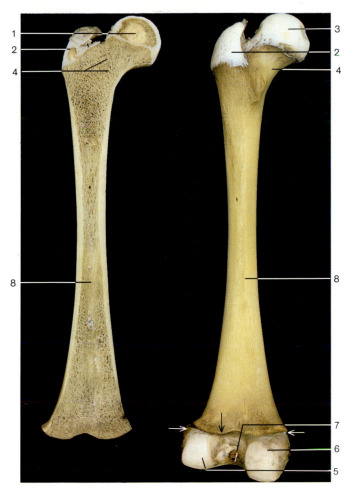

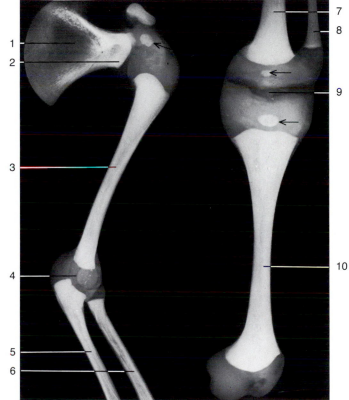

1 Ossification center in the head of the femur
2 Greater trochanter
3 Head of the femur
4 Neck of the femur
5 Lateral condyle
6 Medial condyle
7 Intercondylar notch
8 Diaphysis

Ossification of the femur. Left: coronal section; right: posterior view of the femur; arrows: distal epiphysis.

X-ray of the upper and lower limb of a newborn child. Left: upper limb; right: lower limb (note head of femur below, knee joint above); arrows: ossification centers.

1 Scapula   2 Shoulder joint   3 Humerus
4 Elbow joint   5 Ulna   6 Radius   7 Tibia
8 Fibula   9 Knee joint   10 Femur

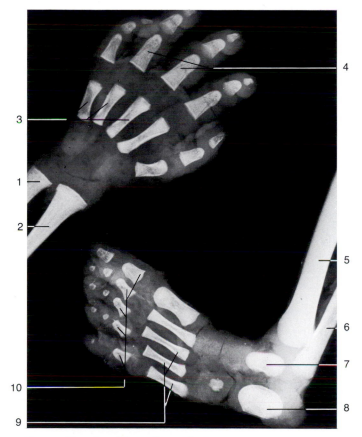

X-ray of hand and foot of a newborn.

1 Ulna
2 Radius
3 Metacarpals
4 Phalanges
5 Tibia
6 Fibula
7 Talus
8 Calcaneus
9 Metatarsals
10 Phalanges

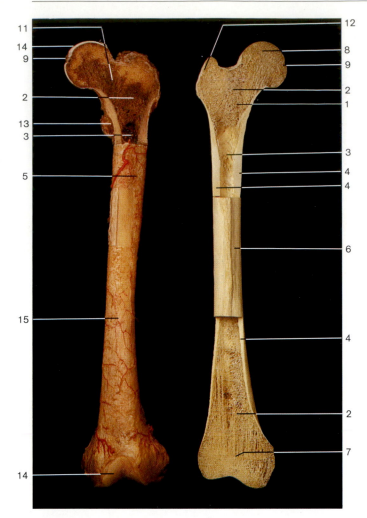

1 Epiphysis
2 Spongy bone
3 Medullary cavity in the diaphysis
4 Compact bone
5 Nutrient canal
6 Diaphysis
7 Epiphyseal line (remnants of the epiphyseal plate)
8 Head of the femur
9 Fovea of head
10 Trabeculae of spongy bone
11 Neck of the femur
12 Greater trochanter
13 Lesser trochanter
14 Articular surface
15 Periosteum

Femur of the adult. Right: coronal section of the proximal and distal epiphyses to display the spongy bone and the medullary cavity; left: the periosteum and the nutrient vessels are preserved.

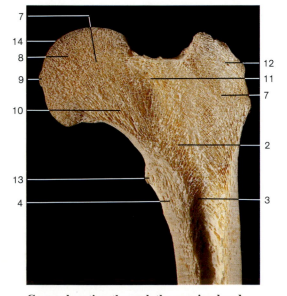

Coronal section through the proximal end of the adult femur, revealing the characteristic trajectorial structure of the spongy bone.

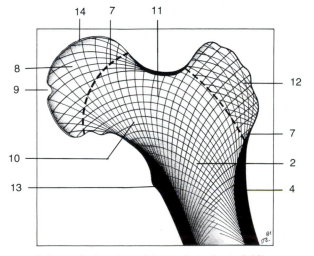

Schematic drawing of the main trajectorial lines of the femoral head.

The **bones** support and protect not only the soft tissue of the body so that the erect posture can be maintained but also serve as levers to which muscles are attached, enabling various kinds of movements. Furthermore, the production of blood cells takes place in the bone marrow which is located in the medullary cavity between the **spongy bone trabeculae.** The spongy bone is highly adapted to the forces acting on the skeleton due to erect posture and movement, while the compact bone is not. Therefore the spongy bone trabeculae reveal, in contrast to the compact bone, a trajectorial structure which reflects the direction of the mechanical forces applied to it. The **periosteum** is an essential structure for bone nutrition and innervation, the blood supply of the bone marrow, as well as the growth and repair of bone tissue. It is continuous with the fibrous capsule of the joints.

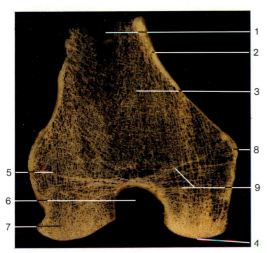

Coronal section through the distal epiphysis of the adult femur. The trajectorial structure of the spongy bone is clearly recognizable.

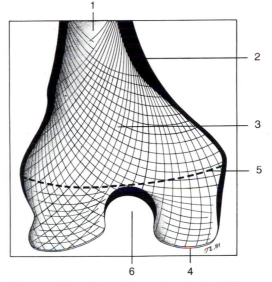

Schematic drawing of the main trajectorial lines, seen in the distal epiphysis of the femur (Tr.).

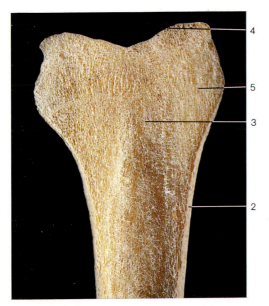

Coronal section through the proximal epiphysis of the adult tibia. Note the structure of the spongy bone and the zone of dense bone at the site of the former epiphyseal plate.

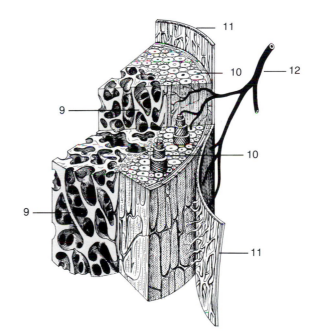

Schematic drawing of the **bone structure** (after BENNINGHOFF).

1 Medullary cavity	8 Femoral epicondyle
2 Compact bone	9 Spongy bone trabeculae
3 Spongy bone	10 Compact bone revealing a lamellar structure (Haversian lamellae and canals)
4 Articular surface (normally covered by articular cartilage)	11 Periosteum
5 Former epiphyseal plate	12 Blood vessel of bone
6 Intercondylar notch	
7 Femoral condyle	

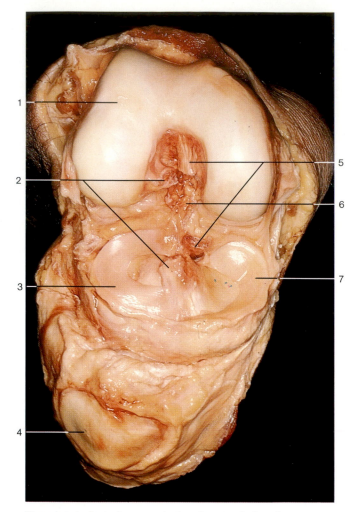

Knee joint. Anterior aspect, showing menisci and cruciate ligaments (cut).

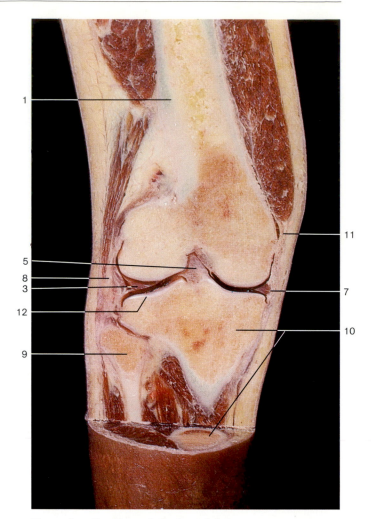

Coronal section through the knee joint. Anterior aspect of the right joint in extension.

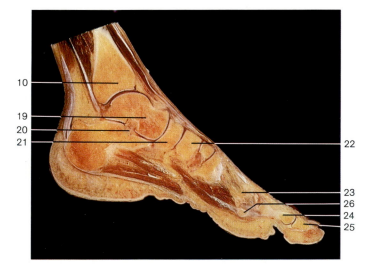

Sagittal section through the lower limb and the foot.

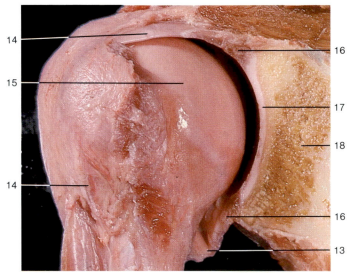

Shoulder joint (anterior view). The anterior part of the articular capsule has been removed.

1	Femur
2	Anterior cruciate ligament
3	Lateral meniscus
4	Patella
5	Posterior cruciate ligament
6	Ligament of Wrisberg
7	Medial meniscus
8	Fibular collateral ligament
9	Fibula
10	Tibia
11	Tibial collateral ligament
12	Articular cartilage
13	Articular capsule
14	Tendon of long head of biceps brachii
15	Head of humerus
16	Glenoid labrum
17	Articular cartilage of glenoid cavity
18	Scapula
19	Talus
20	Interosseous talocalcaneal ligament
21	Navicular bone
22	Medial cuneiform bone
23	First metatarsal bone
24	Proximal phalanx of the hallux (great toe)
25	Distal phalanx of the hallux
26	Sesamoid bone

		Movement	Examples
A	**Fibrous joints**		
1	Sutures	No movements	Sutures of the skull
2	Syndesmoses	No movements	Distal tibiofibular joint
3	Gomphosis	No movements	Roots of teeth in alveolar process
B	**Cartilaginous joints**		
1	Synchondroses	No movements	Epiphyseal plates
2	Symphyses	Slight movement	Symphysis pubis, intervertebral discs
C	**Synovial joints**		
1	Gliding	Monaxial	Intercarpal joint Intertarsal joint Sacroiliacal joint
2	Hinge	Monaxial	Interphalangeal joint Humeroulnar joint Talocrural joint
3	Pivot	Monaxial	Atlantoaxial joint Radioulnar joint
4	Ellipsoidal	Biaxial	Radiocarpal joint
5	Saddle	Biaxial	Carpometacarpal joint of the thumb
6	Ball-and-socket	Multiaxial	Shoulder and hip joint

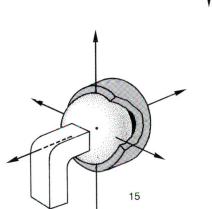

Main types of joints. Arrows: axes of movement.

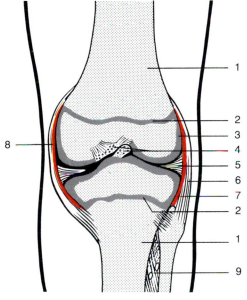

General architecture of a synovial joint with 2 articulating bones and a synovial cavity. Red = synovial membrane (coronal section through the knee joint).

1 Articulating bones
2 Epiphyseal plate
3 Articular cartilage
4 Intraarticular ligaments (e. g. cruciate ligaments)
5 Fibrocartilaginous plates (menisci or intraarticular discs)
6 Collateral ligaments
7 Articular capsule
8 Synovial membrane
9 Interosseous membrane

Fibrous joints (synarthroses)
10 Serrate suture
11 Syndesmosis

Synovial joints (diarthroses)
12 Hinge joints (monaxial) ginglymus
  A Extension
  B Flexion
13 Saddle joint (biaxial)
14 Pivot joint (monaxial, rotation)
15 Ball-and-socket joint (multiaxial)

11

Principal Joints (Immovable)

An articulation or joint is the functional connection between two or more bones. Joints can be divided into two categories depending upon whether the articulating surfaces of the bones are separated by a real cavity (joint cavity) so that they are movable against each other **(synovial joints)** or whether the bones are firmly connected by fibrous or cartilaginous tissue and practically immovable **(fibrous joints, cartilaginous joints, symphysis, etc.).** Synovial joints always possess a joint capsule (with a vascularized synovial membrane), articular cartilages, and a joint cavity. They are grouped according to the degree of movement they permit. A hinge joint (ginglymus) permits movement in only one plane about a single axis **(uniaxial),** an ellipsoidal joint permits movements in two planes **(biaxial),** and ball-and-socket joints permit a range of movements around several axes **(multiaxial).** The following survey gives a few examples of these types of articulation.

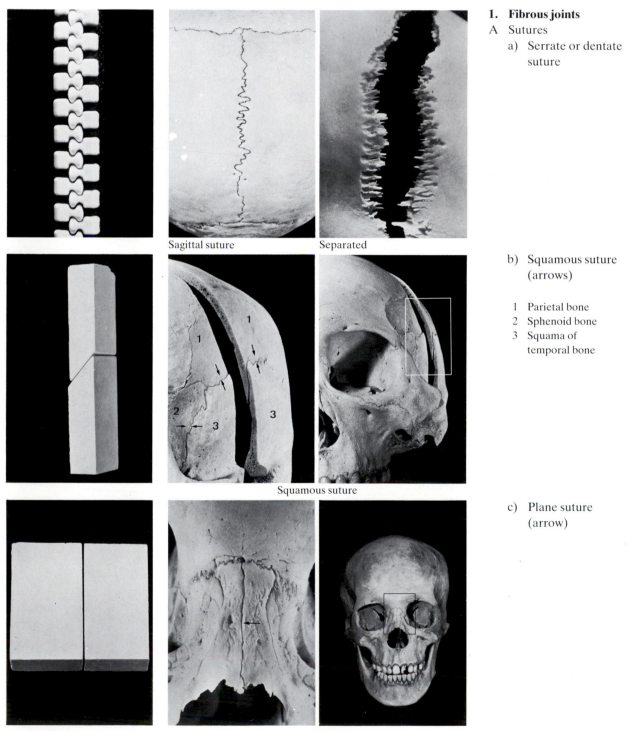

Sagittal suture   Separated

Squamous suture

Nasal bones

1. **Fibrous joints**
A   Sutures
    a) Serrate or dentate suture

b) Squamous suture (arrows)

1 Parietal bone
2 Sphenoid bone
3 Squama of temporal bone

c) Plane suture (arrow)

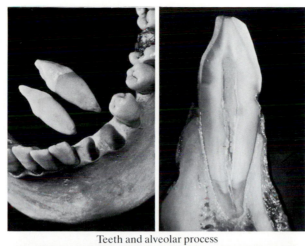

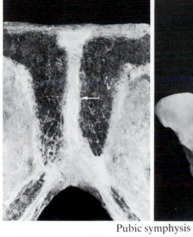

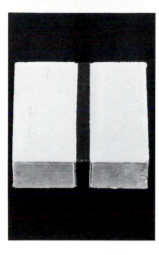

B   Peg suture
    (Gomphosis)

Teeth and alveolar process

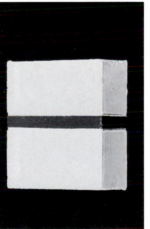

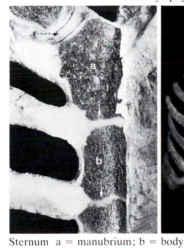

2. Cartilaginous joints
   a) Symphysis
       (fibrocartilage)

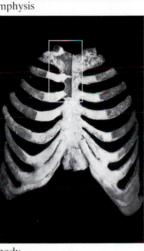

Pubic symphysis

b) Synchondrosis
    (hyaline cartilage)

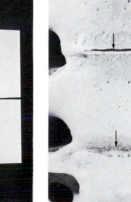

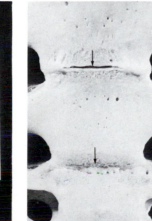

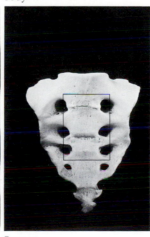

Sternum a = manubrium; b = body

3. Osseous joints
    (synostosis)

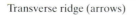

Transverse ridge (arrows)   Sacrum

*   Articular disc
    (sternoclavicular joint)

13

Synovial Joints (Movable)

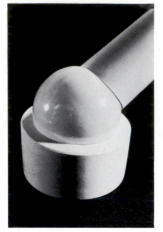

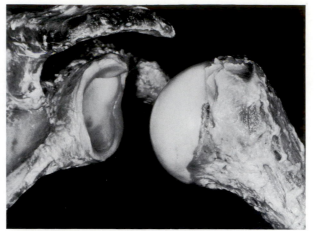

Shoulder joint

1. Ball-and-socket joint

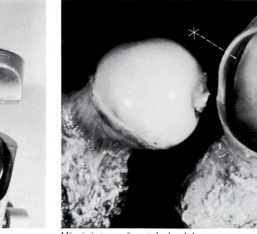

Hip joint   *acetabular labrum

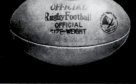

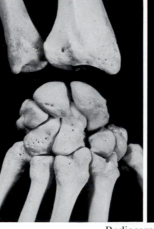

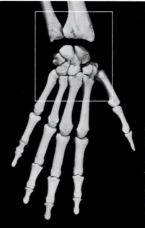

Radiocarpal joint

2. Ellipsoid joint

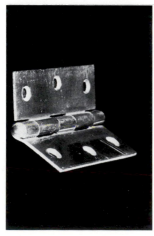

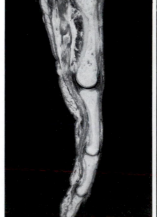

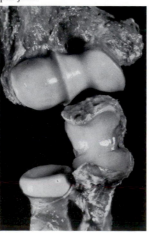

Interphalangeal joint   Elbow joint (humeroulnar joint)

3. Hinge joint

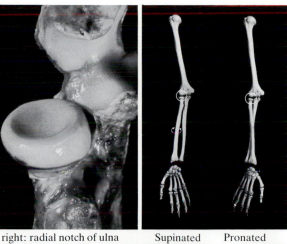

4. Pivot joint

Radioulnar joint; left: head of radius, right: radial notch of ulna   Supinated   Pronated

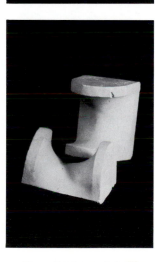
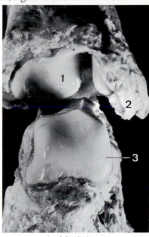

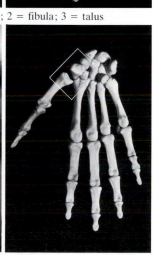

5. Hinge joint
(but a gradually
tilting axis produces
a slight spiral motion)

Ankle joint: 1 = tibia; 2 = fibula; 3 = talus

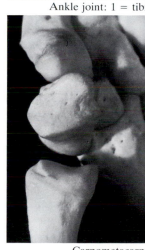

6. Saddle joint

Carpometacarpal joint of the thumb

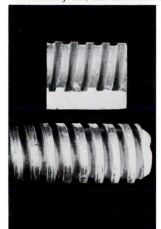
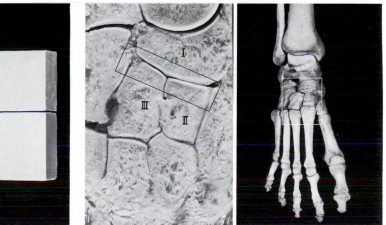

7. Plane joint

I = navicular; **II** = intermediate cuneiform; **III** = lateral cuneiform

The Shapes of Muscles

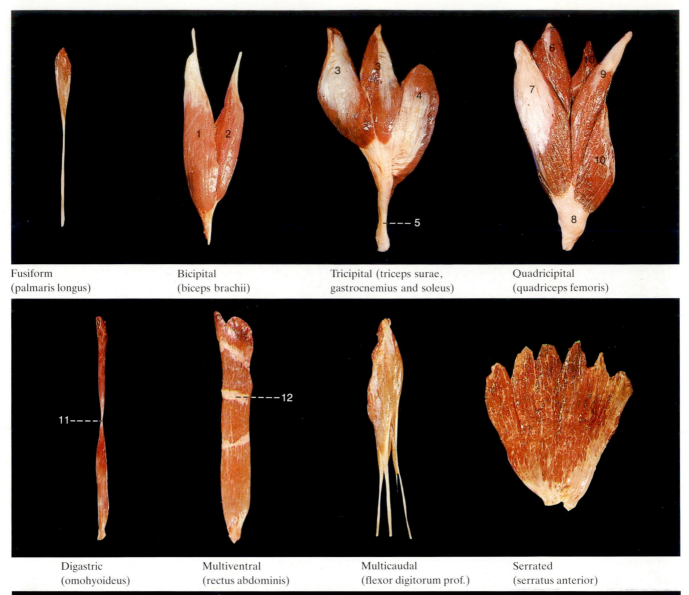

Fusiform
(palmaris longus)

Bicipital
(biceps brachii)

Tricipital (triceps surae,
gastrocnemius and soleus)

Quadricipital
(quadriceps femoris)

Digastric
(omohyoideus)

Multiventral
(rectus abdominis)

Multicaudal
(flexor digitorum prof.)

Serrated
(serratus anterior)

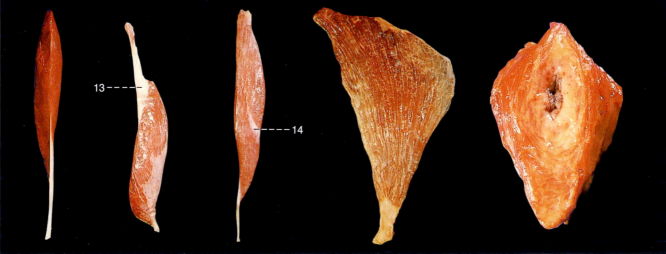

Bipennate
(tibialis anterior)

Unipennate
(semimembranosus)

Semitendinous
(semitendinosus)

Broad, flat muscle
(latissimus dorsi)

Ring-like
(sphincter ani externus)

1 Long head	4 Soleus	8 Patella	12 Tendinous intersection
2 Short head	5 Achilles tendon	9 Rectus femoris	13 Aponeurosis
3 Gastrocnemius	6 Vastus intermedius	10 Vastus lateralis	14 Tendinous intersection
(medial head, lateral head)	7 Vastus medialis	11 Intermediate tendon	

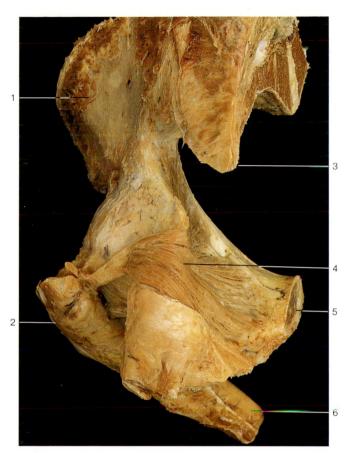

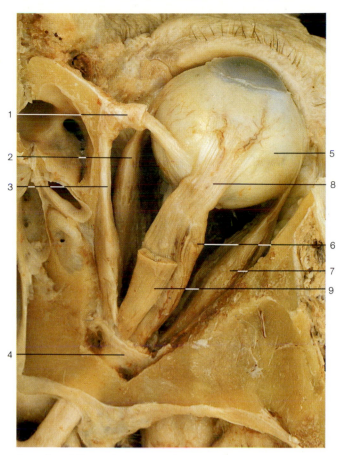

Left half of the pelvis (internal aspect).
M. obturator internus as an example of a muscle the tendon of which does not act in the direction of the main muscle fibers. Its fibers originate at the obturator foramen, turn around the posterior rim of the ischium and insert at the greater trochanter of the femur. The ischium thereby serves as a pulley.

1	Ilium	3	Coccyx	5	Pubis
2	Greater trochanter	4	Obturator internus	6	Femur

Superior oblique of the eyeball (superior aspect of right eye). The tendon of this muscle bends over the trochlea changing its direction so that it becomes attached to the posterior lateral quadrant of the eyeball.

1	Trochlea	6	Superior rectus
2	Medial rectus	7	Lateral rectus
3	Superior oblique	8	Superior rectus (tendon)
4	Common annular tendon	9	Levator palpebrae superioris
5	Eyeball		(divided)

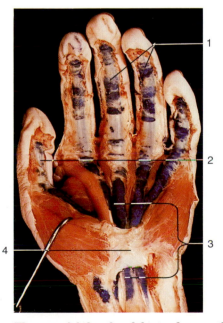

1 Digital synovial sheaths of the tendons of flexor digitorum superficialis and profundus
2 Digital synovial sheaths of the tendon of flexor pollicis longus
3 Common flexor synovial sheaths of flexor digitorum superficialis and profundus
4 Flexor retinaculum

The synovial sheaths of the tendons on the palmar aspect of the left wrist (colored fluid has been injected).

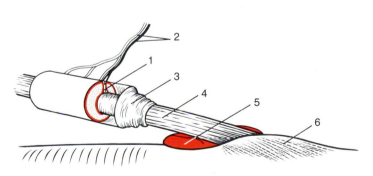

1 Mesotenon
2 Blood vessels
3 Synovial sheath
4 Tendon
5 Synovial bursa
6 Bone (tuberosity)

Structure of a tendon sheath (schematic drawing). The synovial membrane which also forms the mesotenon is indicated in red.

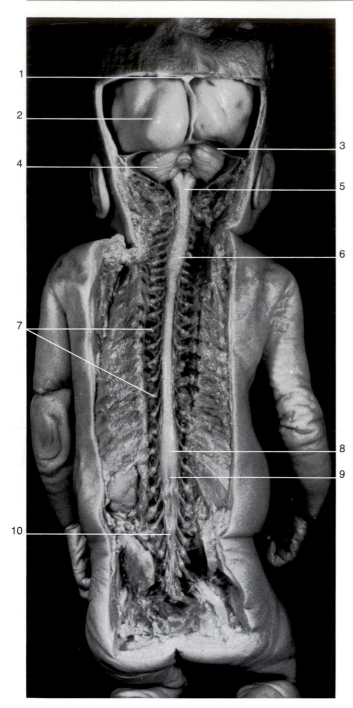

1 Falx cerebri
2 Cerebral hemispheres
3 Tentorium cerebelli
4 Cerebellum
5 Medulla oblongata
6 Spinal cord, cervical enlargement
7 Spinal ganglia
8 Spinal cord, lumbar enlargement
9 Conus medullaris
10 Cauda equina
11 Cervical plexus
12 Brachial plexus
13 Lumbosacral plexus
14 Sympathetic trunk

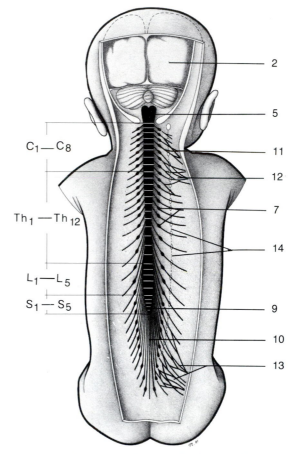

Brain, the **spinal cord** and the **spinal nerves** in the fetus (posterior aspect).

Schematic drawing to illustrate the three main parts of the nervous system in general (Tr.).

The **nervous system** can be divided into three, functionally distinct parts: 1. the cranial part which comprises the great sensory organs and the brain, 2. the spinal cord which shows a segmental structure and serves predominantly as a reflex-organ, and 3. the autonomic nervous system which controls the vegetative processes of organs and functions unconsciously. The vegetative part of the nervous system forms many delicate plexus within the organs. At certain places these plexus contain aggregations of nerve cells (prevertebral and intramural ganglia). The spinal nerves leave the spinal cord at regular intervals, forming the 8 cervical, 12 thoracic, 5 lumbar, 5 sacral and a varying number of coccygeal segments. The ventral rami of the spinal nerves form the cervical (C_1–C_4) and brachial (C_5–T_1) plexus which innervate the anterior part of the neck and the arm, and the lumbosacral plexus (L_1–S_5) which innervates the pelvic and genital organs and the lower extremity.

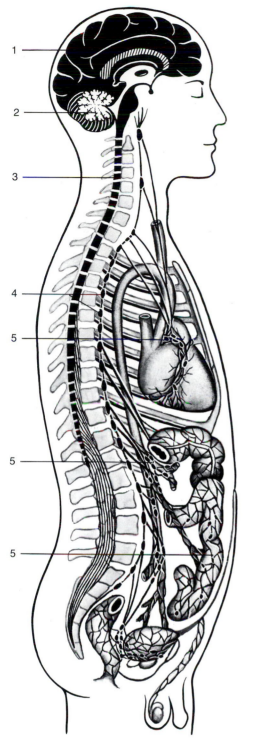

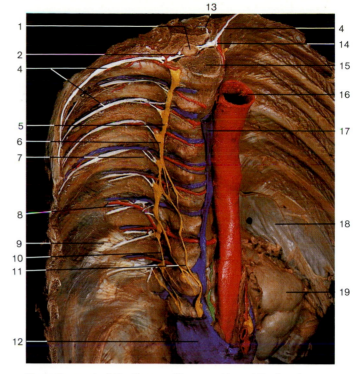

Posterior part of the thorax. Cross-section at the level of the 5th thoracic segment. Spinal nerves and their connections to the sympathetic trunk.

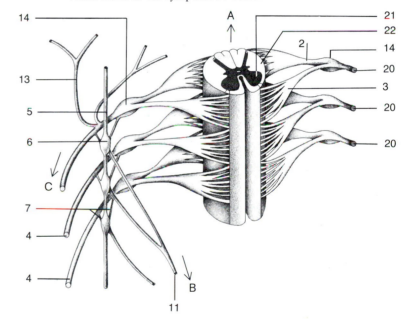

Diagram illustrating the localization of the **three functional portions** of the **nervous system** (brain, spinal cord and autonomic nervous system).

Schematic drawing showing the **organization of the spinal cord** in structurally equal segments which form the paired spinal nerves. A = connections to the brain; B = connections to the autonomic nervous system; C = connections to the trunk and extremities (intercostal nerves and plexus).

1 Cerebrum
2 Cerebellum
3 Spinal cord
4 Sympathetic trunk
5 Plexus and ganglia of the sympathetic nervous system

1	Spinal cord	12	Inferior vena cava
2	Dorsal root	13	Dorsal ramus of spinal nerve
3	Ventral root	14	Spinal ganglion
4	Intercostal nerves	15	Body of the vertebra
5	Sympathetic trunk	16	Aorta
6	Ganglia of the sympathetic trunk	17	Azygos vein
7	Rami communicantes	18	Diaphragm
8	Intercostal artery and vein	19	Left kidney
9	Subcostalis muscle	20	Spinal nerve
10	Lesser splanchnic nerve	21	Gray matter of the spinal cord
11	Greater splanchnic nerve	22	White matter of the spinal cord

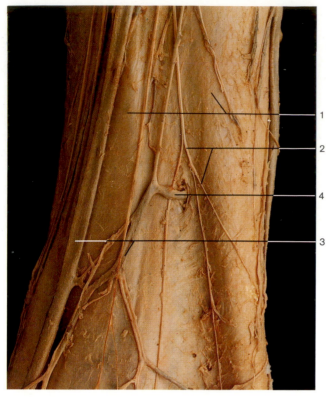

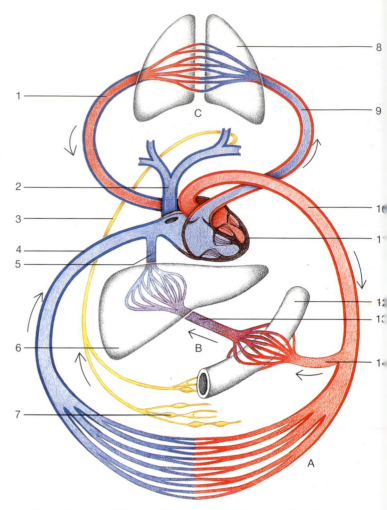

Superficial nerves and vessels of the lower leg, illustrating the structural differences between veins and nerves.

1 Fascia cruris	3 Superficial cutaneous veins
2 Cutaneous nerves	4 Perforating vein

Organization of the circulatory system. Arrows: direction of the blood flow.

Vessel wall in red   = Arteries
Vessel wall in blue = Veins
Yellow   = Lymphatic vessels

A   Systemic circulation
B   Hepatic portal circulation
C   Pulmonary circulation

Superficial nerves and vessels. Temporal region. Note the differences between arteries, veins and nerves.

1 Pulmonary vein	12 Small intestine with capillary network
2 Superior vena cava	
3 Thoracic duct	13 Portal vein
4 Inferior vena cava	14 Mesenteric artery
5 Hepatic vein	15 Superficial temporal artery
6 Liver	16 Superficial temporal vein
7 Lymph nodes and lymphatic vessels	17 Auriculotemporal nerve
	18 Perforating veins for subcutaneous fatty tissue
8 Lung	
9 Pulmonary artery	19 Small artery
10 Aorta	20 Small nerves (branches of facial nerve)
11 Heart	

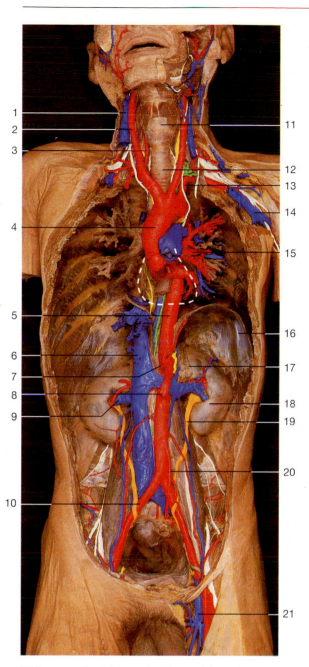

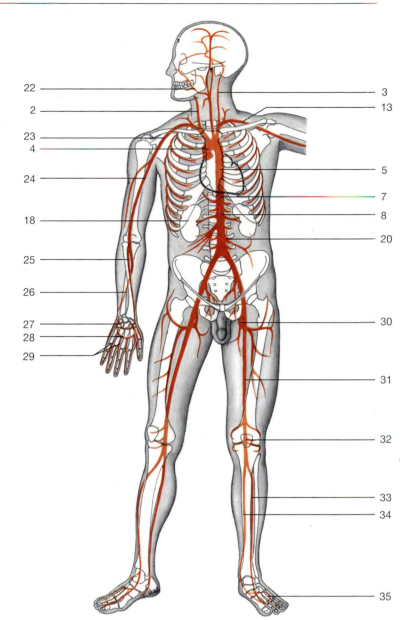

Major vessels of the trunk. The position of the heart is indicated by the dotted line.

Schematic drawing of the **major arteries of the human body** (W.).

1 Internal jugular vein	18 Kidney
2 Common carotid artery	19 Ureter
3 Vertebral artery	20 Inferior mesenteric artery
4 Ascending aorta	21 Femoral vein
5 Descending aorta	22 Facial artery
6 Inferior vena cava	23 Axillary artery
7 Celiac trunk	24 Brachial artery
8 Superior mesenteric artery	25 Radial artery
9 Renal vein	26 Ulnar artery
10 Common iliac artery	27 Deep palmar arch
11 Larynx	28 Superficial palmar arch
12 Trachea	29 Common palmar digital arteries
13 Left subclavian artery	30 Profunda femoris artery
14 Left axillary vein	31 Femoral artery
15 Pulmonary veins	32 Popliteal artery
16 Diaphragm	33 Anterior tibial artery
17 Suprarenal gland	34 Posterior tibial artery
	35 Plantar arch

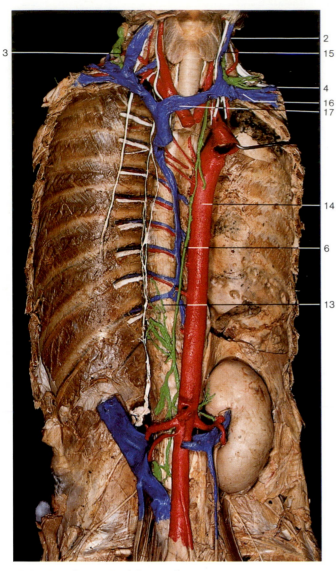

Major lymph vessels of the trunk.

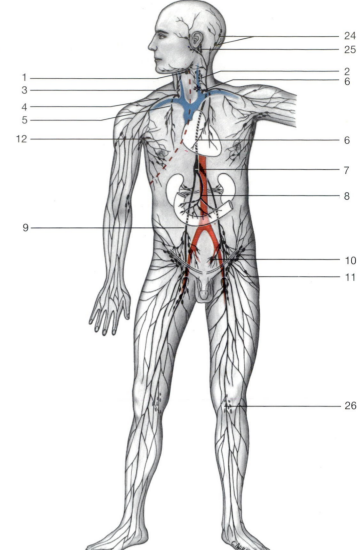

Lymphatic system. Course of the main lymphatic vessels and lymph nodes in the body. Dotted line = border between lymphatic vessels draining towards the right venous angle and towards the left.

1	Submandibular nodes	15	Internal jugular vein
2	Deep cervical nodes	16	Subclavian vein
3	Right jugular trunk	17	Left brachiocephalic vein
4	Subclavian trunk	18	Mandible
5	Right bronchomediastinal trunk	19	Larynx
6	Thoracic duct	20	Internal jugular vein
7	Cisterna chyli	21	Deep cervical nodes
8	Intestinal trunk	22	Cervical nerve plexus
9	Right lumbar trunk	23	Superficial layer of deep fascia
10	Internal iliac nodes	24	Occipital nodes
11	Inguinal nodes	25	Parotid nodes
12	Axillary nodes	26	Popliteal nodes
13	Descending trunk		
14	Descending aorta		

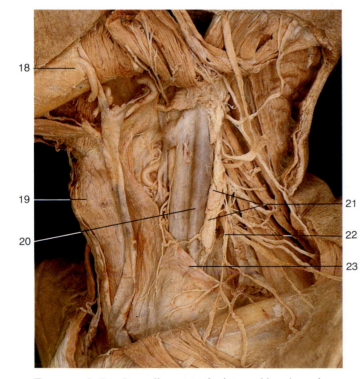

Deep cervical nodes, adjacent to the internal jugular vein.

Lymphatic vessels originate as blind-ending tubes in the tissue spaces (lymph capillaries) and unite to form larger vessels (lymphatics). These resemble veins but have a much thinner wall, more valves and are interrupted by lymph nodes at various intervals. Large groups of lymph nodes are located in the inguinal and axillary regions, deep to the mandible and sternocleidomastoid muscle and within the root of the mesentery of the intestine.

Chapter II
Head

The Bones of the Skull

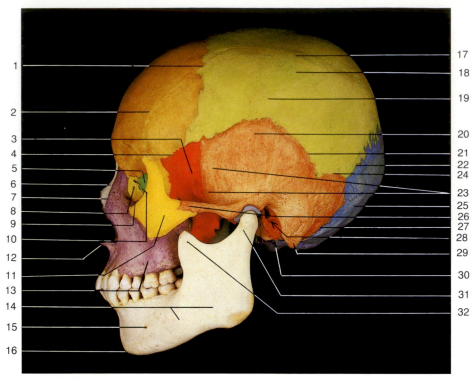

1	Coronal suture
2	Frontal bone
3	Sphenoid bone
4	Sphenofrontal suture
5	Ethmoid bone
6	Nasal bone
7	Nasomaxillary suture
8	Lacrimal bone
9	Lacrimomaxillary suture
10	Lacrimoethmoid suture
11	Zygomatic bone
12	Anterior nasal spine
13	Maxilla
14	Mandible
15	Mental foramen
16	Mental protuberance
17	Superior temporal line
18	Inferior temporal line
19	Parietal bone
20	Temporal bone
21	Squamous suture
22	Lambdoid suture
23	Temporal fossa
24	Parietomastoid suture
25	Occipital bone
26	Zygomatic arch
27	Occipitomastoid suture
28	External acoustic meatus
29	Mastoid process
30	Tympanic portion of temporal bone
31	Condyle of mandible
32	Coronoid process of mandible

General architecture of the skull (lateral aspect). The different bones are indicated in color (numbers cf. table).

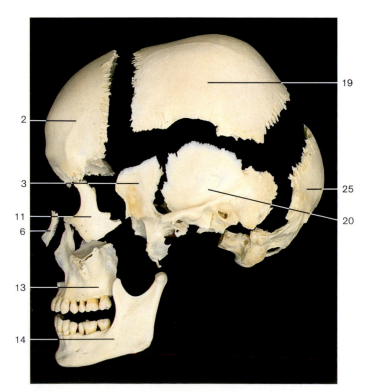

2	Frontal bone (orange)	Cranial bones
19	Parietal bone (light green)	
3	Greater wing of sphenoid bone (red)	
25	Squama of occipital bone (blue)	
20	Squama of temporal bone (brown)	
5	Ethmoid bone (dark green)	Base of skull
3	Sphenoid bone (red)	
	Temporal bone excluding squama (brown)	
30	Tympanic portion of temporal bone (dark brown)	
	Occipital bone excluding squama (blue)	
6	Nasal bone (white)	Facial bones
8	Lacrimal bone (yellow)	
	Inferior nasal concha	
	Vomer	
11	Zygomatic bone (light yellow)	
	Palatine bone	
13	Maxilla (violet)	
14	Mandible (white)	
	Malleus	Auditory ossicles
	Incus } within petrous portion of	
	Stapes temporal bone	
	Hyoid	

Lateral aspect of the disarticulated skull (palatine bone, lacrimal bone, ethmoid bone and vomer are not depicted).

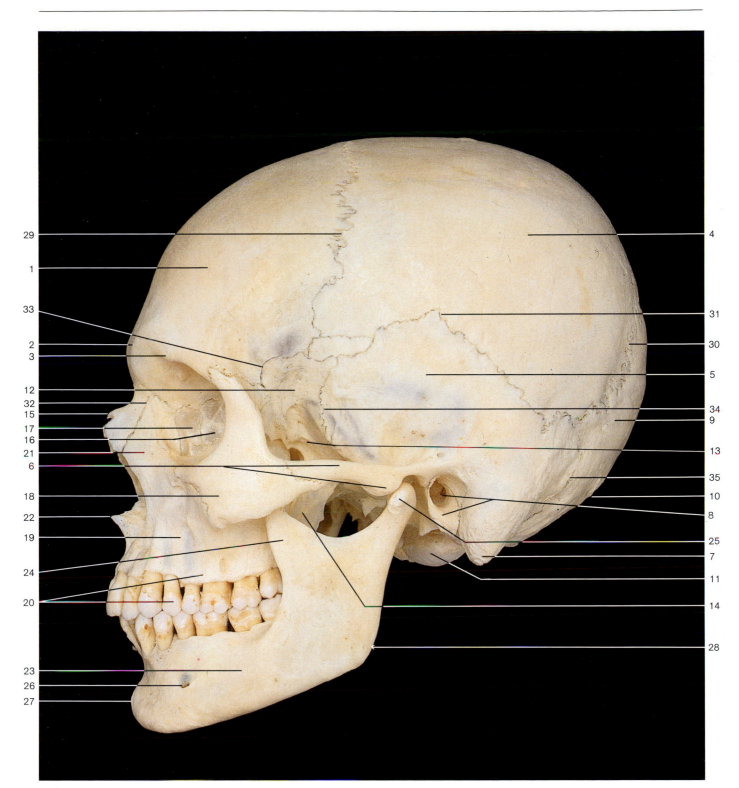

Lateral aspect of the skull.

1 **Frontal bone**
2 Glabella
3 Supraorbital margin
4 **Parietal bone**
5 **Temporal bone** (squamous part)
6 Zygomatic process,
   articular tubercle
7 Mastoid process
8 Tympanic part (tympanic plate)
   and external acoustic meatus
9 **Occipital bone** (squamous part)
10 External occipital protuberance

11 Occipital condyle
12 **Sphenoid bone,** greater wing of sphenoid
   bone
13 Infratemporal crest of sphenoid
14 Pterygoid process, lateral pterygoid plate
15 **Nasal bone**
16 **Ethmoid bone** (orbital part)
17 **Lacrimal bone**
18 **Zygomatic bone**
19 **Maxilla** (body)
20 Alveolar process and teeth
21 Frontal process
22 Anterior nasal spine
23 **Mandible** (body)

24 Coronoid process
25 Condyloid process
26 Mental foramen
27 Mental protuberance
28 Angle of the mandible

Sutures
29 Coronal suture
30 Lambdoid suture
31 Squamous suture
32 Nasomaxillary suture
33 Frontosphenoid suture
34 Sphenosquamosal suture
35 Occipitomastoid suture

The Facial Bones

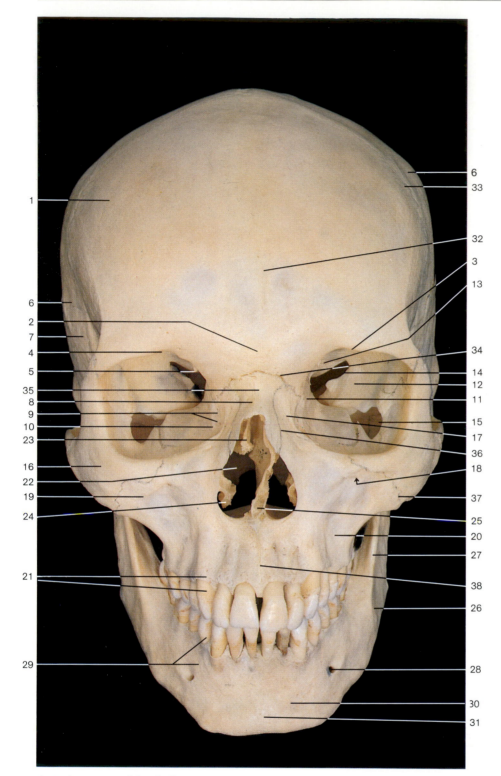

1	**Frontal bone**
2	Glabella
3	Supraorbital margin
4	Supraorbital notch
5	Trochlear spine
6	**Parietal bone**
7	**Temporal bone**
8	**Nasal bone**

Orbit
9	Lacrimal bone
10	Posterior lacrimal crest
11	Ethmoid bone

Sphenoid bone
12	Greater wing of sphenoid bone
13	Lesser wing of sphenoid bone
14	Superior orbital fissure
15	Inferior orbital fissure
16	**Zygomatic bone**

Maxilla
17	Frontal process
18	Infraorbital foramen
19	Zygomatic process
20	Body of maxilla
21	Alveolar process with teeth

Nasal cavity
22	Anterior nasal aperture
23	Middle nasal concha
24	Inferior nasal concha
25	Nasal septum, vomer

Mandible
26	Body of mandible
27	Ramus of mandible
28	Mental foramen
29	Alveolar part with teeth
30	Base of mandible
31	Mental protuberance

Sutures
32	Frontal suture
33	Coronal suture
34	Frontonasal suture
35	Internasal suture
36	Nasomaxillary suture
37	Zygomaticomaxillary suture
38	Intermaxillary suture

Anterior aspect of the skull.

The skull comprises a mosaic of numerous complicated bones which form the cranial cavity protecting the brain (**neurocranium**) and several cavities such as nasal and oral cavities in the facial region. The neurocranium consists of large bony plates which develop directly from the surrounding sheets of connective tissue (**desmocranium**). The bones of the skull base are formed out of cartilaginous tissue (**chondrocranium**) which ossifies secondarily. The **visceral skeleton** which, in fish, gives rise to the gills, has in higher vertebrates been transformed into the bones of the masticatory and auditory apparatus (maxilla, mandible, auditory ossicles and hyoid bone).

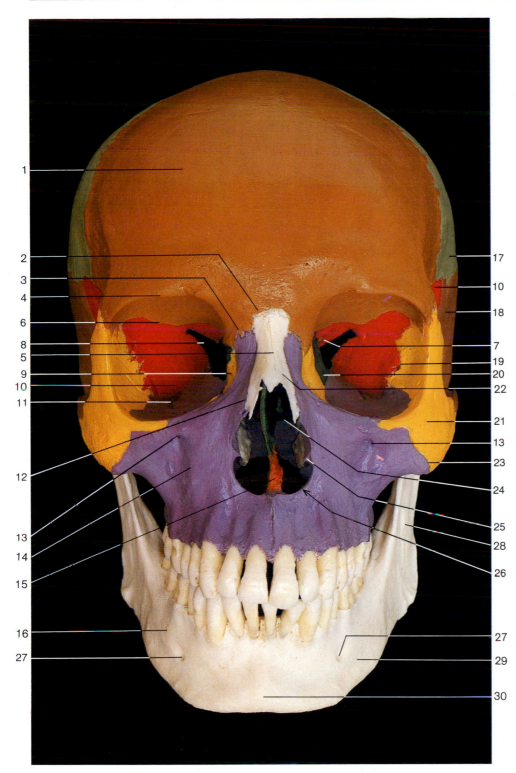

1	Frontal bone
2	Frontonasal suture
3	Frontomaxillary suture
4	Supraorbital notch
5	Internasal suture
6	Sphenofrontal suture
7	Optic canal in smaller wing of sphenoid bone
8	Superior orbital fissure
9	Lacrimal bone
10	Sphenoid bone (greater wing)
11	Inferior orbital fissure
12	Nasomaxillary suture
13	Infraorbital foramen
14	Maxilla
15	Vomer
16	Body of mandible
17	Parietal bone
18	Temporal bone
19	Sphenozygomatic suture
20	Ethmoid bone
21	Zygomatic bone
22	Nasal bone
23	Zygomaticomaxillary suture
24	Middle nasal concha
25	Inferior nasal concha
26	Anterior nasal aperture
27	Mental foramen
28	Ramus of mandible
29	Base of mandible
30	Mental protuberance

Bones

Frontal bone (brown)
Parietal bone (light green)
Temporal bone (dark brown)
Sphenoidal bone (red)
Zygomatic bone (yellow)
Ethmoid bone (dark green)
Lacrimal bone (yellow)
Vomer (orange)
Maxilla (violet)
Nasal bone (white)
Mandible (white)

Anterior aspect of the skull (individual bones indicated by color).

The following series of figures are arranged so that the mosaic-like pattern of the skull becomes understandable. It starts with the bones of the **skull base** (sphenoid and occipital) to which the other bones are added step by step. The facial skeleton is built up by the ethmoid bone to which the palatine bone and maxilla are attached laterally; the small nasal and lacrimal bones fill the remaining spaces. Cartilages remain only in the external part of the nose.

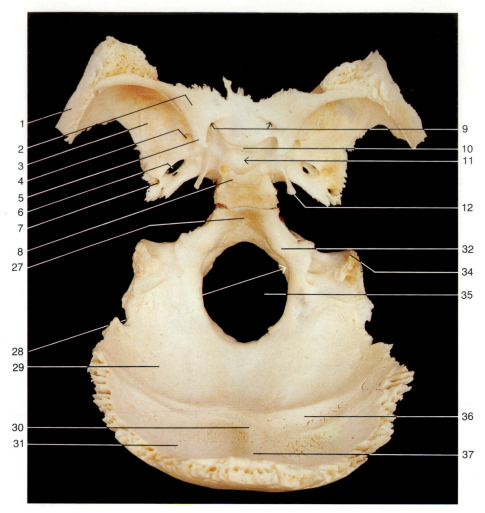

Sphenoid and occipital bone (from above).

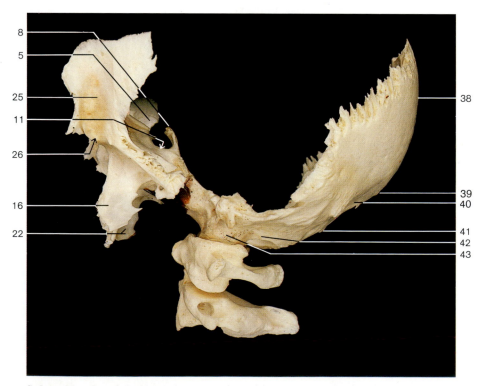

Sphenoid and occipital bone in connection with the atlas and axis
(1st and 2nd cervical vertebrae) (left lateral view).

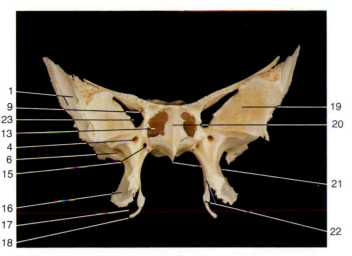

Sphenoid bone (anterior aspect).

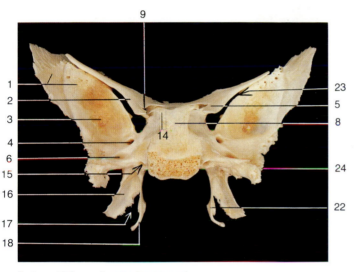

Sphenoid bone (posterior aspect).

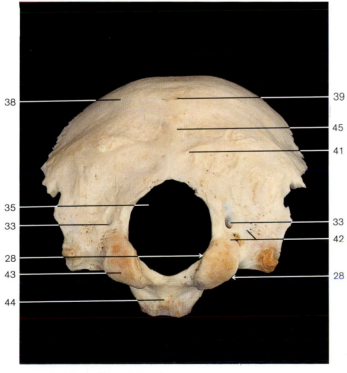

Occipital bone (from below).

Sphenoid bone

1 Greater wing
2 Lesser wing
3 Cerebral or superior surface of greater wing
4 Foramen rotundum
5 Anterior clinoid process
6 Foramen ovale
7 Foramen spinosum
8 Dorsum sellae
9 Optic canal
10 Chiasmatic groove, sulcus chiasmatis
11 Hypophysial fossa
12 Lingula
13 Opening of sphenoidal sinus
14 Posterior clinoid process
15 Pterygoid canal
16 Lateral pterygoid plate
17 Pterygoid notch
18 Pterygoid hamulus
19 Orbital surface of greater wing
20 Sphenoid crest
21 Sphenoid rostrum
22 Medial pterygoid plate
23 Superior orbital fissure
24 Spine of sphenoid
25 Temporal surface of greater wing
26 Infratemporal crest

Occipital bone

27 Clivus
28 Hypoglossal canal
29 Fossa for cerebellar hemisphere
30 Internal occipital protuberance
31 Fossa for cerebral hemisphere
32 Jugular tubercle
33 Condylar canal
34 Jugular process
35 Foramen magnum
36 Groove for transverse sinus
37 Groove for superior sagittal sinus
38 Squamous part of the occipital bone
39 External occipital protuberance
40 Superior nuchal line
41 Inferior nuchal line
42 Condylar fossa
43 Condyle
44 Pharyngeal tubercle
45 External occipital crest

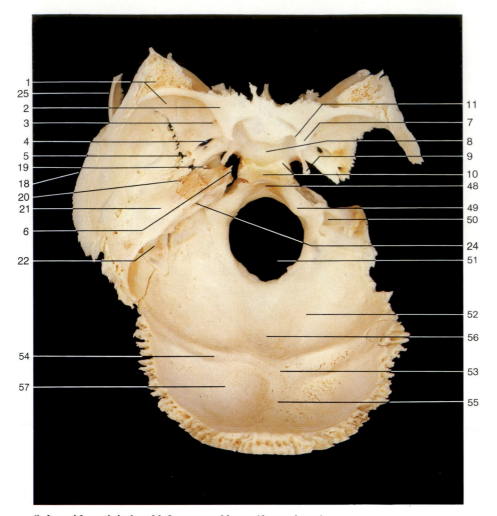

Sphenoid, occipital and left temporal bone (from above).
Internal aspect of the base of the skull. The left temporal
bone has been added to the foregoing figure.

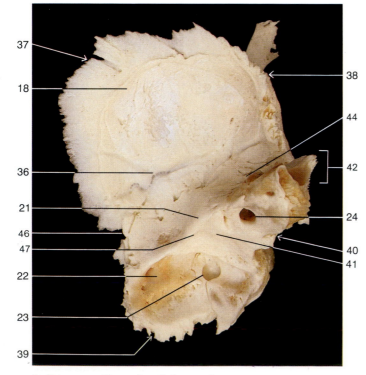

Left temporal bone (medial aspect).

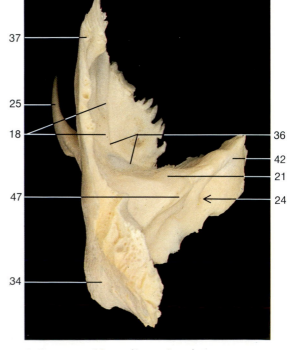

Left temporal bone (from above).

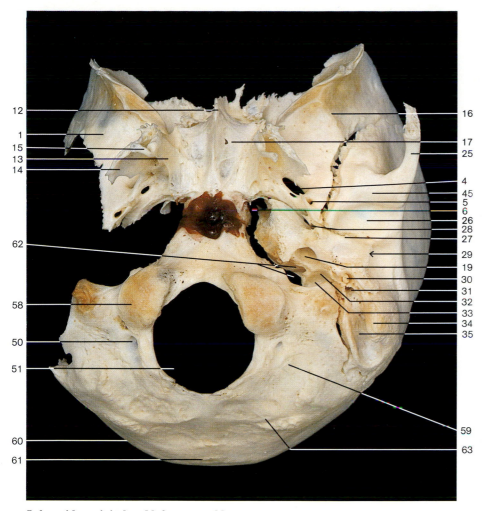

Sphenoid, occipital and left temporal bone.
Base of the skull (external aspect).

Temporal bone
18 Squamous part
19 Carotid canal
20 Hiatus for the greater petrosal nerve
21 Arcuate eminence
22 Groove for the sigmoid sinus
23 Mastoid foramen
24 Internal acoustic meatus
25 Zygomatic process
26 Mandibular fossa
27 Petrotympanic fissure
28 Canalis musculotubarius
29 External acoustic meatus
30 Styloid process (remnant only)
31 Stylomastoid foramen
32 Mastoid canaliculus
33 Jugular fossa
34 Mastoid process
35 Mastoid notch
36 Groove for middle meningeal vessels
37 Parietal margin
38 Sphenoid margin
39 Occipital margin
40 Cochlear canaliculus
41 Aqueduct of the vestibule
42 Apex of the petrous part
43 Tympanic part
44 Trigeminal impression
45 Articular tubercle
46 Parietal notch
47 Groove for the superior petrosal sinus

Occipital bone
48 Clivus
49 Jugular tubercle
50 Condylar canal
51 Foramen magnum
52 Lower part of squamous occipital bone
   (cerebellar fossa)
53 Internal occipital protuberance
54 Groove for the transverse sinus
55 Groove for the superior sagittal sinus
56 Internal occipital crest
57 Upper part of squamous occipital bone
   (cerebral fossa)
58 Condyle
59 Nuchal plane
60 Superior nuchal line
61 External occipital protuberance
62 Jugular foramen
63 Inferior nuchal line

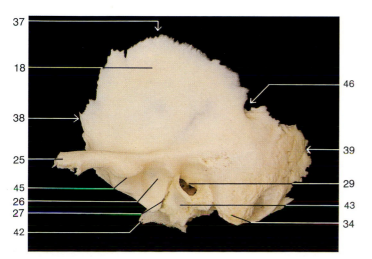

Left temporal bone (lateral aspect).

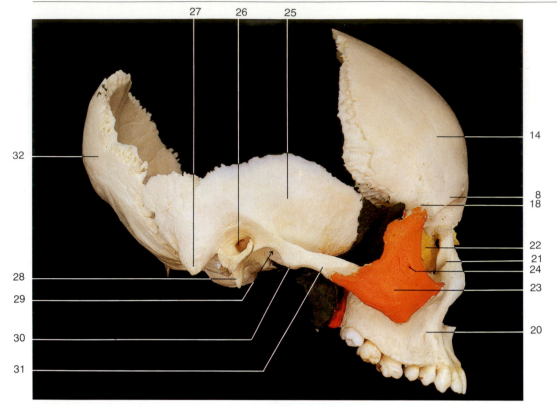

Part of a disarticulated skull (right lateral aspect).
The **frontal bone** and the maxilla are connected with
the temporal bone by the zygomatic bone (orange).

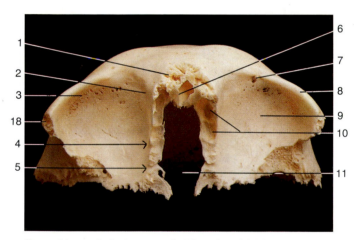

Frontal bone (inferior aspect). The ethmoidal foveolae
cover the ethmoidal cavities of the ethmoid bone.

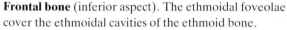

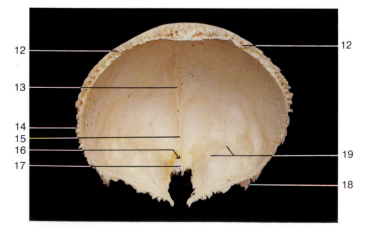

Frontal bone (posterior aspect).

Frontal bone
1 Nasal margin
2 Trochlear fossa
3 Fossa for lacrimal gland
4 Anterior ethmoidal foramen
5 Posterior ethmoidal foramen
6 Nasal spine
7 Supraorbital notch
8 Supraorbital margin
9 Orbital plate
10 Roofs of the ethmoidal air cells
11 Ethmoidal notch
12 Parietal margin
13 Groove for superior sagittal sinus
14 Squamous part of frontal bone
15 Frontal crest
16 Foramen cecum
17 Nasal spine
18 Zygomatic process
19 Juga cerebralia

20 **Maxilla**
21 Frontal process
22 **Lacrimal bone**
23 **Zygomatic bone**
24 Zygomaticofacial foramen

Temporal bone
25 Squamous part of temporal bone
26 External acoustic meatus
27 Mastoid process
28 Styloid process
29 Mandibular fossa
30 Articular tubercle
31 Zygomatic process

Occipital bone
32 Squamous part of occipital bone

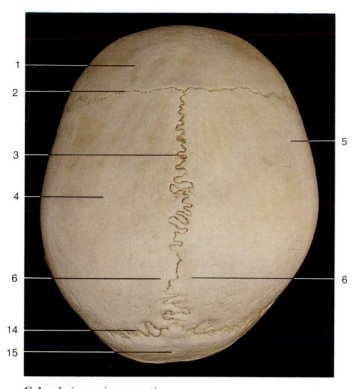

Calvaria (superior aspect).

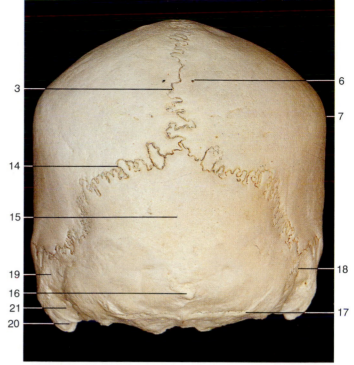

Calvaria (posterior aspect).

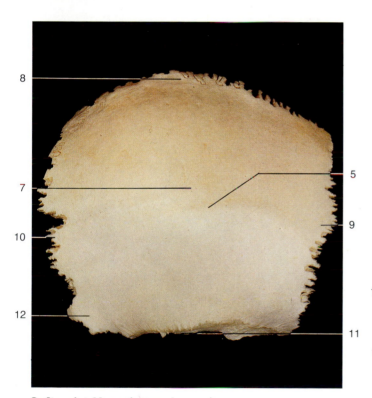

Left parietal bone (external aspect).

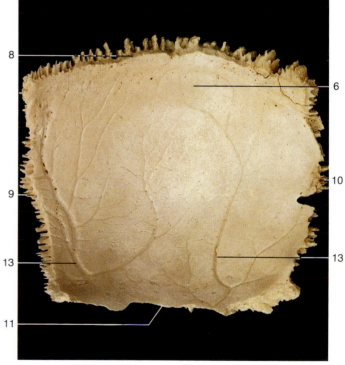

Left parietal bone (internal aspect).

1	**Frontal bone**	8	Sagittal margin	15	**Occipital bone**	
2	Coronal suture	9	Occipital margin	16	External occipital protuberance	
3	Sagittal suture	10	Frontal margin	17	Inferior nuchal line	
4	**Parietal bone**	11	Squamous margin	18	Occipitomastoid suture	
5	Superior temporal line	12	Sphenoidal angle	19	**Temporal bone**	
6	Parietal foramen	13	Groove for middle meningeal artery	20	Mastoid process	
7	Parietal tuber or eminence	14	Lambdoid suture	21	Mastoid notch	

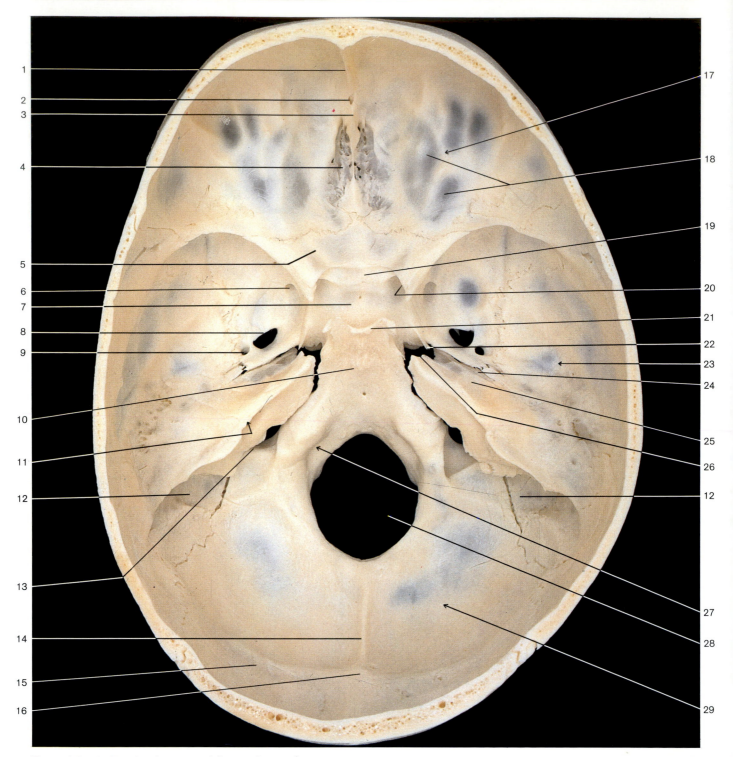

Base of the skull, calvaria removed (internal aspect).

1	Frontal crest	11	Internal acoustic meatus	21	Dorsum sellae
2	Foramen cecum	12	Groove for sigmoid sinus	22	Lingula of the sphenoid
3	Crista galli	13	Jugular foramen	23	**Middle cranial fossa**
4	Cribriform plate of ethmoid bone	14	Internal occipital crest	24	Groove for greater petrosal nerve
5	Lesser wing of sphenoid bone	15	Groove for transverse sinus	25	Superior margin of the petrous temporal bone
6	Foramen rotundum	16	Internal occipital protuberance	26	Foramen lacerum
7	Hypophysial fossa	17	**Anterior cranial fossa**	27	Hypoglossal canal
8	Foramen ovale	18	Finger-like impressions	28	Foramen magnum
9	Foramen spinosum	19	Chiasmatic sulcus	29	**Posterior cranial fossa**
10	Clivus	20	Optic canal		

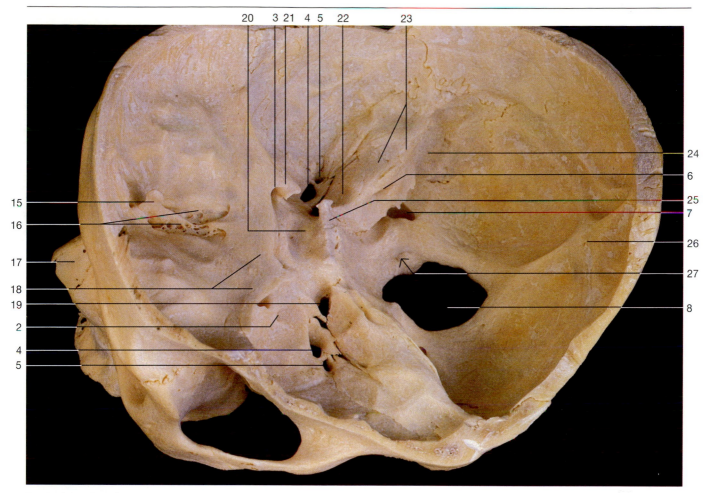

Base of the skull (oblique lateral aspect from left side).

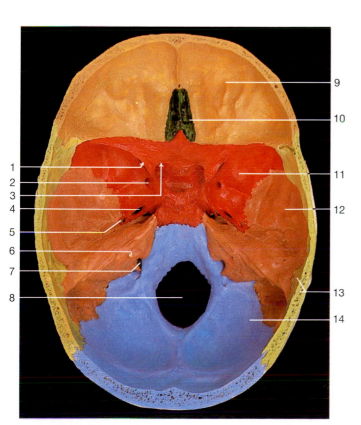

Base of the skull (superior aspect).
Individual bones indicated by color.

Canals, fissures and foramina of the base of the skull

1 Superior orbital fissure
2 Foramen rotundum
3 Optic canal
4 Foramen ovale
5 Foramen spinosum
6 Internal acoustic meatus
7 Jugular foramen
8 Foramen magnum

Bones

9 Frontal bone (orange)
10 Ethmoid bone (dark green)
11 Sphenoid bone (red)
12 Temporal bone (brown)
13 Parietal bone (light green)
14 Occipital bone (blue)

Details of bones

15 Crista galli
16 Cribriform plate
17 Nasal bone
18 Lesser wing of sphenoid bone
19 Foramen lacerum
20 Hypophysial fossa
21 Anterior clinoid process
22 Depression for trigeminal ganglion
23 Petrous part of temporal bone
24 Groove for sigmoid sinus
25 Dorsum sellae
26 Internal occipital protuberance
27 Hypoglossal canal

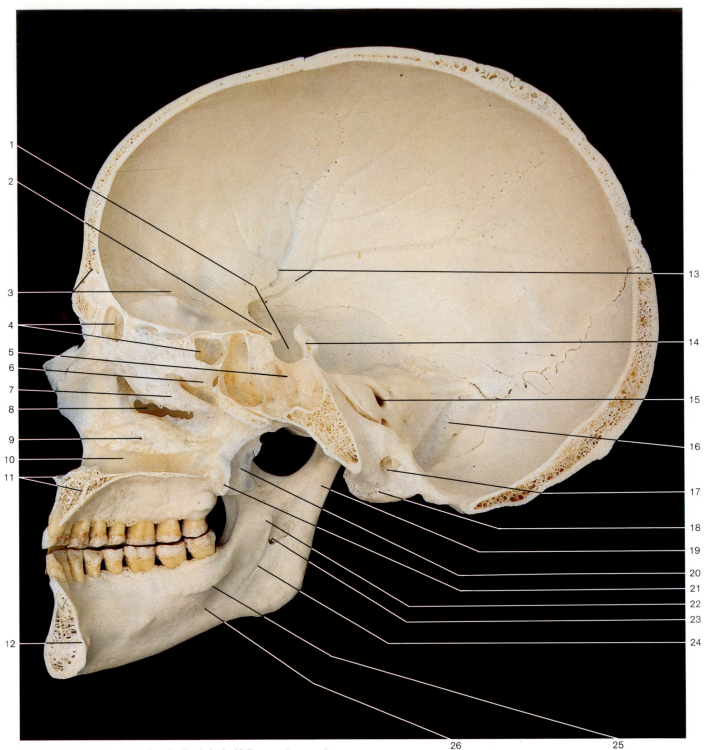

Median section through the skull, right half (internal aspect).

1 Hypophysial fossa
2 Anterior clinoid process
3 Frontal bone
4 Ethmoidal air cells
5 Sphenoidal sinus
6 Superior concha
7 Middle concha
8 Maxillary hiatus
9 Inferior concha
10 Inferior meatus
11 Anterior nasal spine and maxilla
12 Mental spine or genial tubercle
13 Groove for middle meningeal artery

14 Dorsum sellae
15 Internal acoustic meatus
16 Groove for sigmoid sinus
17 Hypoglossal canal
18 Occipital condyle
19 Condylar process
20 Lateral pterygoid plate
21 Medial pterygoid plate
22 Lingula of mandible
23 Mandibular foramen
24 Mylohyoid groove
25 Mylohyoid line
26 Submandibular fovea

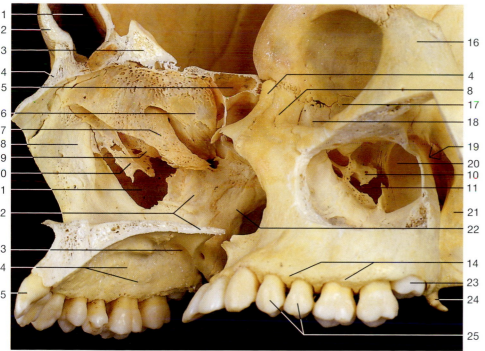

1	Frontal sinus
2	Frontal bone
3	Crista galli
4	Nasal bone
5	Sphenoidal sinus
6	Superior concha ⎱ of ethmoid
7	Middle concha ⎰ bone
8	Frontal process of maxilla
9	Ethmoidal bulla
10	Uncinate process
11	Maxillary hiatus
12	Palatine bone
13	Greater palatine foramen
14	Alveolar process of maxilla
15	Central incisor
16	Zygomatic bone
17	Ethmoid bone
18	Lacrimal bone
19	Pterygopalatine fossa
20	Maxillary sinus
21	Lateral pterygoid plate
22	Medial pterygoid plate
23	Third molar tooth
24	Pterygoid hamulus
25	Two premolar teeth

Facial part of the skull (viscerocranium), divided in two halves (lateral and medial aspect). Right inferior concha has been removed to show the maxillary hiatus. Left maxillary sinus opened.

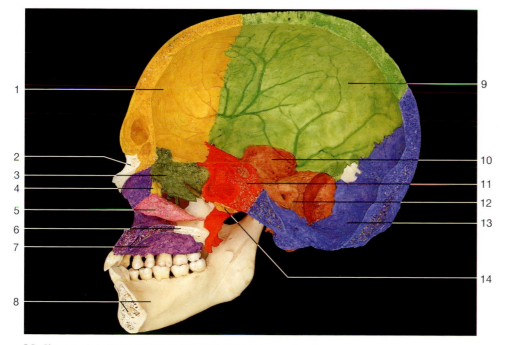

Bones (indicated by colors)
1 Frontal bone (yellow)
2 Nasal bone (white)
3 Ethmoid bone (dark green)
4 Lacrimal bone (yellow)
5 Inferior nasal concha (pink)
6 Palatine bone (white)
7 Maxilla (violet)
8 Mandible (white)
9 Parietal bone (light green)
10 Temporal bone (brown)
11 Sphenoid bone (red)
12 Petrous part of temporal bone (brown)
13 Occipital bone (blue)
14 Ala of vomer (light brown)

Median section through the skull. The nasal septum has been removed. Bones indicated by colors.

Because of the upright posture which man developed in the course of evolution, the cranial cavity greatly increased in size whereas the facial skeleton decreased. As a result, the base of the skull developed an angulation of about 120° between the clivus and the cribriform plate. The hypophysial fossa containing the pituitary gland lies at the angle formed between these two planes.

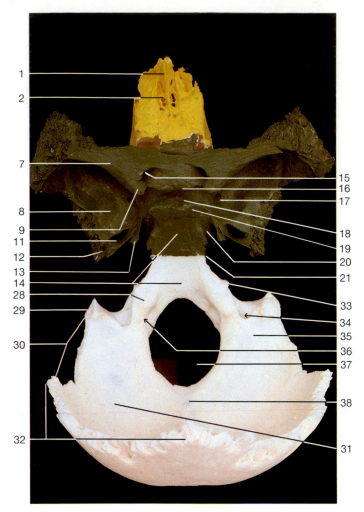

Ethmoid bone
1 Crista galli
2 Cribriform plate
3 Ethmoidal air cells
4 Middle concha
5 Perpendicular plate (part of nasal septum)
6 Orbital plate

Sphenoid bone
7 Lesser wing
8 Greater wing
9 Anterior clinoid process
10 Posterior clinoid process
11 Foramen ovale
12 Foramen spinosum
13 Lingula of the sphenoid
14 Clivus
15 Optic canal
16 Tuberculum sellae
17 Foramen rotundum (right side)
18 Hypophysial fossa
19 Dorsum sellae
20 Carotid sulcus
21 Sphenooccipital synchondrosis
22 Lateral pterygoid plate
23 Greater wing of sphenoid bone (orbital surface)
24 Greater wing of sphenoid bone (maxillary surface)
25 Foramen rotundum (left side)
26 Superior orbital fissure
27 Infratemporal crest of the greater wing

Part of the disarticulated base of the skull.
Ethmoid, sphenoid and occipital bones (from above).
Green = sphenoid bone; yellow = ethmoid bone.

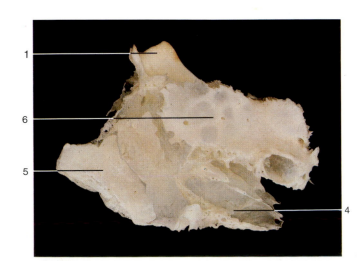

Ethmoid bone (lateral aspect), posterior portion to the right.

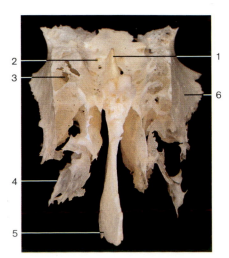

Ethmoid bone (anterior aspect).

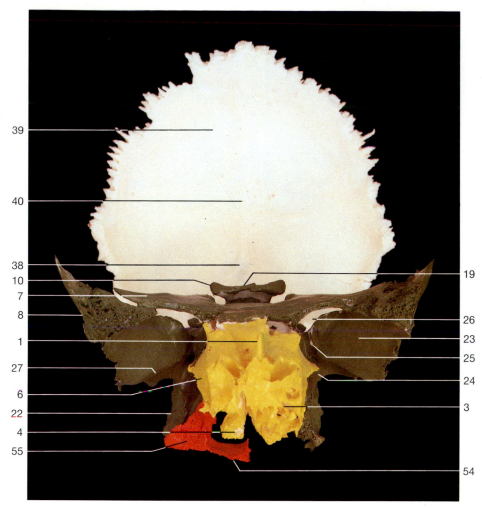

Disarticulated base of the skull (anterior aspect).
Green = sphenoid bone; yellow = ethmoid bone; red = palatine bone.

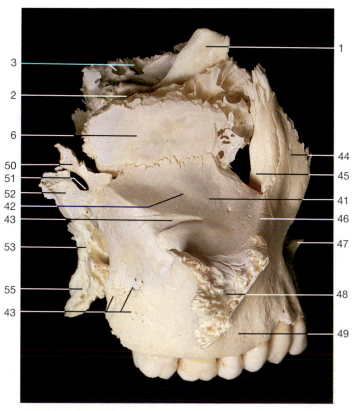

Right maxilla, ethmoid and palatine bone (lateral aspect).

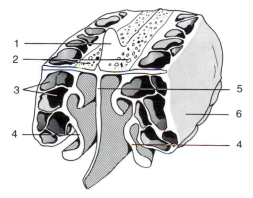

Schematic drawing of the **ethmoid bone**
(oblique anterior aspect).

39

The Palatine Bone

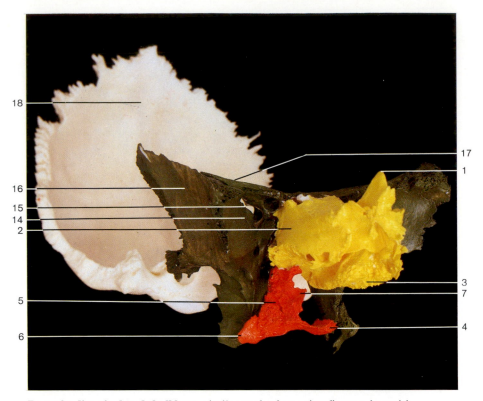

Part of a disarticulated skull base, similar to the foregoing figures, but with palatine bone. Green = sphenoid bone; yellow = ethmoid bone; red = palatine bone.

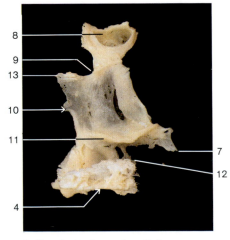

Left palatine bone (medial aspect, posterior aspect to the left).

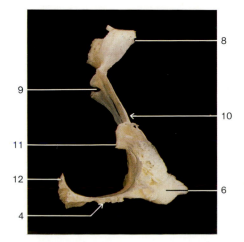

Left palatine bone (anterior aspect).

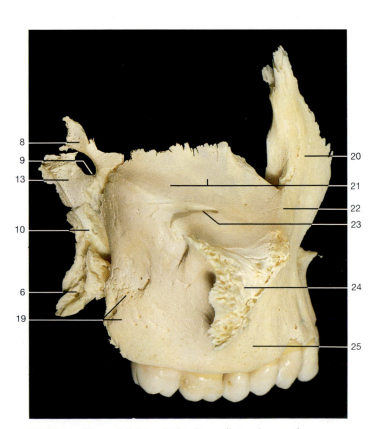

Right maxilla and right palatine bone (lateral aspect).

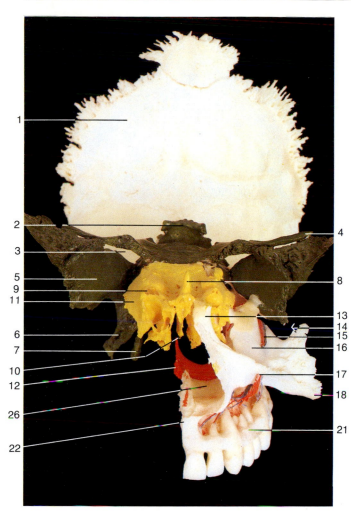

Occipital bone
1 Squamous part

Sphenoid bone
2 Dorsum sellae
3 Superior orbital fissure
4 Lesser wing
5 Greater wing (orbital surface)
6 Lateral pterygoid plate
7 Medial pterygoid plate

Ethmoid bone
8 Crista galli
9 Ethmoidal air cells
10 Perpendicular plate
11 Orbital plate

Palatine bone
12 Horizontal plate (nasal crest)

Maxilla
13 Frontal process
14 Inferior orbital fissure
15 Infraorbital groove with artificial vessels and nerves
16 Orbital surface
17 Infraorbital foramen with artificial vessels and nerves
18 Zygomatic process
19 Anterior lacrimal crest
20 Canine fossa
21 Alveolar process with teeth
22 Anterior nasal spine
23 Juga alveolaria (elevations formed by roots of teeth)
24 Lacrimal groove
25 Maxillary tuberosity with alveolar foramina
26 Palatine process

Part of a disarticulated skull.
The **maxilla** is added to the preceding specimen.

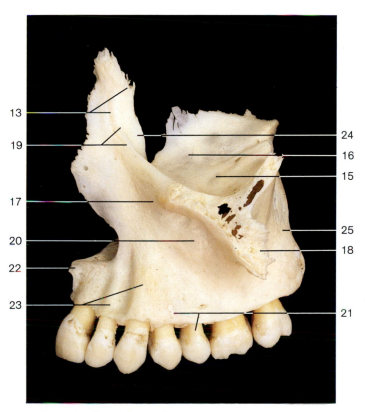

Left maxilla (lateral aspect).

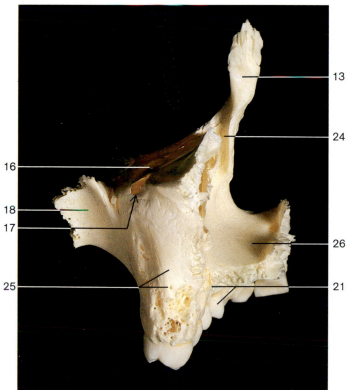

Left maxilla (posterior aspect).

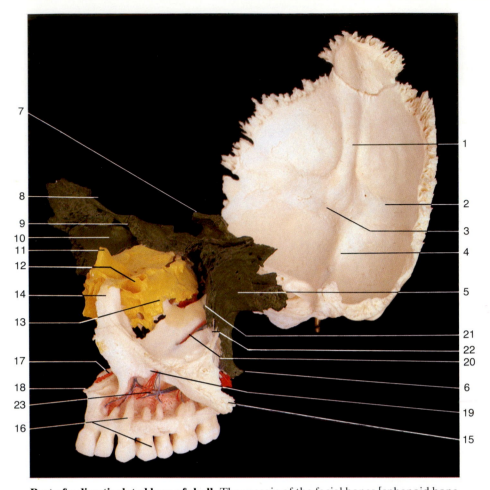

Occipital bone

1 Groove for superior sagittal sinus
2 Groove for transverse sinus
3 Internal occipital protuberance
4 Internal occipital crest

Sphenoid bone

5 Greater wing (temporal surface)
6 Lateral pterygoid plate
7 Dorsum sellae
8 Lesser wing
9 Superior orbital fissure
10 Greater wing (orbital surface)

Ethmoid bone

11 Crista galli
12 Ethmoidal air cells
13 Orbital plate

Maxilla

14 Frontal process
15 Zygomatic process
16 Alveolar process with teeth
17 Palatine process
18 Anterior nasal spine
19 Infraorbital foramen
20 Infraorbital groove
21 Inferior orbital fissure
22 Posterior superior alveolar nerves
23 Superior dental plexus
24 Maxillary hiatus
    (leading to maxillary sinus)
25 Greater palatine groove
26 Lacrimal groove
27 Conchal crest
28 Body of maxilla (nasal surface)
29 Nasal crest
30 Incisive canal

Palatine bone

31 Orbital process
32 Sphenopalatine notch
33 Sphenoidal process
34 Perpendicular plate
35 Conchal crest
36 Horizontal plate
37 Pyramidal process

Part of a disarticulated base of skull. The mosaic of the facial bones [sphenoid bone (green), ethmoid bone (yellow), and palatine bone (red)] is seen from the lateral aspect. Part of the body of the maxilla has been removed to show the dental plexus and the roots of the teeth.

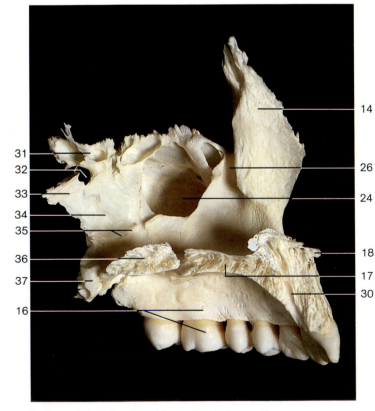

Left maxilla and palatine bone (medial aspect).

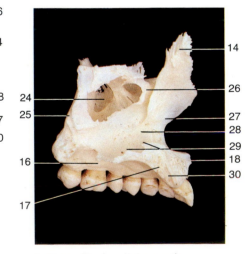

Left maxilla (medial aspect).

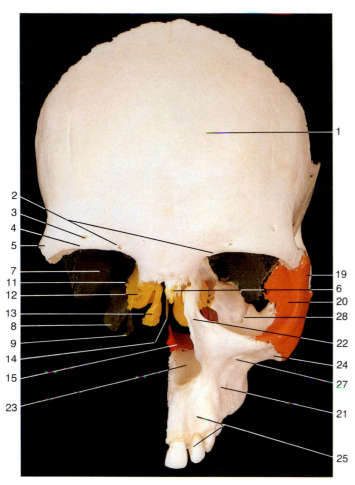

Frontal bone
1 Squamous part
2 Frontal foramen or notch
3 Supraorbital foramen
4 Supraorbital margin
5 Zygomatic process
6 Frontal spine

Sphenoid bone
7 Greater wing (orbital surface)
8 Lateral pterygoid plate
9 Medial pterygoid plate
10 Pterygoid hamulus

Ethmoid bone
11 Orbital plate
12 Ethmoidal air cells
13 Middle concha
14 Perpendicular plate

Palatine bone
15 Horizontal plate
16 Pyramidal process
17 Lesser palatine foramen
18 Greater palatine foramen

Zygomatic bone
19 Frontal process
20 Orbital surface

Maxilla
21 Canine fossa
22 Frontal process
23 Palatine process
24 Zygomatic process
25 Alveolar process and teeth
26 Juga alveolaria
27 Infraorbital foramen
28 Infraorbital groove
29 Anterior nasal aperture
30 Anterior nasal spine

Incisive bone
31 Central incisor and incisive bone or premaxilla
32 Incisive fossa

Vomer
33 Ala of the vomer

Sutures and choanae
34 Intermaxillary suture
35 Palatomaxillary suture
36 Choanae

Anterior view of a disarticulated skull, showing the connection of the maxilla with the frontal and zygomatic bone. Orange = zygomatic bone; yellow = ethmoid bone; red = palatine bone; green = sphenoid bone.

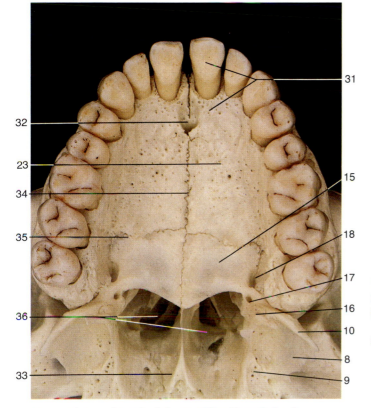

Bony palate and teeth of the maxillae (from below).

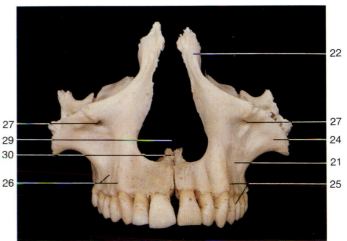

Anterior view of both maxillae, forming the anterior bony aperture of the nose.

43

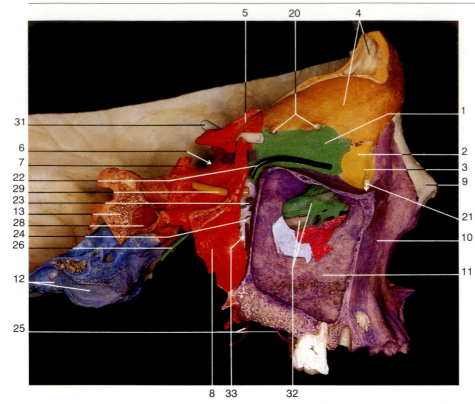

1 **Ethmoid bone** (green)
2 **Lacrimal bone** (yellow)
3 Posterior lacrimal crest
4 **Frontal bone** and frontal sinus (orange)
5 **Sphenoid bone** (lesser wing) (red)
6 Hypophysial fossa
7 Dorsum sellae
8 Pterygoid process (red)
9 **Nasal bone** (white)
10 **Maxilla** (violet)
11 Maxillary sinus
12 **Occipital bone** (blue)
13 **Temporal bone** (petrous part)
14 Zygomatic process
15 Mastoid process
16 Articular tubercle
17 **Zygomatic bone**
18 **Vomer**

Fossae, foramina and canals
19 Condylar fossa
20 Anterior and posterior ethmoidal foramina
21 Nasolacrimal canal
22 Inferior orbital fissure, entrance to the pterygopalatine fossa (black probe)
23 Sphenopalatine foramen
24 **Pterygopalatine fossa**
25 Greater and lesser palatine foramen continuous with greater palatine canal (brown probe)
26 Pterygoid canal (green probe)
27 Foramen ovale
28 Carotid canal
29 Foramen rotundum (yellow probe)
30 Internal acoustic meatus
31 Optic foramen or canal (white probe)
32 Maxillary hiatus and uncinate process of ethmoid bone (green)
33 Pterygomaxillary fissure
34 Tympanomastoid fissure
35 Petrotympanic fissure
36 External acoustic meatus
37 Temporal fossa
38 Mandibular fossa
39 Lesser palatine foramina

Paramedian section through the skull (lateral aspect). **Facial skeleton.**
Maxillary sinus, orbit and pterygopalatine fossa. Maxillary sinus opened from the lateral side. Maxillary hiatus is narrowed by palatine bone (light blue), uncinate process (green) and inferior nasal concha (red).

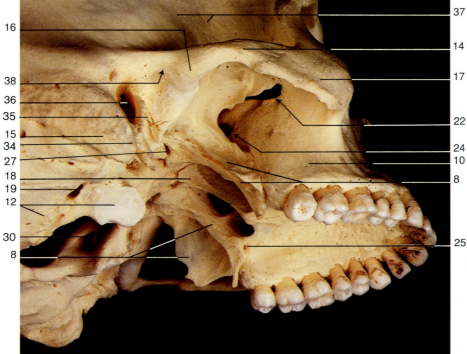

Base of the skull (oblique lateral aspect). **Facial skeleton.**

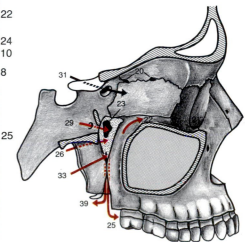

Openings and canals of the pterygopalatine fossa. (Schematic drawing.)

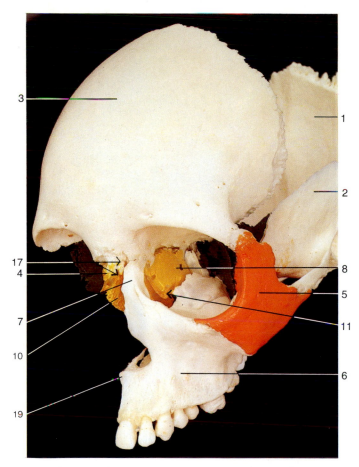

1 **Occipital bone**
2 **Temporal bone**
3 **Frontal bone**
4 Nasal spine of frontal bone
5 **Zygomatic bone**
6 **Maxilla**
7 Frontal process of maxilla
8 **Ethmoid bone**
9 Orbital plate of ethmoid bone
10 Perpendicular plate of ethmoid bone
11 Site of **lacrimal bone**
12 Lacrimal groove of lacrimal bone
13 Posterior lacrimal crest
14 Fossa for lacrimal sac
15 Lacrimal hamulus
16 Nasolacrimal canal
17 Site of **nasal bone**
18 Nasal foramina of nasal bone
19 Anterior nasal spine of maxilla
20 **Vomer**
21 Greater wing of sphenoid bone
22 Anterior and posterior ethmoidal foramina
23 Optic canal
24 Superior orbital fissure
25 Inferior orbital fissure
26 Infraorbital groove
27 Infraorbital foramen

Anterior part of a disarticulated skull, nearly complete. Orange = zygomatic bone; yellow = ethmoidal bone; green = sphenoidal bone. The arrows indicate the locations of the lacrimal bone (11) and the nasal bone (17).

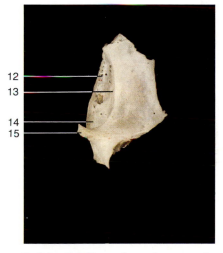

Left lacrimal bone (anterior aspect).

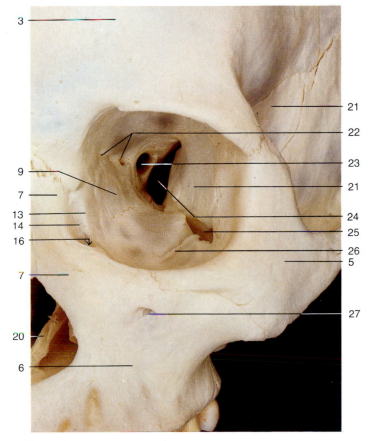

Left orbit (anterior aspect).

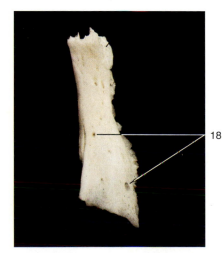

Left nasal bone (anterior aspect).

45

The Bones of the Nasal Cavity

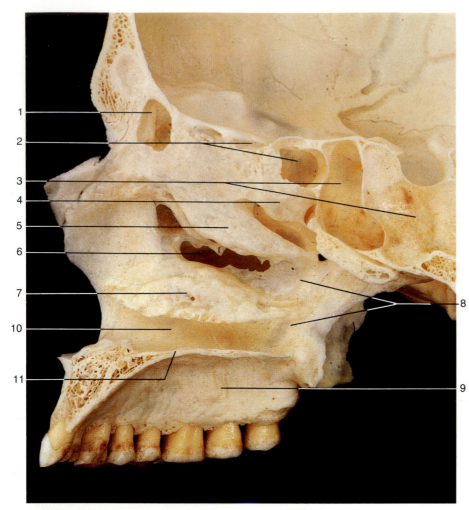

1 Frontal sinus
2 Ethmoid air cells
3 Sphenoid sinus
4 Superior nasal concha
5 Middle nasal concha
6 Maxillary hiatus
7 Inferior nasal concha
8 Palatine bone
9 Maxilla
10 Inferior meatus
11 Palatine process of the maxilla

Lateral wall of the nasal cavity. Median section through the skull.

▷
To page 47:

Blue   = Occipital bone
Light green   = Parietal bone
Light brown   = Frontal bone
Dark brown   = Temporal bone
Red   = Sphenoid bone
Dark green   = Ethmoid bone
Light blue   = Nasal bone
Pink   = Inferior concha
Orange   = Vomer
Violet   = Maxilla
White   = Palatine bone
White   = Mandible

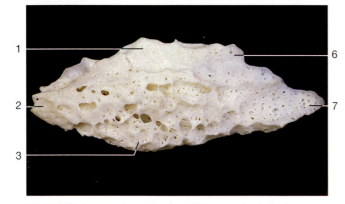

Right inferior nasal concha (medial aspect). Anterior part to the left.

Inferior Concha and Vomer

1 Ethmoidal process
2 Anterior part of concha
3 Inferior border
4 Ala of vomer
5 Posterior border of nasal septum
6 Lacrimal process
7 Posterior part of concha
8 Maxillary process

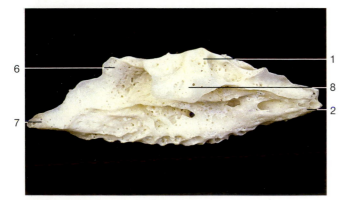

Right inferior nasal concha (lateral aspect). Anterior part to the right.

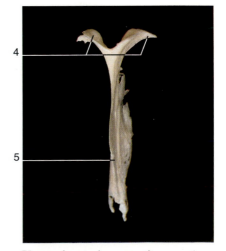

Vomer (posterior aspect).

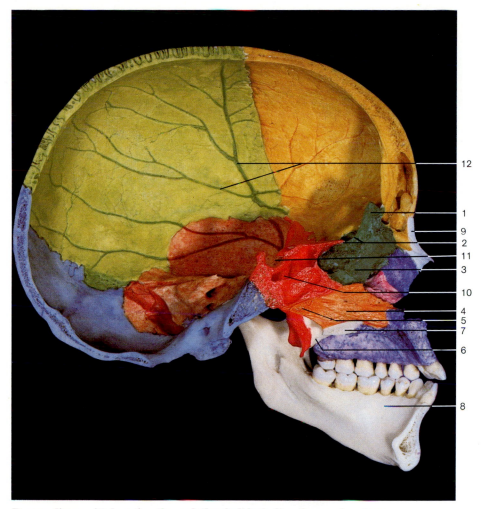

1 Crista galli
2 Cribriform plate
  of ethmoid bone
3 Perpendicular plate
  of ethmoid bone
4 Vomer
5 Ala of the vomer
6 Palatine bone,
  perpendicular process
7 Palatine bone, horizontal plate
8 Mandible
9 Nasal bone
10 Sphenoidal sinus
11 Sella turcica
12 Grooves for the middle
   meningeal artery

Cartilages of the nose

13 Lateral nasal cartilages
14 Greater alar cartilage
15 Lesser alar cartilages
16 Septal cartilage
17 Nasal bone

Bones of nasal cavity

18 Middle nasal concha
19 Frontal process of maxilla
20 Inferior nasal concha
21 Palatine process of maxilla
22 Maxillary hiatus
23 Medial pterygoid plate
24 Pterygoid hamulus

Paramedian sagittal section through the skull including the nasal septum.

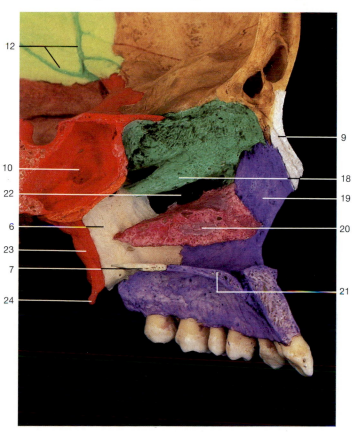

Bones of left nasal cavity (medial aspect).

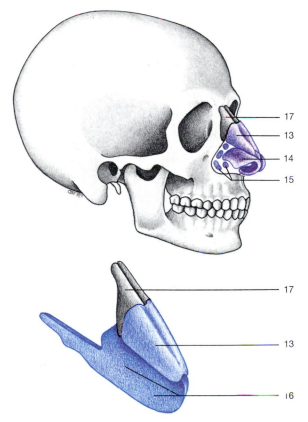

Cartilages of the nose.
Schematic diagram of the external nose (O.).

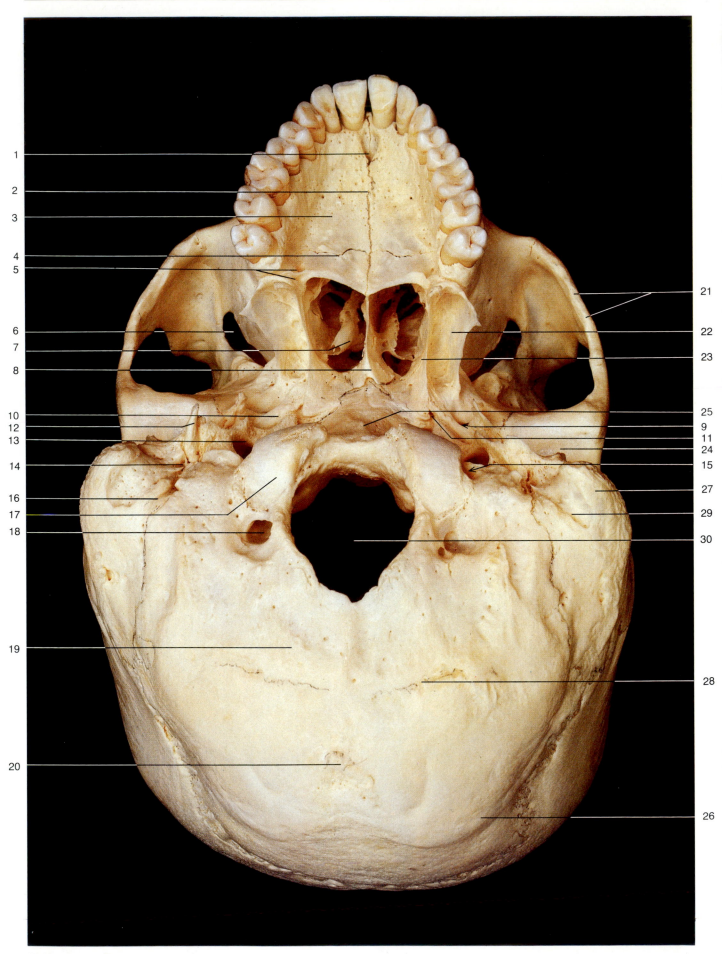

Base of the skull (inferior aspect).

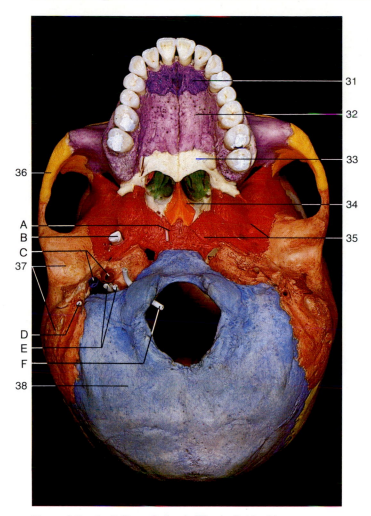

Base of the skull (from below). The individual bones are indicated by different colours.

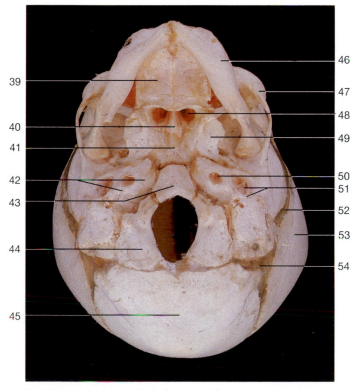

Skull of the newborn (inferior aspect).

A Pterygoid canal
B Foramen ovale
C Internal carotid artery within carotid canal, internal jugular vein within the venous part of jugular foramen
D Stylomastoid foramen (facial nerve)
E Jugular foramen (glossopharyngeal, vagus and accessory nerves)
F Hypoglossal canal (hypoglossal nerve)

1   Incisive canal
2   Median palatine suture
3   Bony palate
4   Palatomaxillary suture
5   Greater and lesser palatine foramina
6   Inferior orbital fissure
7   Middle concha (ethmoid bone)
8   Vomer
9   Foramen ovale
10 Groove for auditory tube
11 Pterygoid canal
12 Styloid process
13 Carotid canal
14 Stylomastoid foramen
15 Jugular foramen
16 Groove for occipital artery
17 Occipital condyle
18 Condylar canal
19 Nuchal plane
20 External occipital protuberance
21 Zygomatic arch
22 Lateral pterygoid plate
23 Medial pterygoid plate
24 Mandibular fossa
25 Pharyngeal tubercle
26 Superior nuchal line
27 Mastoid process
28 Inferior nuchal line
29 Mastoid notch
30 Foramen magnum
31 Incisive bone or premaxilla (dark violet)
32 Maxilla (violet)
33 Palatine bone (white)
34 Vomer (orange)
35 Sphenoid bone (red)
36 Zygomatic bone (yellow)
37 Temporal bone (brown)
38 Occipital bone (blue)
39 Palatine process of maxilla
40 Vomer
41 Sphenoid bone
42 Petrous part of temporal bone
43 Basilar part ⎫
44 Lateral part ⎬ of occipital bone
45 Squamous part ⎭
46 Mandible
47 Zygomatic arch
48 Choana
49 Pterygoid process of sphenoid bone
50 Carotid canal
51 External acoustic meatus, tympanic annulus
52 Sphenoidal fontanelle
53 Parietal bone
54 Mastoid fontanelle

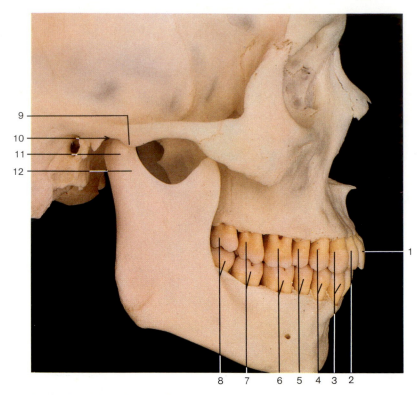

1 Central incisor
2 Lateral incisor
3 Canines
4 First premolars or bicuspids
5 Second premolars or bicuspids
6 First molars
7 Second molars
8 Third molars
9 Articular tubercle
10 Mandibular fossa
11 Head of mandible
12 Condylar process

Normal position of teeth. Dentition in centric occlusion (lateral view).

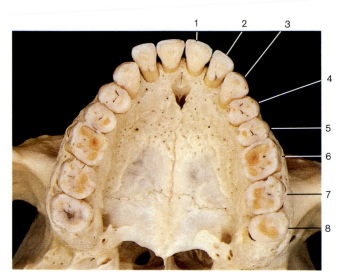

Upper teeth of the adult (inferior aspect).

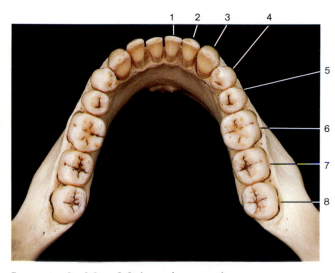

Lower teeth of the adult (superior aspect).

Table of dentition. Eruption of deciduous and permanent teeth (after C. Röse according to A. Kröncke).

Primary dentition (Deciduous teeth)	Maxilla months post partum	Mandible months
1. Central incisor	10.3	8.6
2. Lateral incisor	12.2	14.4
3. Cuspid incisor	19.5	20.1
4. First molar	15.5	16.5
5. Second molar	24.8	24.5

Secondary dentition (Permanent teeth)	years and months ♂	years and months ♀	years and months ♂	years and months ♀
1. Central incisor	7/8	7/5	6/10	6/7
2. Lateral incisor	8/11	8/6	7/11	7/7
3. Cuspid incisor	12/2	11/7	11/12	10/3
4. First premolar	10/5	10/1	11/3	10/8
5. Second premolar	11/4	11/1	12/0	11/7
6. First molar	6/7	6/6	6/5	6/3
7. Second molar	12/9	12/5	12/3	11/9

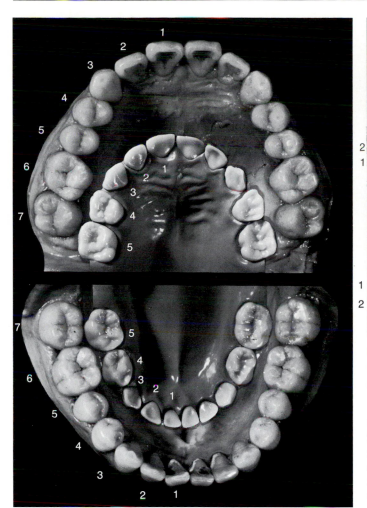

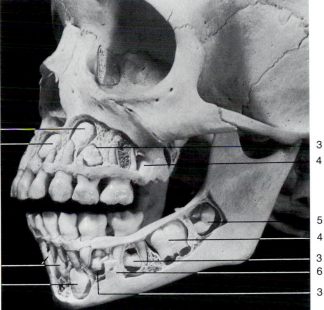

Deciduous teeth in child's skull. The developing crowns of the permanent teeth are displayed in their sockets in the maxilla and mandible.

△

1 Permanent incisors
2 Permanent canine
3 Premolars
4 First permanent molar
5 Second permanent molar
6 Mental foramen

Comparison of the deciduous and permanent teeth.
Notice that the breadth of the alveolar arch of the child's mandible and maxilla holding the deciduous teeth is nearly the same as the comparable portion in the jaws of the adult. Note the unerupted third molars.

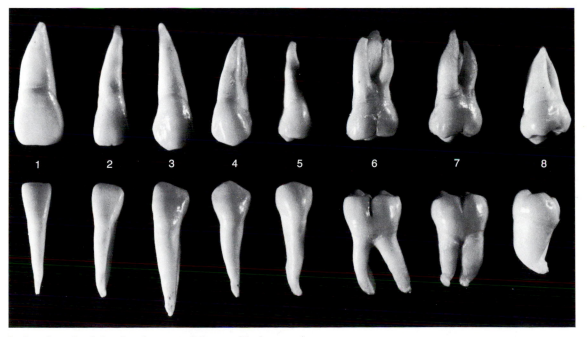

Isolated teeth of the alveolar part of the maxilla (top row) and the mandible (lower row), labial surface of the teeth.

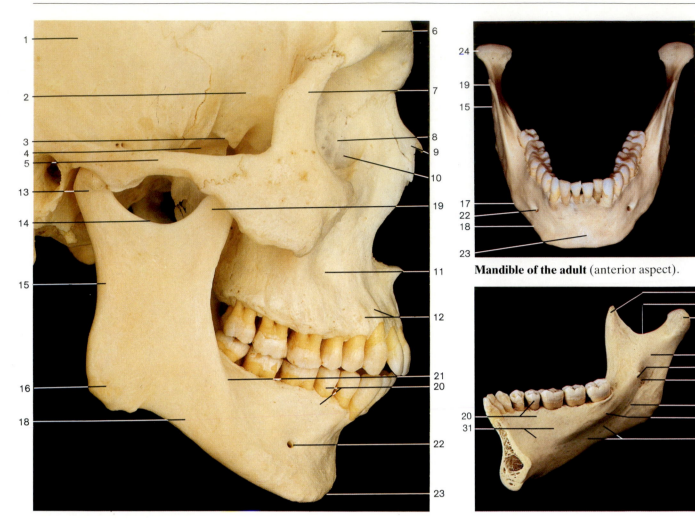

Lateral aspect of the facial bones. Mandible and teeth in the position of occlusion. Upper and lower jaw occluded.

Mandible of the adult (anterior aspect).

Right half of mandible (medial aspect).

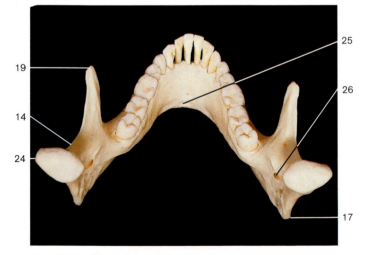

Mandible of the adult (posterior aspect).

1 **Temporal bone**
2 Temporal fossa, greater wing of sphenoid bone
3 Infratemporal crest
4 Infratemporal fossa
5 Zygomatic arch
6 **Frontal bone**
7 **Zygomatic bone,** frontal process
8 **Lacrimal bone**

9 **Nasal bone**
10 Lacrimal groove
11 **Maxilla,** canine fossa
12 Alveolar juga

Mandible
13 Condylar process
14 Mandibular notch
15 Ramus of the mandible
16 Masseteric tuberosity
17 Angle of the mandible
18 Body of the mandible
19 Coronoid process
20 Alveolar process including teeth
21 Oblique line
22 Mental foramen
23 Mental protuberance
24 Head of the mandible
25 Genial tubercle or mental spine
26 Mandibular foramen
27 Lingula
28 Mylohyoid sulcus
29 Mylohyoid line
30 Submandibular fossa
31 Sublingual fossa

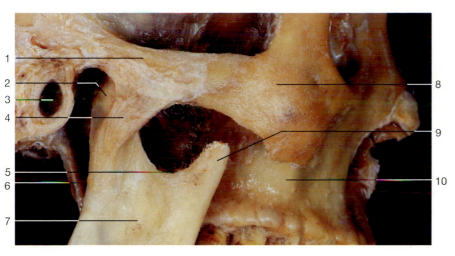

Temporomandibular joint with ligaments.

1 Zygomatic arch
2 Articular capsule
3 External acoustic meatus
4 **Lateral ligament**
5 Mandibular notch
6 **Stylomandibular ligament**
7 Ramus of the mandible
8 Zygomatic bone
9 Coronoid process
10 Maxilla
11 Articular cartilage of
   condylar process
12 Styloid process
13 Mandibular fossa
14 **Articular disc**
15 Articular tubercle
16 Lateral pterygoid muscle
17 Condylar process of mandible

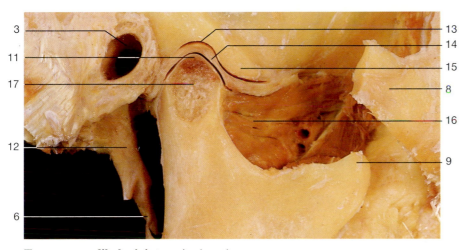

Temporomandibular joint, sagittal section.

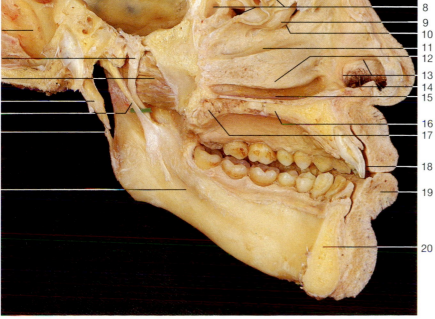

Ligaments of temporomandibular joint. Left half of the head (medial aspect).

1 Groove for sigmoid sinus
2 Mandibular nerve
3 Lateral pterygoid muscle
4 Styloid process
5 Sphenomandibular ligament
6 Stylomandibular ligament
7 Mylohyoid groove
8 Ethmoidal air cells
9 Ethmoidal bulla
10 Hiatus semilunaris
11 Middle meatus
12 Inferior nasal concha
13 Limen nasi
14 Vestibule with hairs
15 Inferior meatus
16 Hard palate
17 Soft palate
18 Vestibule of oral cavity
19 Lower lip
20 Mandible

The Temporomandibular Joint

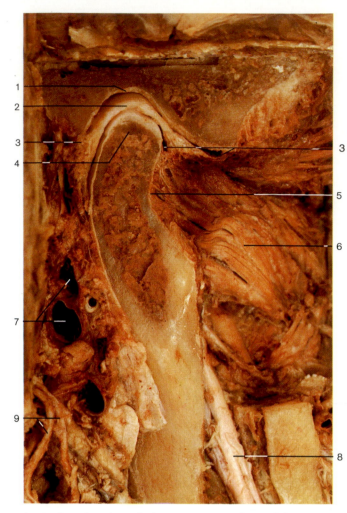

Sagittal section through the **temporomandibular joint.**

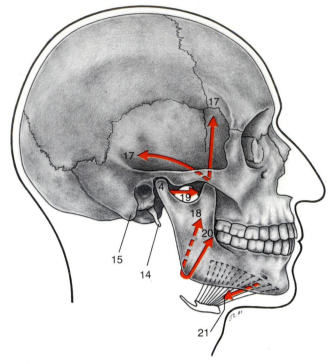

Effect of the muscles of mastication on the temporomandibular joint (Tr.).

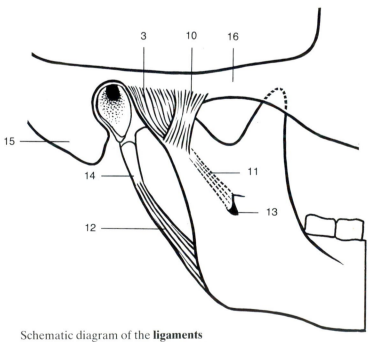

Schematic diagram of the **ligaments** related to the **temporomandibular joint.**

1 Mandibular fossa
2 Articular disc
3 Articular capsule
4 Head of the mandible
5 Depression for the lateral pterygoid muscle
6 Lateral pterygoid muscle
7 Retroarticular venous plexus
8 Mandibular canal with inferior alveolar nerve
9 Facial nerve
10 Lateral ligament
11 Sphenomandibular ligament
12 Stylomandibular ligament
13 Mandibular foramen
14 Styloid process
15 Mastoid process
16 Zygomatic arch
17 Temporalis muscle
18 Medial pterygoid muscle
19 Lateral pterygoid muscle
20 Masseter muscle
21 Mylohyoid muscle

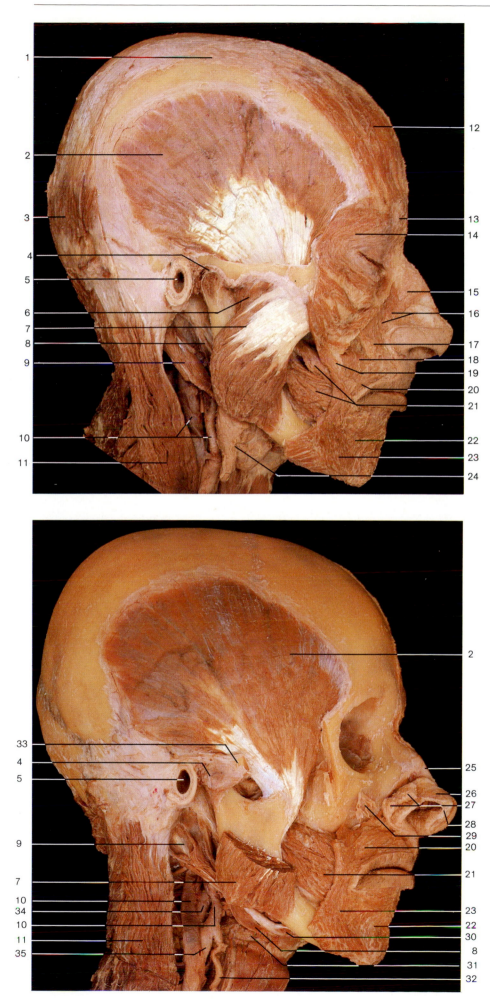

Temporalis and masseter.
The temporal fascia has been removed, the temporomandibular joint severed and the zygomatic arch displayed.

1　Galea aponeurotica
2　Temporalis
3　Occipital belly of occipitofrontalis
4　Temporomandibular joint
5　External acoustic meatus
6　Deep layer of masseter
7　Superficial layer of masseter
8　Stylohyoid muscle
9　Posterior belly of digastric muscle
10　Internal jugular vein and external carotid artery
11　Sternocleidomastoid muscle
12　Frontal belly of occipitofrontalis
13　Depressor supercilii
14　Orbicularis oculi
15　Transverse part of nasalis
16　Levator labii superioris alaeque nasi
17　Levator labii superioris
18　Levator anguli oris
19　Zygomaticus major
20　Orbicularis oris
21　Buccinator
22　Depressor labii inferioris
23　Depressor anguli oris
24　Submandibular gland
25　Lateral nasal cartilage
26　Greater alar cartilage, lateral part
27　Lesser alar cartilages
28　Greater alar cartilage, medial part
29　Infraorbital nerve
30　Anterior belly of digastric muscle
31　Hypoglossal nerve, hyoglossus
32　Superior thyroid artery
33　Zygomatic arch
34　Internal carotid artery
35　Common carotid artery

Temporalis and temporomandibular joint. The zygomatic arch and the masseter have been partially severed to display the insertion of the temporalis.

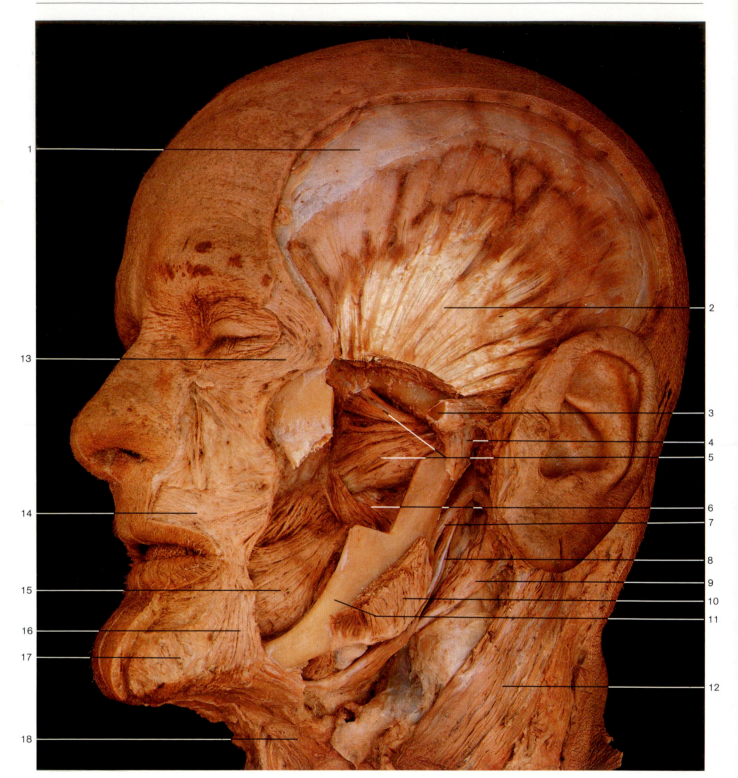

Medial and lateral pterygoid muscles. A portion of the mandible and the zygomatic arch has been removed revealing the pterygoid region or infratemporal fossa.

1　Periosteum
2　**Temporalis**
3　Zygomatic arch
4　Articular capsule of temporomandibular joint
5　**Lateral pterygoid**
　　Upper head
　　Lower head

6　**Medial pterygoid**
7　Styloglossus
8　Stylohyoid
9　Posterior belly of digastric muscle
10　**Masseter** (severed)
11　Mandible
12　Sternocleidomastoid

13　Orbicularis oculi
14　Orbicularis oris
15　Buccinator
16　Depressor anguli oris
17　Depressor labii inferioris
18　Platysma

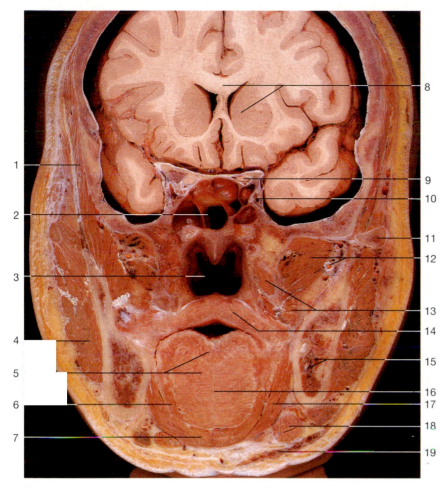

1 Temporalis muscle
2 Sphenoidal sinus
3 Nasopharynx
4 Masseter muscle
5 Superior longitudinal, transverse and vertical muscles of tongue
6 Hyoglossus muscle
7 Geniohyoid
8 Corpus callosum, caudate nucleus
9 Optic nerve
10 Cavernous sinus
11 Zygomatic arch
12 Cross section of lateral pterygoid muscle, maxillary artery
13 Section of medial pterygoid muscle
14 Soft palate
15 Mandible, inferior alveolar nerve
16 Septum of the tongue
17 Mylohyoid muscle
18 Submandibular gland
19 Platysma
20 Foramen magnum, vertebral artery and spinal cord
21 Internal carotid artery
22 Head of mandible
23 Styloid process
24 Inferior alveolar nerve
25 Lingual nerve and chorda tympani nerve
26 Medial pterygoid muscle
27 Uvula
28 Anterior belly of digastric muscle (cut)
29 Condyle of occipital bone
30 Mastoid process
31 Lateral pterygoid muscle
32 Auditory tube and levator veli palatini
33 Tensor veli palatini

Coronal section through cranial, nasal and oral cavity at the level of sphenoidal sinus.

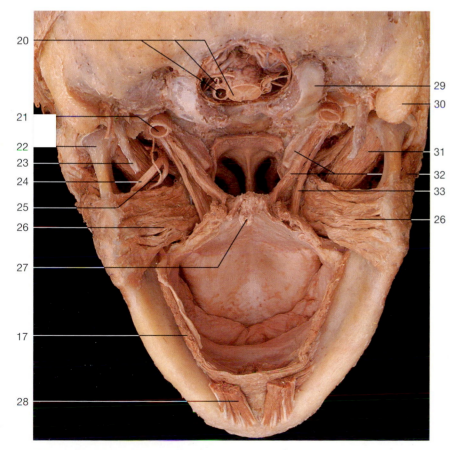

Pterygoid and palatine muscles (posterior aspect).

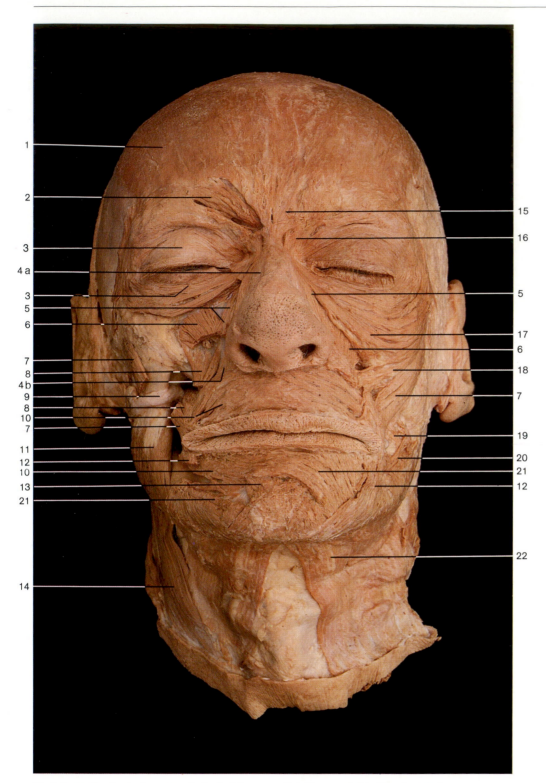

Facial muscles (anterior aspect). Left side: superficial layer; right side: deeper layer.

1	Frontal belly of occipitofrontalis	10	Orbicularis oris	20	Risorius
2	Corrugator supercilii	11	Masseter	21	Depressor labii inferioris
3	Palpebral part of orbicularis oculi	12	Depressor anguli oris	22	Platysma
4a	Transverse part of nasalis	13	Mentalis	23	Galea aponeurotica
4b	Alar part of nasalis	14	Sternocleidomastoid	24	Temporoparietalis
5	Levator labii superioris alaeque nasi	15	Procerus	25	Occipital belly of occipitofrontalis
6	Levator labii superioris	16	Depressor supercilii	26	Parotid gland
7	Zygomaticus major	17	Orbital part of orbicularis oculi	27	Temporal fascia
8	Levator anguli oris	18	Zygomaticus minor	28	Orbicularis oculi
9	Parotid duct	19	Buccinator	29	Parotid duct, masseter

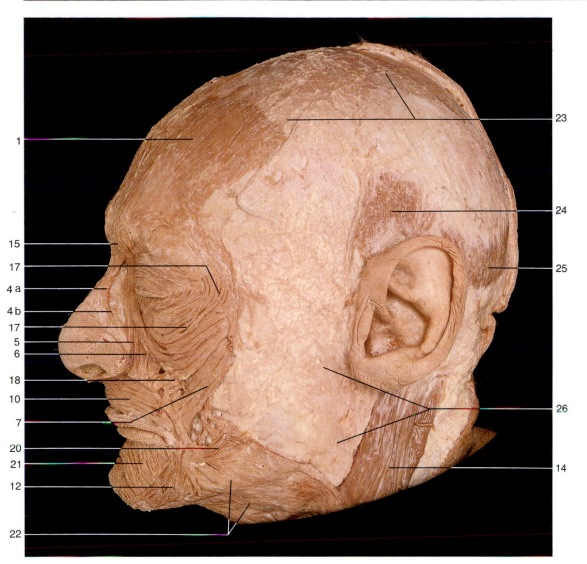

Facial muscles (lateral aspect).

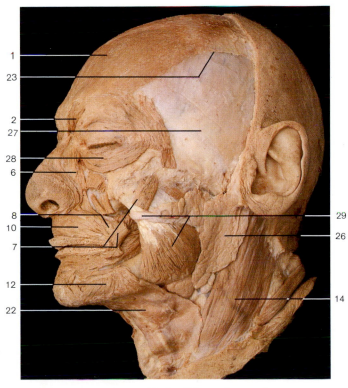

Facial muscles and parotid gland (lateral aspect).

The facial muscles are cutaneous muscles whose tendons end in the skin. They serve primarily as a means of closing or opening the orifices of the head (e. g. of the mouth, eyelids, nose or ear), but, in addition, they are of great importance for facial expression. There are sphincter-like muscles (orbicularis muscles), capable of closing the orifices, and radially arranged muscles (levators, depressors, zygomatic muscles) for opening them. The buccinator continues posteriorly into the pharynx, the occipitofrontalis muscle stretches from the forehead to the occipital region, so that the scalp is moveable as a whole.

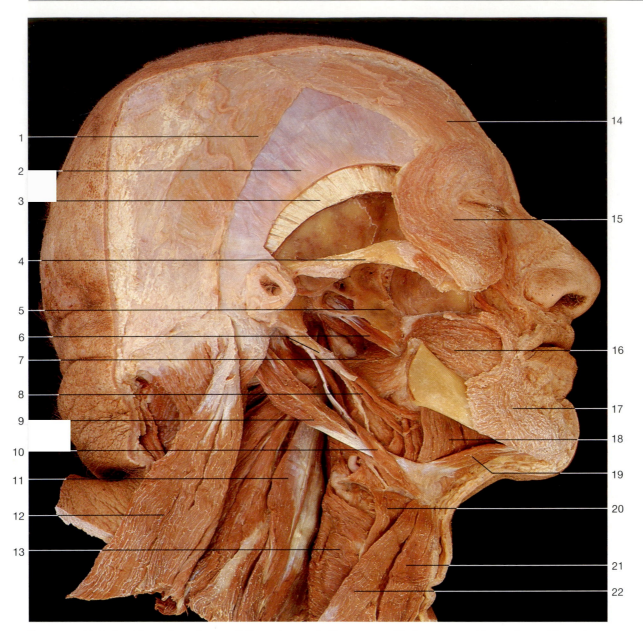

Supra- and infrahyoid muscles, pharynx I (lateral aspect). Ramus mandibulae, pterygoid muscles and insertion of temporal muscle removed.

1	Galea aponeurotica	13	Inferior constrictor of pharynx
2	Temporal fascia	14	Frontal belly of occipito-frontalis muscle
3	Tendon of temporalis muscle	15	Orbital part of orbicularis oculi
4	Zygomatic arch	16	Buccinator
5	Lateral pterygoid plate	17	Depressor anguli oris
6	Tensor veli palatini, styloid process	18	Mylohyoid muscle
7	Superior constrictor of pharynx	19	Anterior belly of digastric muscle
8	Styloglossus muscle	20	Thyrohyoid muscle
9	Posterior belly of digastric muscle	21	Sternohyoid muscle
10	Stylohyoid muscle	22	Omohyoid muscle
11	Longus capitis		
12	Sternocleidomastoid (reflected)		

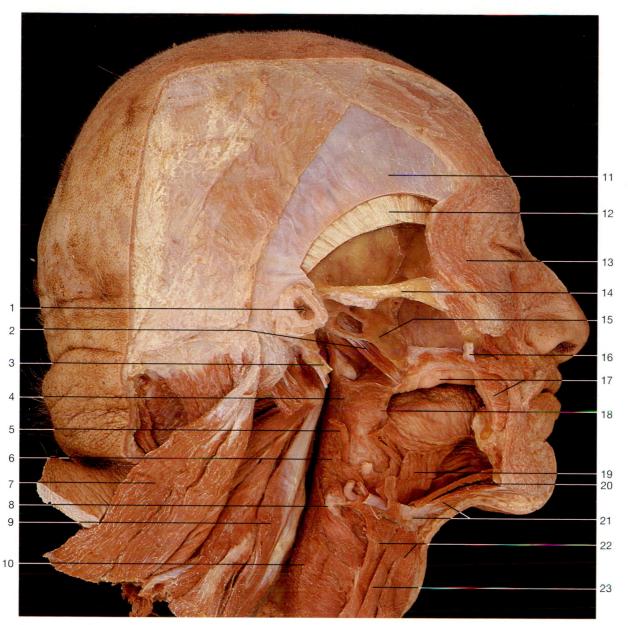

Supra- and infrahyoid muscles, pharynx II. Buccinator removed; oral cavity opened.

1 External acoustic meatus	13 Orbicularis oculi
2 Tensor veli palatini	14 Zygomatic arch
3 Styloid process	15 Lateral pterygoid plate
4 Superior constrictor muscle of pharynx	16 Parotid duct
5 Stylopharyngeus muscle (divided)	17 Gingiva of upper jaw (without teeth), buccinator muscle (divided)
6 Middle constrictor muscle of pharynx	18 Pterygomandibular raphe
7 Sternocleidomastoid	19 Hyoglossus muscle
8 Greater horn of hyoid bone	20 Mylohyoid muscle
9 Longus capitis	21 Anterior belly of digastric muscle, hyoid bone
10 Inferior constrictor of pharynx	22 Sternohyoid and thyrohyoid muscles
11 Temporal fascia	23 Omohyoid muscle
12 Tendon of temporalis muscle	

The Skull of the Newborn

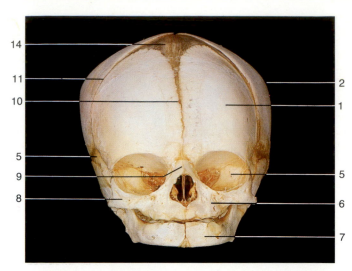

Skull of the newborn (anterior aspect).

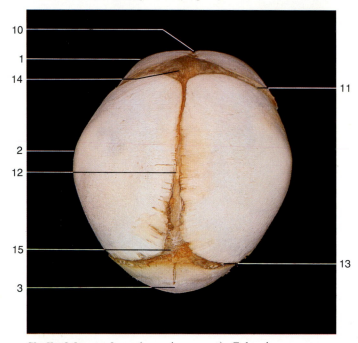

Skull of the newborn (superior aspect). Calvaria.

Cranial skeleton
1 Frontal tuber or eminence
2 Parietal tuber or eminence
3 Occipital tuber or eminence
4 Squamous part of temporal bone
5 Greater wing of sphenoid bone

Facial skeleton
6 Maxilla
7 Mandible
8 Zygomatic bone
9 Nasal bone

Sutures and fontanelles
10 Frontal suture
11 Coronal suture
12 Sagittal suture
13 Lambdoid suture
14 Anterior fontanelle
15 Posterior fontanelle
16 Sphenoidal fontanelle
17 Mastoid fontanelle

Base of the skull
18 Frontal bone
19 Ethmoid bone
20 Sphenoid bone
21 Hypophysial fossa
22 Dorsum sellae
23 Temporal bone
24 Mastoid fontanelle
25 Occipital bone

In the newborn the facial skeleton, in contrast to the cranial skeleton, appears relatively small. There are no teeth presenting. The bones of the cranium are separated by wide fontanelles.

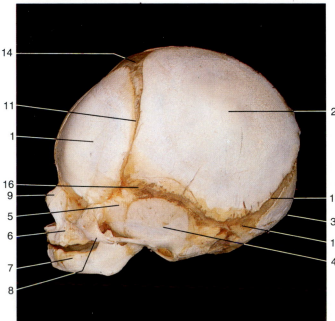

Skull of the newborn (lateral aspect).

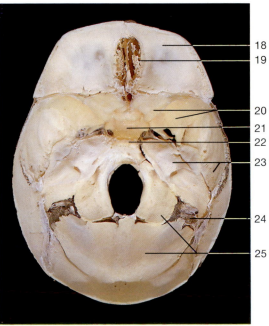

Base of the skull of the newborn (internal aspect).

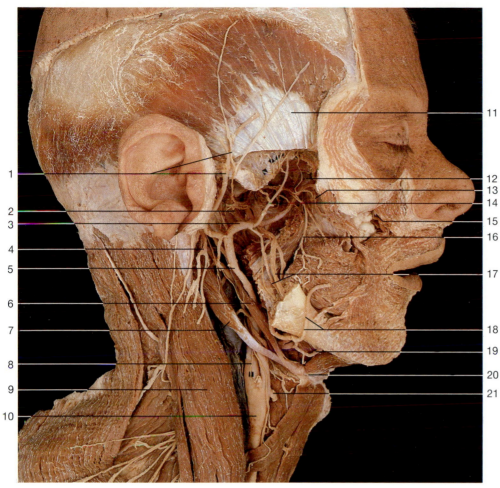

1 Superficial temporal artery, auriculotemporal nerve
2 Middle meningeal artery
3 **Maxillary artery**
4 Facial nerve (divided and reflected)
5 **External carotid artery**
6 Stylohyoid muscle
7 Digastric muscle (posterior belly)
8 Internal carotid artery, carotid sinus branch of glossopharyngeal nerve
9 Sternocleidomastoid
10 Common carotid artery
11 Temporalis
12 Pterygopalatine fossa
13 Posterior superior alveolar artery
14 Deep temporal artery
15 Infraorbital artery
16 Buccal nerve
17 Inferior alveolar artery and nerve
18 **Facial artery**
19 Submental artery
20 Hyoid bone
21 Superior thyroid artery (divided)

Dissection of maxillary artery. Mandible and lateral pterygoid muscle partly removed.

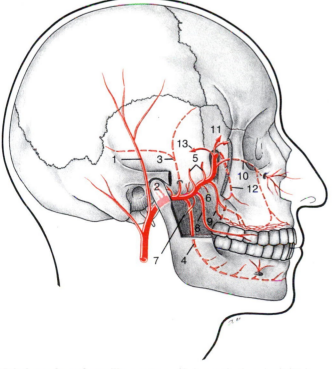

1 Superficial temporal artery

Branches of the first part
2 Deep auricular artery and anterior tympanic artery
3 Middle meningeal artery
4 Inferior alveolar artery

Branches of the second part
5 Deep temporal branches
6 Pterygoid branches
7 Masseteric artery
8 Buccal artery

Branches of the third part
9 Posterior superior alveolar artery
10 Infraorbital artery
11 Sphenopalatine artery and branches to the nasal cavity
12 Descending palatine artery
13 Artery of the pterygoid canal

Main branches of maxillary artery. (Schematic drawing) (Tr.).

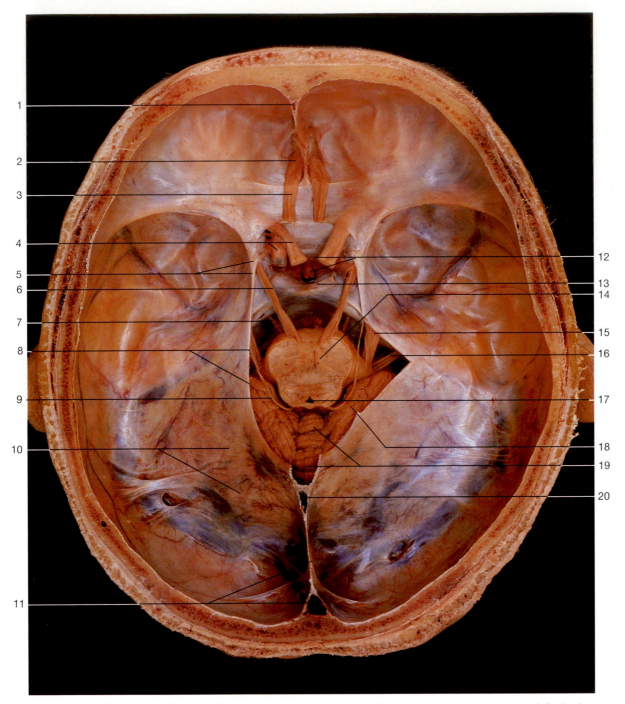

Base of the skull with cranial nerves (internal aspect). Both cerebral hemispheres and upper part of the brain stem removed. Incision on the right tentorium cerebelli to display the cranial nerves of the infratentorial space.

1 Superior sagittal sinus with falx cerebri
2 Olfactory bulb
3 Olfactory tract
4 Optic nerve, internal carotid artery
5 Anterior clinoid process, anterior attachment of tentorium cerebelli
6 Oculomotor nerve (n. III)
7 Abducens nerve (n. VI)
8 Tentorial notch (incisura tentorii)
9 Trochlear nerve (n. IV)
10 Tentorium cerebelli
11 Falx cerebri, confluence of sinuses

12 Hypophysial fossa, infundibulum, diaphragma sellae
13 Dorsum sellae
14 Midbrain (divided)
15 Trigeminal nerve (n. V)
16 Facial nerve (n. VII), vestibulocochlear nerve (n. VIII)
17 Aqueduct
18 Right hemisphere of cerebellum
19 Vermis of cerebellum
20 Inferior sagittal sinus

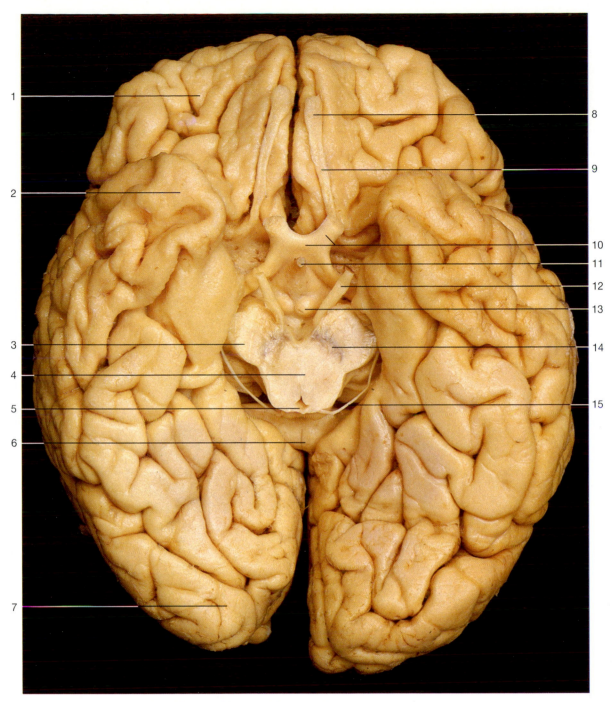

Inferior aspect of the brain with cranial nerves. Midbrain divided.

1 Frontal lobe
2 Temporal lobe
3 Crus cerebri
4 Midbrain (divided)
5 Aqueduct
6 Splenium of corpus callosum
7 Occipital lobe
8 Olfactory bulb
9 Olfactory tract
10 Optic nerve, optic chiasma
11 Infundibulum
12 Oculomotor nerve (n. III)
13 Mamillary body
14 Substantia nigra
15 Trochlear nerve (n. IV)

Cranial Nerves	
I = Olfactory nerves	VII = Facial nerve
II = Optic nerve	VIII = Vestibulocochlear nerve
III = Oculomotor nerve	IX = Glossopharyngeal nerve
IV = Trochlear nerve	X = Vagus nerve
V = Trigeminal nerve	XI = Accessory nerve
VI = Abducens nerve	XII = Hypoglossal nerve

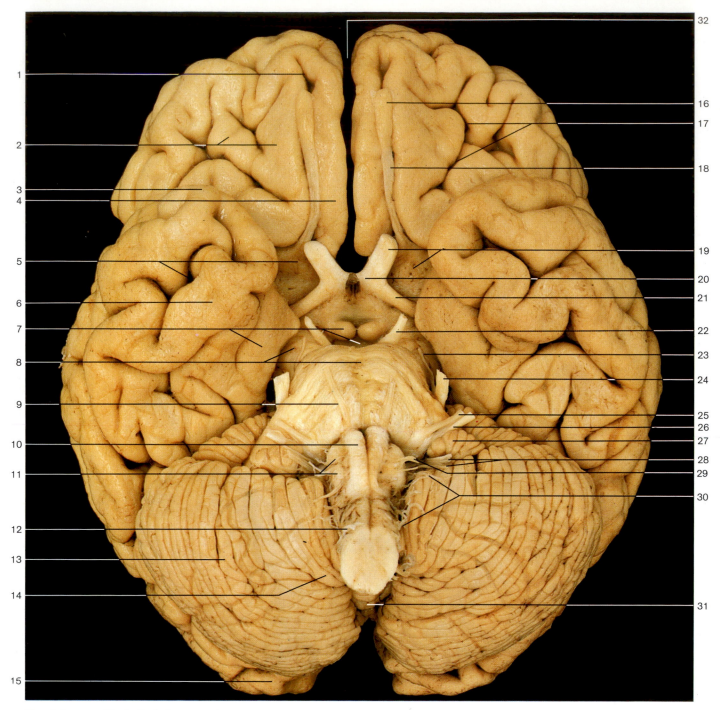

Cranial nerves. Brain (inferior aspect).

1 Olfactory sulcus (termination)
2 Orbital gyri
3 Temporal lobe
4 Straight gyrus
5 Olfactory trigone, inferior temporal sulcus
6 Medial occipitotemporal gyrus
7 Parahippocampal gyrus, mamillary body, interpeduncular fossa
8 Pons and cerebral peduncle
9 Abducens nerve
10 Pyramid
11 Lower part of olive
12 Cervical spinal nerves
13 Cerebellum
14 Tonsil of cerebellum
15 Occipital lobe, posterior pole
16 Olfactory bulb
17 Orbital sulci of frontal lobe
18 Olfactory tract
19 Optic nerve (n. II) and anterior perforated substance
20 Optic chiasma
21 Optic tract
22 Oculomotor nerve (n. III)
23 Trochlear nerve (n. IV)
24 Trigeminal nerve (n. V)
25 Facial nerve (n. VII)
26 Vestibulocochlear nerve (n. VIII)
27 Flocculus of cerebellum
28 Glossopharyngeal (n. IX) and vagus nerve (n. X)
29 Hypoglossal nerve (n. XII)
30 Accessory nerve (n. XI)
31 Vermis of cerebellum
32 Longitudinal fissure

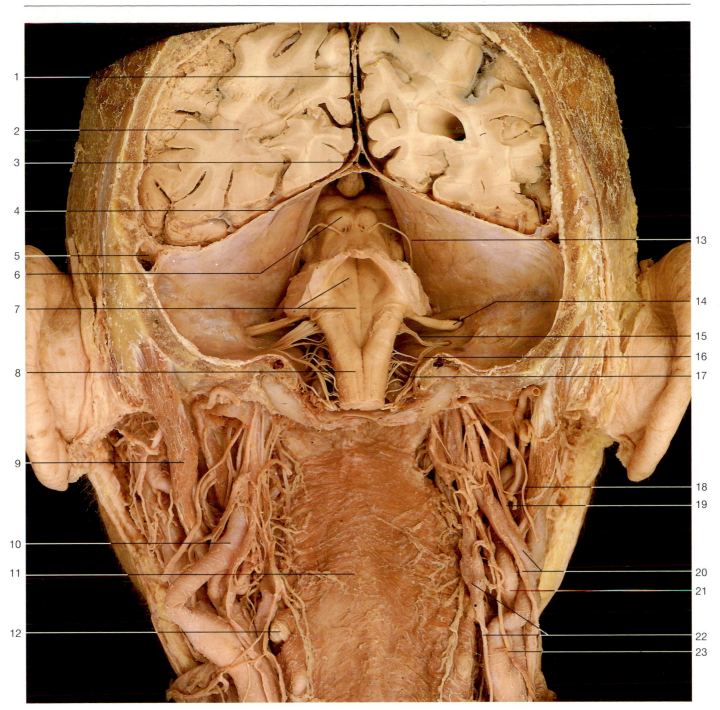

Brain stem and pharynx with cranial nerves (posterior aspect). Cranial cavity opened and cerebellum removed.

1 Falx cerebri
2 Occipital lobe
3 Straight sinus
4 Tentorium cerebelli
5 Transverse sinus
6 Inferior colliculus of midbrain
7 **Rhomboid fossa**
8 Medulla oblongata
9 Posterior belly of digastric muscle
10 Internal carotid artery
11 Pharynx (middle constrictor muscle)
12 Hyoid bone, greater horn
13 **Trochlear nerve** (n. IV)
14 **Facial nerve** (n. VII),
   Vestibulocochlear nerve (n. VIII)

15 **Glossopharyngeal nerve** (n. IX)
16 **Accessory nerve** (intracranial portion)
   (n. XI)
17 **Hypoglossal nerve** (intracranial portion)
   (n. XII)
18 **Accessory nerve** (n. XI)
19 **Hypoglossal nerve** (n. XII)
20 **Vagus nerve** (n. X), internal carotid
   artery
21 External carotid artery
22 **Sympathetic trunk,** superior cervical
   ganglion
23 Ansa cervicalis

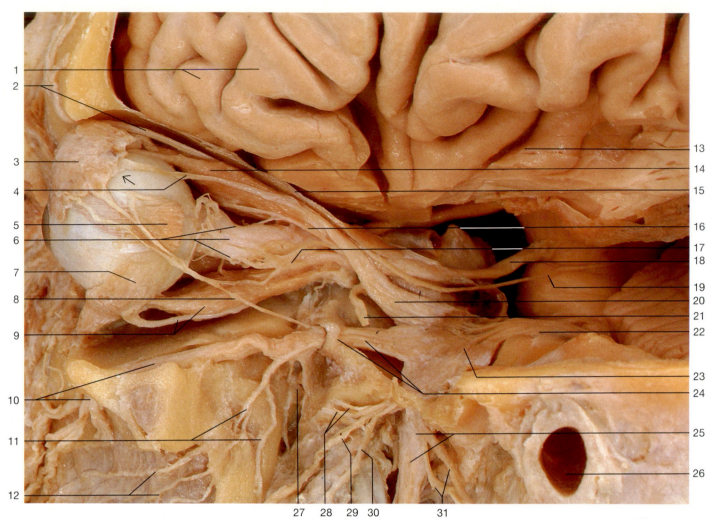

Cranial nerves of the orbit and pterygopalatine fossa. Left orbit (lateral aspect).
Note the zygomaticolacrimal anastomosis (arrow).

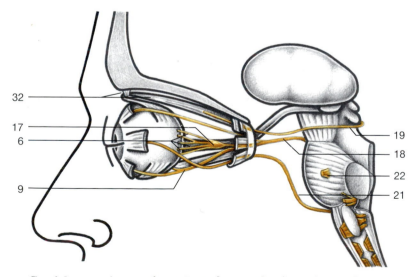

Cranial nerves innervating extraocular muscles (lateral aspect).
(Schematic drawing) (O.).

1 Frontal lobe
2 Supraorbital nerve
3 Lacrimal gland
4 Lacrimal nerve
5 Lateral rectus (divided)
6 **Optic nerve,** short ciliary nerves
7 Inferior oblique muscle
8 Zygomatic nerve
9 Inferior branch of oculomotor nerve, inferior rectus
10 Infraorbital nerve
11 Posterior superior alveolar nerves
12 Branches of superior alveolar plexus adjacent to mucous membrane of maxillary sinus
13 Central sulcus of insula
14 Superior rectus
15 Periorbita, roof of orbit
16 Nasociliary nerve
17 Ciliary ganglion
18 **Oculomotor nerve** (n. III)
19 **Trochlear nerve** (n. IV)
20 **Ophthalmic nerve** (n. V₁)

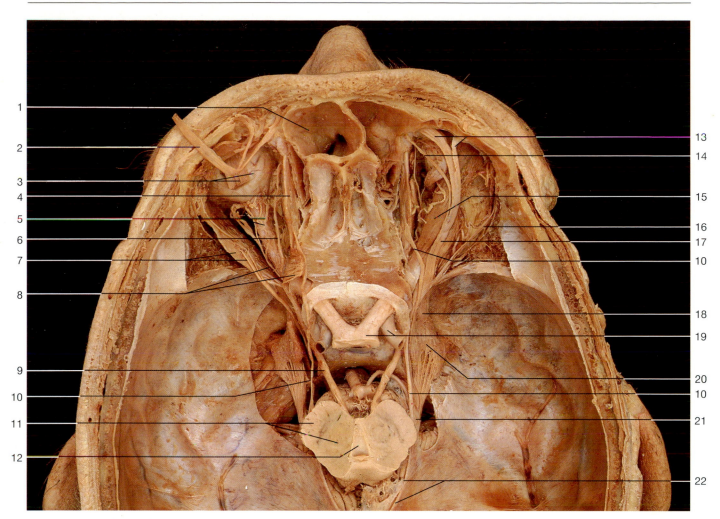

Cranial nerves of the orbit (superior aspect). Right side: superficial layer; left side: middle layer of the orbit (superior rectus and frontal nerve divided and reflected). Tentorium and dura mater partly removed.

◁ **to page 68**

21 **Abducens nerve** (n. VI) (divided)
22 **Trigeminal nerve** (n. V)
23 Trigeminal ganglion
24 **Maxillary nerve** (n. V₂), foramen rotundum
25 **Mandibular nerve** (n. V₃)
26 External acoustic meatus
27 Pterygopalatine nerves
28 Deep temporal nerves
29 Buccal nerve
30 Masseteric nerve
31 Auriculotemporal nerve
32 Trochlea, superior oblique

1 Frontal sinus (enlarged)
2 Frontal nerve (divided and reflected)
3 Superior rectus (divided), eyeball
4 Superior oblique muscle
5 Short ciliary nerves, optic nerve (n. II)
6 Nasociliary nerve
7 **Abducens nerve** (n. VI), lateral rectus
8 Ciliary ganglion, superior rectus (reflected)
9 **Oculomotor nerve** (n. III)
10 **Trochlear nerve** (n. IV)
11 Crus cerebri, midbrain
12 Inferior wall of IIIrd ventricle connected with aqueduct
13 Lateral and medial branch of supraorbital nerve
14 Supratrochlear nerve
15 Superior rectus
16 Lacrimal nerve
17 Frontal nerve
18 **Ophthalmic nerve** (n. V₁)
19 Optic chiasma, internal carotid artery
20 Trigeminal ganglion
21 **Trigeminal nerve** (n. V)
22 Tentorial notch

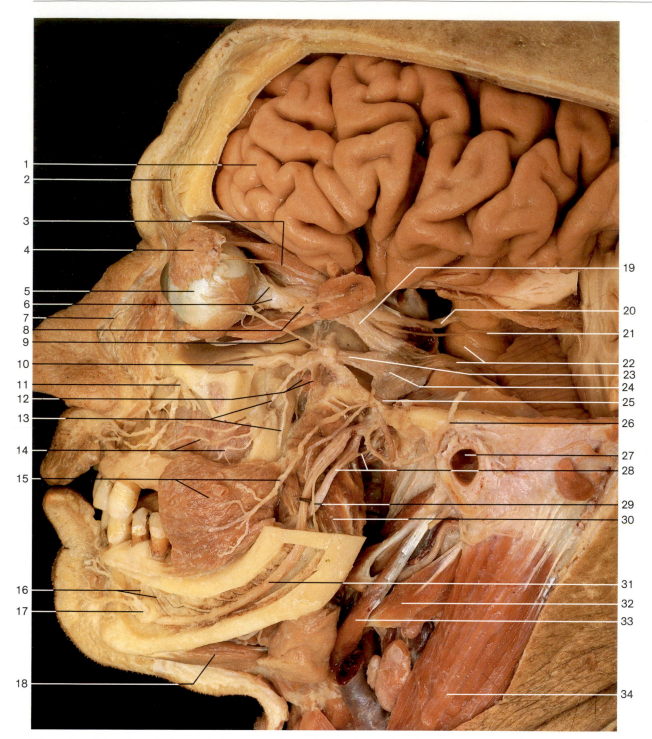

Dissection of the trigeminal nerve in its entirety. Lateral wall of cranial cavity, lateral wall of orbit, zygomatic arch and ramus of the mandible have been removed and the mandibular canal opened.

1 Frontal lobe of cerebrum	12 Pterygopalatine ganglion, pterygopalatine nerves	23 **Maxillary nerve** (n. V₂)
2 Supraorbital nerve		24 Trigeminal ganglion
3 Lacrimal nerve	13 Posterior superior alveolar nerves	25 **Mandibular nerve** (n. V₃)
4 Lacrimal gland	14 Superior dental plexus	26 Auriculotemporal nerve
5 Eyeball	15 Buccinator muscle, buccal nerve	27 External acoustic meatus (divided)
6 Optic nerve, short ciliary nerves	16 Inferior dental plexus	28 Lingual nerve, chorda tympani
7 External nasal branch of anterior ethmoidal nerve	17 Mental foramen, mental nerve	29 Mylohyoid nerve
8 Ciliary ganglion	18 Anterior belly of digastric muscle	30 Medial pterygoid muscle
9 Zygomatic nerve	19 **Ophthalmic nerve** (n. V₁)	31 Inferior alveolar nerve
10 Infraorbital nerve	20 **Oculomotor nerve** (n. III)	32 Posterior belly of digastric muscle
11 Infraorbital foramen, terminal branches of infraorbital nerve	21 **Trochlear nerve** (n. IV)	33 Stylohyoid
	22 Trigeminal nerve, pons	34 Sternocleidomastoid

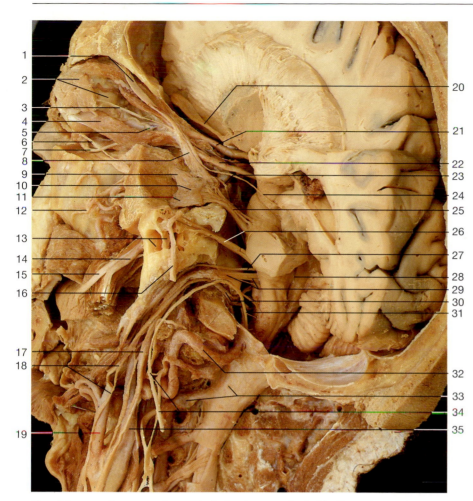

1 Frontal nerve
2 Lacrimal gland, eyeball
3 Lacrimal nerve
4 Lateral rectus
5 **Ciliary ganglion** lateral to optic nerve
6 Zygomatic nerve
7 Inferior branch of oculomotor nerve
8 **Ophthalmic nerve** (n. V₁)
9 **Maxillary nerve** (n. V₂)
10 **Trigeminal ganglion**
11 **Mandibular nerve** (n. V₃)
12 Posterior superior alveolar nerves
13 Tympanic cavity, external acoustic meatus, tympanic membrane
14 Inferior alveolar nerve
15 Lingual nerve
16 **Facial nerve** (n. VII)
17 **Vagus nerve** (n. X)
18 **Hypoglossal nerve** (n. XII), superior root of ansa cervicalis
19 External carotid artery
20 **Olfactory tract** (n. I)
21 **Optic nerve** (n. II), intracranial part
22 **Oculomotor nerve** (n. III)
23 **Abducens nerve** (n. VI)
24 **Trochlear nerve** (n. IV)
25 **Trigeminal nerve** (n. V)
26 **Vestibulocochlear nerve** (n. VIII), **Facial nerve** (VII)
27 **Glossopharyngeal nerve** (n. IX), leaving brain stem
28 Rhomboid fossa
29 **Vagus nerve** (n. X), leaving brain stem
30 **Hypoglossal nerve** (n. XII), leaving medulla oblongata
31 **Accessory nerve** (n. XI), ascending from foramen magnum
32 Vertebral artery
33 Spinal ganglion, dura mater of spinal cord
34 Accessory nerve (n. XI)
35 Internal carotid artery
36 Lateral and medial branch of supraorbital nerve
37 Supratrochlear nerve
38 Infraorbital nerve
39 **Pterygopalatine ganglion,** middle superior alveolar nerve
40 Middle superior alveolar nerves, entering superior dental plexus
41 Buccal nerve
42 Mental nerve, mental foramen
43 Auriculotemporal nerve
44 Otic ganglion (dotted line)
45 Chorda tympani
46 Mylohyoid nerve
47 Submandibular gland
48 Hyoid bone

Cranial nerves in connection with the brain stem. Left side (lateral superior aspect). Left half of brain and head partly removed. Notice the location of trigeminal ganglion.

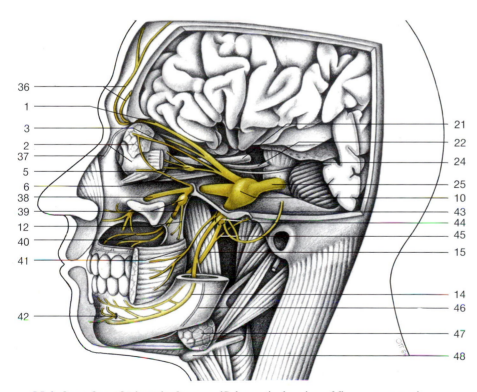

Main branches of trigeminal nerve. (Schematic drawing of figure on opposite page) (O.).

71

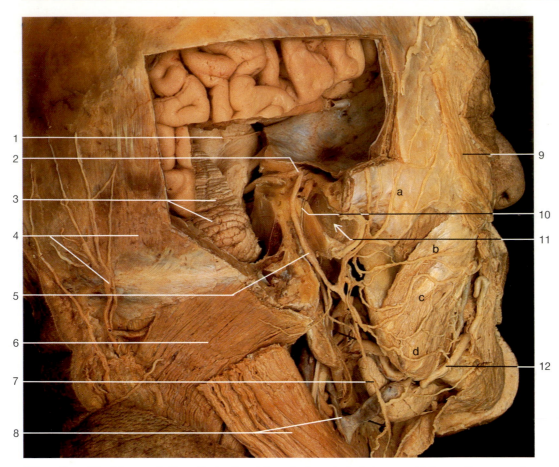

Dissection of facial nerve in its entirety. Cranial cavity fenestrated; temporal lobe partly removed. Facial canal and tympanic cavity opened, posterior wall of external acoustic meatus removed.
Branches of facial nerve: a = temporal branch; b = zygomatic branches; c = buccal branches; d = marginal mandibular branch.

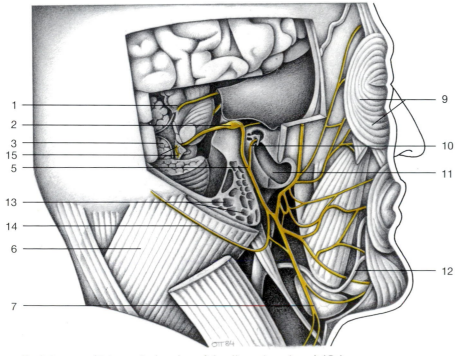

Facial nerve. (Schematic drawing of the dissection above) (O.).

1 Trochlear nerve
2 Facial nerve with geniculate ganglion
3 Cerebellum, right hemisphere
4 Occipital belly of occipitofrontalis, greater occipital nerve
5 Facial nerve at stylomastoid foramen
6 Splenius capitis
7 Cervical branch of facial nerve
8 Sternocleidomastoid, retromandibular vein
9 Orbicularis oculi
10 Chorda tympani
11 External acoustic meatus
12 Facial artery
13 Mastoid air cells
14 Posterior auricular nerve
15 Nucleus and genu of facial nerve

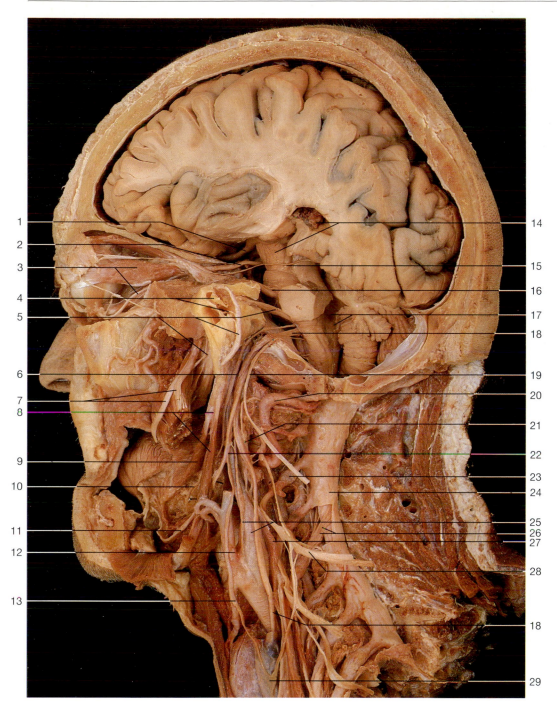

Cranial nerves in connection with the brain stem (oblique-lateral aspect). Lateral portion of the skull, brain, neck and facial structures, lateral wall of orbit and oral cavity have been removed. The tympanic cavity has been opened. The mandible has been divided and the muscles of mastication have been removed.

1 Optic tract
2 **Oculomotor nerve** (n. III)
3 Lateral rectus, inferior branch of oculomotor nerve
4 Malleus, chorda tympani
5 Chorda tympani, **facial nerve** (n. VII), **vestibulocochlear nerve** (n. VIII)
6 **Glossopharyngeal nerve** (n. XI)
7 Lingual nerve, inferior alveolar nerve
8 Styloid process, stylohyoid muscle
9 Styloglossus muscle
10 Lingual branches of glossopharyngeal nerve

11 Lingual branch of hypoglossal nerve
12 External carotid artery
13 Superior root of ansa cervicalis (branch of hypoglossal nerve)
14 Lateral ventricle with choroid plexus, cerebral peduncle
15 **Trochlear nerve** (n. IV)
16 **Trigeminal nerve** (n. V)
17 Fourth ventricle, rhomboid fossa
18 **Vagus nerve** (n. X)
19 **Accessory nerve** (n. XI)
20 Vertebral artery
21 Superior cervical ganglion

22 **Hypoglossal nerve** (n. XII)
23 Spinal ganglion with dural sheath
24 Dura mater of spinal cord
25 Internal carotid artery, carotid sinus branch of glossopharyngeal nerve
26 Dorsal roots of spinal nerve
27 Sympathetic trunk
28 Cervical plexus
29 Ansa cervicalis

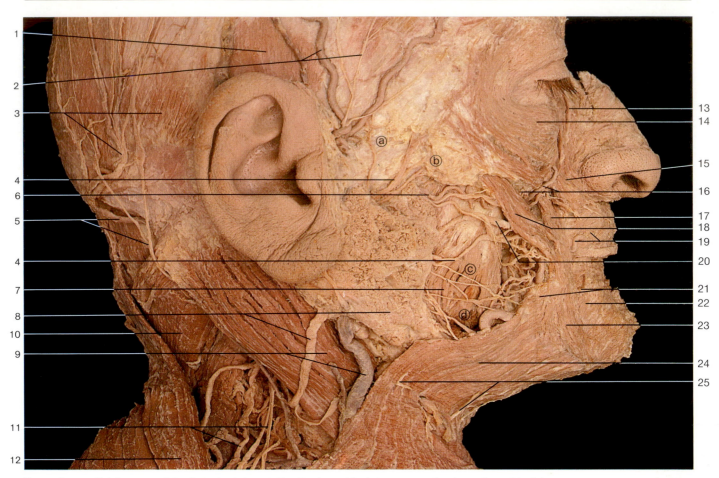

Lateral superficial aspect of the face. Peripheral distribution of facial nerve. a–d = branches of facial nerve: a = temporal branch; b = zygomatic branches; c = buccal branches; d = marginal mandibular branch.

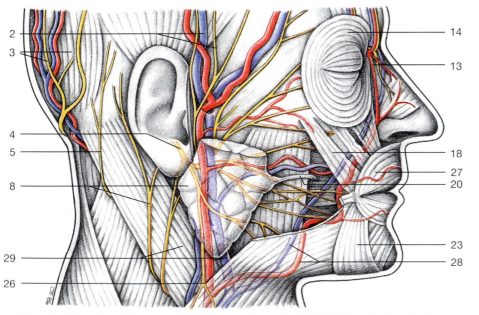

Superficial region of the face. (Semischematic drawing) (O.). Note the facial plexus within the parotid gland.

1 Temporoparietalis
2 Parietal branch of **superficial temporal artery,** auriculotemporal nerve
3 Occipital belly of occipitofrontalis, greater occipital nerve
4 **Facial nerve**
5 Lesser occipital nerve, occipital artery
6 Transverse facial artery
7 Masseter
8 **Parotid gland,** great auricular nerve
9 Sternocleidomastoid, external jugular vein
10 Splenius capitis
11 Cervical plexus
12 Trapezius
13 Angular artery (terminal portion of facial artery)
14 Orbicularis oculi
15 Levator labii superioris alaeque nasi
16 **Facial artery,** zygomaticus minor
17 Levator anguli oris
18 Zygomaticus major
19 Orbicularis oris, superior labial artery
20 Parotid duct
21 Risorius, inferior labial artery

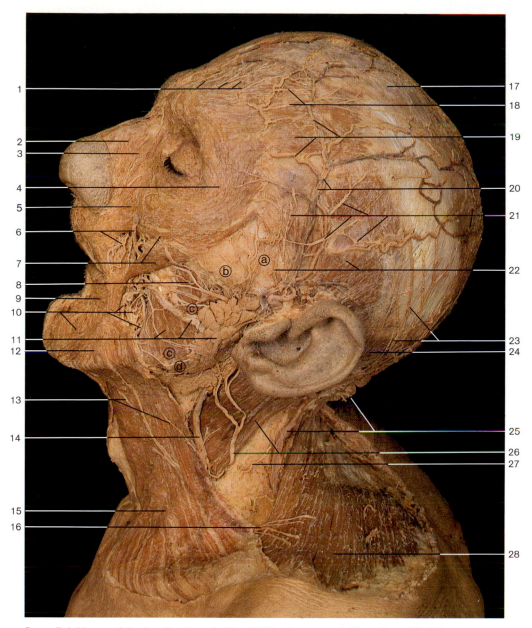

1. Medial branch of supraorbital nerve
2. Nasalis
3. Levator labii superioris alaeque nasi
4. Orbicularis oculi
5. Levator labii superioris
6. Facial artery and vein
7. Zygomaticus minor and major
8. Transverse facial artery
9. Orbicularis oris
10. Buccal nerves, depressor labii inferioris, facial artery and vein
11. Parotid gland and duct, masseter
12. Depressor anguli oris
13. Transverse cervical nerve
14. External jugular vein
15. Platysma
16. Supraclavicular nerve
17. Galea aponeurotica
18. Lateral branches of the supraorbital nerve
19. Frontal belly of occipitofrontalis; branches of superficial temporal vein and artery
20. Superficial temporal artery and vein
21. Auriculotemporal nerve
22. Zygomaticoorbital artery, temporoparietalis muscle
23. Lesser occipital nerve
24. Occipital belly of occipitofrontalis
25. Occipital vein, occipital artery
26. Great auricular nerve, sternocleidomastoid
27. Lesser occipital nerve
28. Trapezius

Superficial layer of the head and neck. Parotid fascia removed. Branches of facial nerve: a = temporal branch; b = zygomatic branches; c = buccal branches; d = marginal mandibular branch.

◁ **to page 74**

22. Depressor labii inferioris
23. Depressor anguli oris
24. Platysma
25. Terminal branches of transverse cervical nerve
26. Cervical branch of facial nerve
27. Orbicularis oris
28. Facial artery and vein
29. Sternocleidomastoid, retromandibular vein

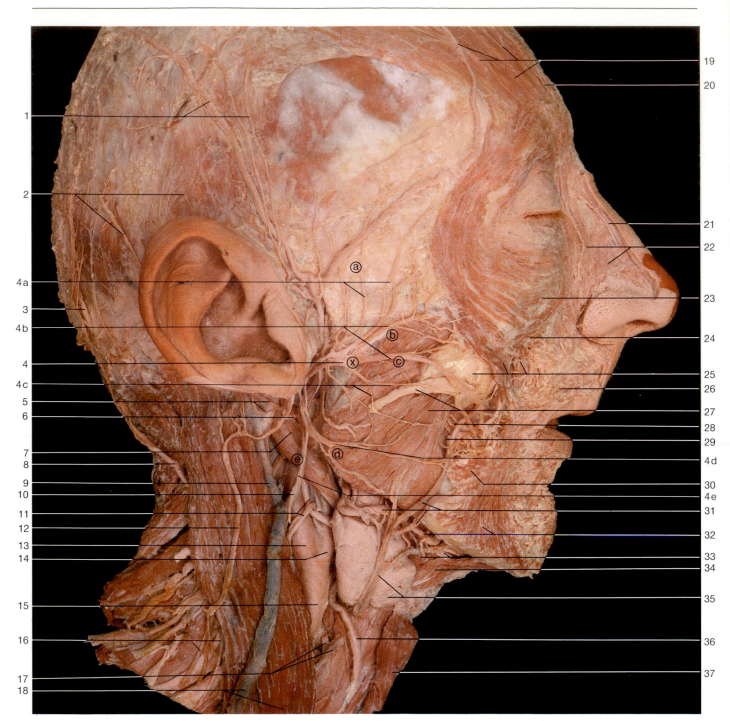

Lateral superficial aspect of the face. The parotid gland has been removed to display the parotid plexus of the facial nerve. a–e = branches of facial nerve: a = temporal branch; b = zygomatic branches; c = buccal branches; d = marginal mandibular branch; e = cervical branch.

1 Superficial temporal artery, auriculotemporal nerve
2 Posterior auricular artery and nerve, temporoparietalis
3 Occipital artery
4 Facial nerve (n. VII), parotid plexus (x)
   a Temporal branches
   b Zygomatic branches
   c Buccal branches
   d Marginal mandibular branch
   e Cervical branch
5 Posterior auricular nerve
6 Posterior auricular artery
7 Digastric muscle, posterior belly
8 Lesser occipital nerve
9 Posterior auricular vein

10 Retromandibular vein
11 Hypoglossal nerve and sternocleidomastoid artery
12 Great auricular nerve
13 Internal carotid artery
14 External carotid artery
15 Common carotid artery
16 Cervical plexus
17 Superior laryngeal artery and vein
18 External jugular vein, sternocleidomastoid
19 Frontal branch of superficial temporal artery, lateral branch of supraorbital nerve and frontal belly of occipitofrontalis
20 Medial branch of supraorbital nerve
21 Dorsal nasal artery
22 Angular artery, nasalis

23 Orbicularis oculi
24 Zygomaticus minor
25 Fatty tissue of the cheek, zygomaticus major, infraorbital nerve
26 Orbicularis oris
27 Parotid duct, masseter
28 Buccal artery and nerve
29 Buccinator
30 Risorius
31 Facial artery and vein
32 Submental artery, depressor anguli oris
33 Mylohyoid nerve and mylohyoid muscle
34 Digastric muscle, anterior belly
35 Facial vein, submandibular gland
36 Superior thyroid artery
37 Sternohyoid

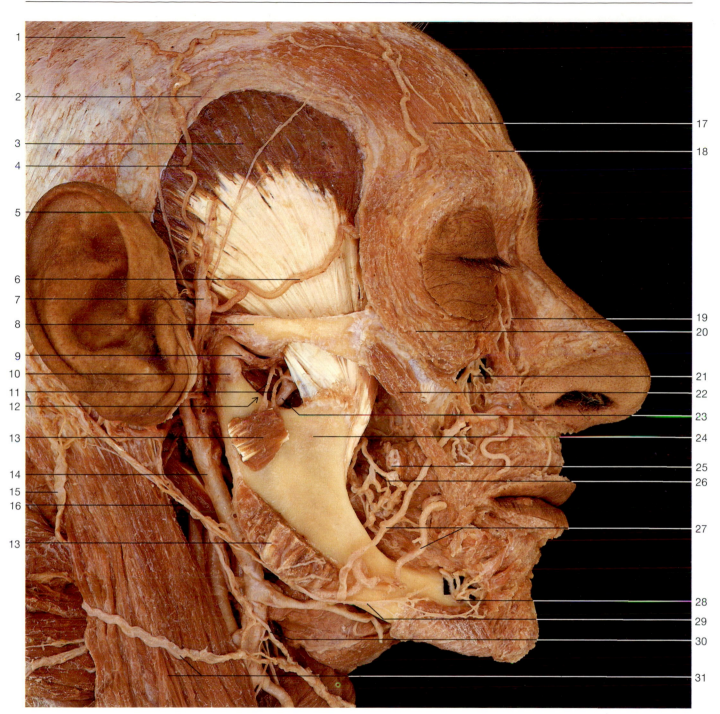

Lateral superficial aspect of the face. Masseter and temporal fascia have been partly removed to display the masseteric artery and nerve.

1 Galea aponeurotica
2 Temporal fascia
3 Temporalis muscle
4 Parietal branch of superficial temporal artery
5 Auriculotemporal nerve
6 Frontal branch of superficial temporal artery
7 Superficial temporal vein
8 Zygomatic arch
9 Articular disc of temporomandibular joint
10 Condylar process
11 Masseteric artery and nerve
12 Mandibular notch
13 Masseter muscle (divided)
14 External carotid artery
15 Great auricular nerve
16 Facial nerve (reflected)
17 Frontal belly of occipitofrontalis muscle
18 Medial branch of supraorbital nerve
19 Angular artery
20 Orbicularis oculi
21 Infraorbital nerve
22 Zygomaticus major muscle
23 Maxillary artery
24 Coronoid process
25 Parotid duct (divided)
26 Buccal nerve
27 Facial artery and vein
28 Mental nerve
29 Mandibular branch of facial nerve
30 Cervical branch of facial nerve
31 Transverse cervical nerve, communicating branch with facial nerve, sternocleidomastoid

The Retromandibular Region

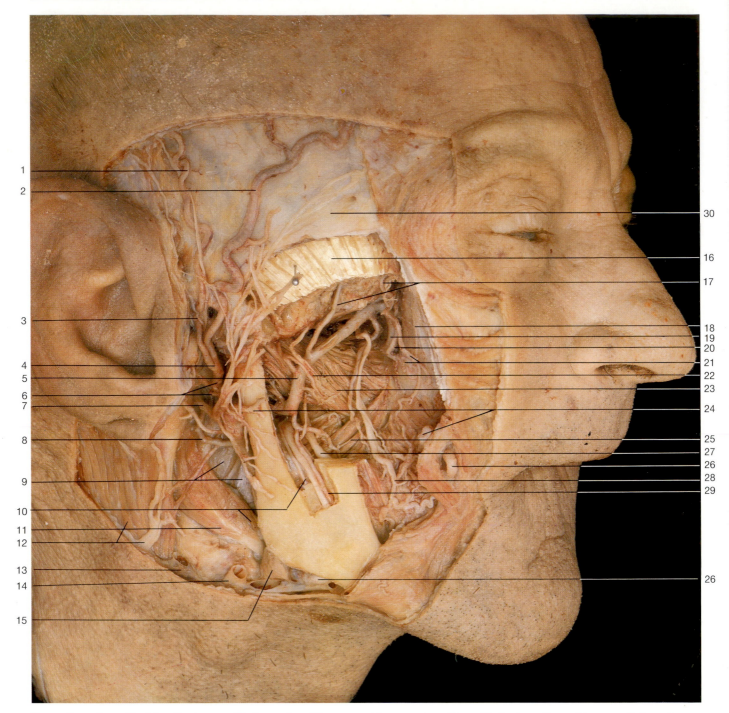

Deep dissection of facial and retromandibular region. The coronoid process together with the insertions of temporalis have been removed to display the maxillary artery. The mandibular canal has been partly opened.

1   Parietal branch of the superficial
    temporal artery
2   Frontal branch of the superficial
    temporal artery
3   Auriculotemporal nerve
4   Superficial temporal artery
5   Maxillary artery
6   Communicating branches between facial
    and auriculotemporal nerves
7   Facial nerve
8   Posterior auricular artery
9   Internal jugular vein

10 Mylohyoid nerve, stylohyoid
11 Posterior belly of digastric muscle
12 Great auricular nerve,
    sternocleidomastoid
13 External jugular vein
14 Retromandibular vein
15 Submandibular gland
16 Temporalis
17 Deep temporal arteries
18 Posterior superior alveolar nerve
19 Sphenopalatine artery
20 Posterior superior alveolar artery

21 Posterior superior alveolar nerve
22 Masseteric artery and nerve
23 Lateral pterygoid
24 Transverse facial artery, parotid
    duct (divided)
25 Medial pterygoid
26 Facial artery
27 Lingual nerve
28 Buccal nerve and artery
29 Inferior alveolar artery and nerve
    (mandibular canal opened)
30 Temporal fascia

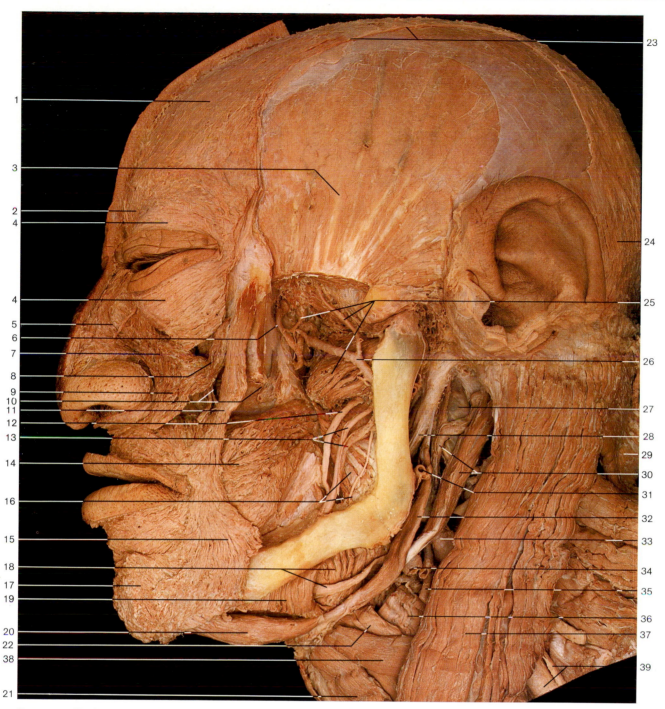

Retromandibular region with maxillary artery and branches of trigeminal nerve (n. V).

1	Frontal belly of occipitofrontalis	14	Buccinator
2	Depressor supercilii	15	Depressor anguli oris
3	Temporalis	16	Medial pterygoid, mylohyoid nerve
4	Orbicularis oculi	17	Depressor labii inferioris
5	Nasalis	18	Hypoglossal nerve, hyoglossus
6	Infraorbital artery	19	Mylohyoid
7	Levator labii superioris alaeque nasi	20	Anterior belly of digastric muscle
8	Zygomaticus minor	21	Sternohyoid
9	Levator labii superioris	22	Thyrohyoid
10	Infraorbital artery and nerve, posterior superior alveolar artery	23	Galea aponeurotica
11	Zygomaticus major	24	Occipital belly of occipitofrontalis
12	Lingual nerve	25	Lateral pterygoid, deep temporal artery
13	Inferior alveolar artery and nerve	26	Maxillary artery
		27	Internal jugular vein

28	Styloglossus
29	Splenius capitis
30	Posterior belly of digastric muscle, occipital artery
31	Superficial temporal artery
32	Stylohyoid
33	External carotid artery
34	Retromandibular vein
35	Superior thyroid artery
36	Inferior constrictor of the pharynx
37	Sternocleidomastoid
38	Omohyoid
39	Common carotid artery and vagus

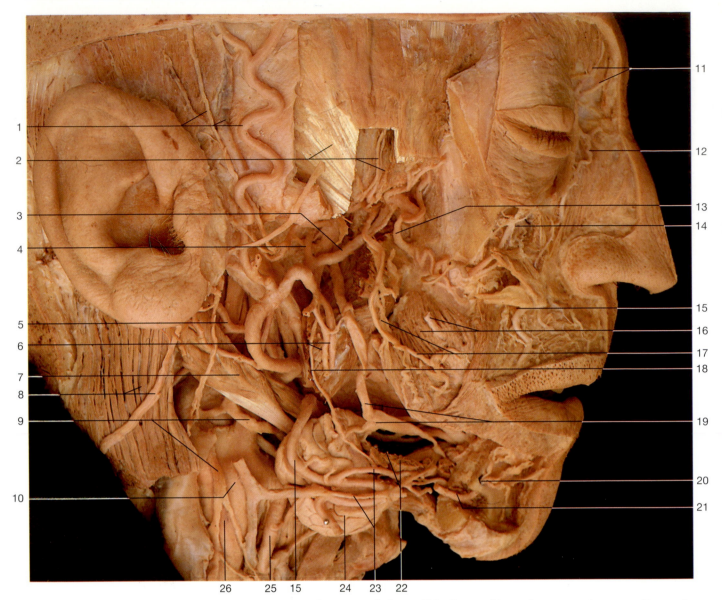

Dissection of deep facial and retromandibular regions after removal of mandible. Pterygoid muscles removed, temporalis muscle fenestrated.

1	**Superficial temporal artery** and vein, auriculotemporal nerve	14	Infraorbital nerve
2	Temporalis muscle, deep temporal nerves and artery	15	**Facial artery**
3	**Maxillary artery**	16	Parotid duct (divided), buccinator
4	Middle meningeal artery	17	Buccal artery and nerve
5	Occipital artery	18	Mylohyoid nerve
6	Inferior alveolar artery and nerve (divided)	19	**Lingual nerve, submandibular ganglion**
7	Posterior belly of digastric muscle	20	Mental nerve, mental foramen
8	Great auricular nerve, sternocleidomastoid	21	Inferior alveolar nerve
9	Hypoglossal nerve, superior root of ansa cervicalis	22	Mylohyoid muscle (divided), hypoglossal nerve
10	**External carotid artery**	23	Submental artery and vein
11	Supratrochlear nerve, medial branch of supraorbital artery	24	Submandibular gland
12	Angular artery	25	Superior thyroid artery
13	Posterior superior alveolar artery	26	Common carotid artery

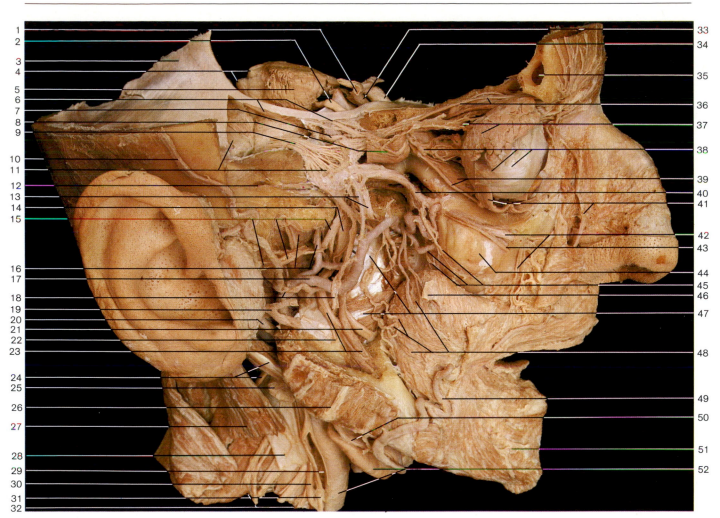

Para- and retropharyngeal regions. The mandible and the lateral wall of the orbit have been removed. The main branches of the trigeminal nerve and its ganglion are displayed.

1 Middle cerebral artery
2 Oculomotor nerve
3 Tentorium cerebelli
4 Tectum of the midbrain
5 Crus cerebri
6 Trochlear nerve
7 Abducens nerve
8 Lateral rectus muscle, abducens nerve
9 **Trigeminal nerve and cerebellum**
10 Superficial temporal artery
11 Trigeminal ganglion
12 Groove for greater petrosal nerve
13 Deep temporal artery and nerve
14 Mandibular nerve
15 Auriculotemporal nerve
16 Middle meningeal artery, sphenomandibular ligament
17 **Maxillary artery**
18 Masseteric artery and nerve, transverse facial artery
19 Facial nerve
20 Occipital artery
21 Lingual nerve
22 Mylohyoid nerve
23 Inferior alveolar artery and nerve
24 Posterior belly of digastric muscle, accessory nerve (n. XI)
25 Submandibular lymph nodes
26 Masseter
27 Sternocleidomastoid

28 Internal jugular vein
29 Thyrohyoid branch of ansa cervicalis
30 Vagus nerve (n. X)
31 Superior root of ansa cervicalis
32 Cervical plexus (C₁–C₅)
33 Internal carotid artery
34 Optic nerve (n. II)
35 Frontal sinus
36 Frontal nerve, levator palpebrae superioris
37 Superior rectus, lacrimal artery and nerve, lacrimal gland
38 Ciliary ganglion, ciliary nerves, optic nerve, eyeball and lateral rectus muscle
39 Inferior rectus and inferior branch of oculomotor nerve
40 Maxillary nerve, sphenopalatine artery
41 Inferior oblique muscle, angular artery
42 Infraorbital nerve and artery
43 Anterior superior alveolar nerve and artery
44 Maxillary sinus (mucous membrane)
45 Posterior superior alveolar nerve and artery
46 Parotid duct
47 Medial pterygoid muscle
48 Buccal artery and nerve, buccinator
49 Facial artery
50 Hypoglossal nerve (n. XII)
51 Mental nerve
52 Submandibular gland, common carotid artery

81

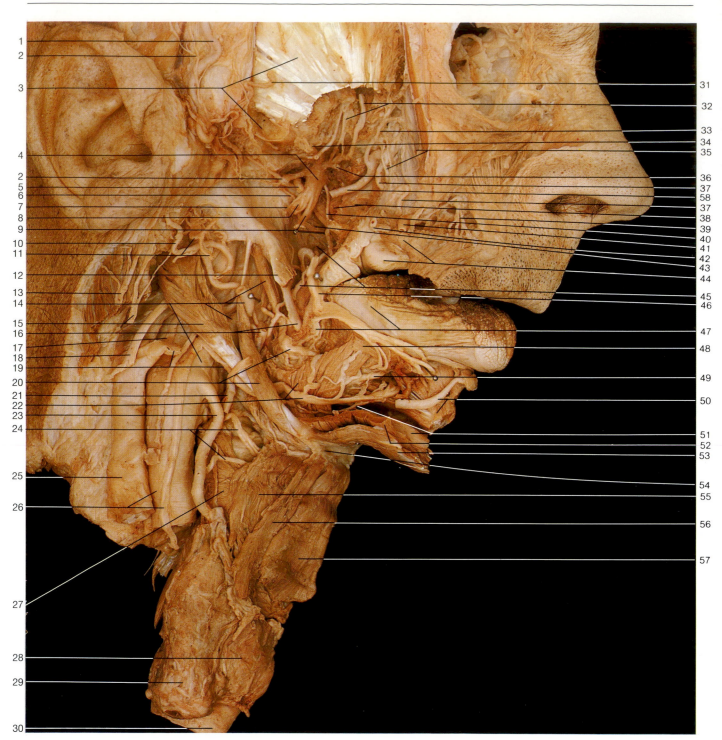

Retropharyngeal and sublingual regions. The mandible has been completely removed.

1 Parietal branch of superficial temporal artery
2 Auriculotemporal nerve
3 Temporalis muscle and zygomatic arch
4 Mandibular nerve (n. V₃)
5 Middle meningeal artery
6 Chorda tympani
7 Mylohyoid nerve
8 Inferior alveolar nerve
9 Lingual nerve
10 Posterior auricular artery
11 Facial nerve
12 Styloglossus muscle
13 Great auricular nerve
14 Maxillary artery, external carotid artery, stylopharyngeus
15 Posterior belly of digastric muscle

16 Styloid process and facial artery
17 Vagus nerve (n. X)
18 Accessory nerve (n. XI)
19 Hypoglossal nerve (n. XII)
20 Stylohyoid muscle, glossopharyngeal nerve (n. IX)
21 Facial vein
22 Hypoglossal nerve (n. XII), hyoglossus muscle
23 Superior thyroid artery
24 Superior laryngeal nerve and artery
25 Internal jugular vein
26 Common carotid artery, superior root of ansa cervicalis
27 Inferior pharyngeal constrictor
28 Thyroid gland
29 Esophagus
30 Trachea

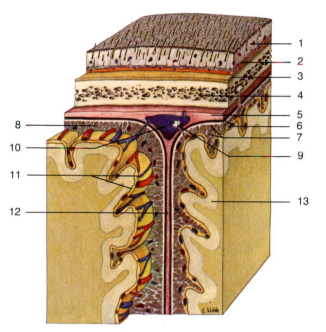

1   Posterior auricular vein
2   Parietal branch of superficial temporal
    artery and auriculotemporal nerve
3   Temporoparietalis
4   Greater occipital nerve
5   Occipital belly of occipitofrontalis
6   Occipital artery
7   Temporal branches of facial nerve
8   Frontal branch of superficial temporal
    artery
9   Lateral and medial branch of supraorbital
    nerve
10 Supratrochlear nerve
11 Angular artery
12 Orbicularis oculi
13 Frontal belly of occipitofrontalis

Nerves and blood vessels of the scalp.

1   Skin
2   Galea aponeurotica
3   Pericranium, periosteum
4   Skull with diploe
5   Dura mater
6   Subdural space
7   Arachnoid mater
8   Subarachnoid space
9   Arachnoid granulations
10 Superior sagittal sinus
11 Pia mater with cerebral vessels
12 Falx cerebri
13 Cerebral cortex

A coronal **section through the vertex of the skull** showing
the arrangement of the meninges and vessels of the brain (W.).
Together the arachnoid mater and the pia mater form the
leptomeninx.

◁   **to page 66**
31 Middle temporal artery
32 Deep temporal nerves and posterior deep temporal artery
33 Anterior deep temporal artery
34 Masseteric nerve
35 Posterior superior alveolar branches of maxillary artery and nerve
36 Pterygoid branches of mandibular nerve
37 Posterior superior alveolar artery
38 Lateral pterygoid plate and medial pterygoid muscle
39 Infraorbital nerve and artery
40 Buccal nerve
41 Facial artery
42 Parotid duct
43 Levator veli palatini
44 Gingiva, buccinator

45 Ascending pharyngeal artery, superior pharyngeal constrictor
    (pterygopharyngeal part)
46 Lingual nerve
47 Submandibular ganglion and tongue
48 Palatoglossus
49 Deep lingual artery
50 Submandibular duct and genioglossus
51 Geniohyoid nerve and muscle
52 Mylohyoid
53 Anterior belly of digastric
54 Hyoid bone
55 Thyrohyoid
56 Omohyoid muscle, superior belly
57 Sternohyoid muscle
58 Maxillary artery

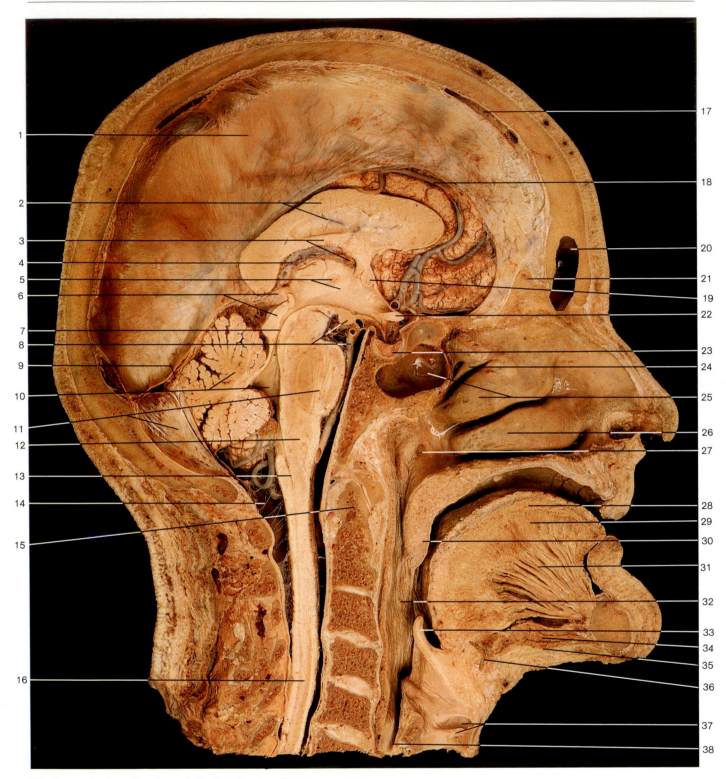

Median sagittal section through the head and neck.

1 Falx cerebri
2 Corpus callosum, septum pellucidum
3 Interventricular foramen and fornix
4 Choroid plexus of third ventricle,
  internal cerebral vein
5 Third ventricle and interthalamic adhesion
6 Pineal body, colliculi of the midbrain
7 Cerebral aqueduct
8 Mamillary body, basilar artery
9 Straight sinus
10 Fourth ventricle and vermis of the cerebellum
11 Pons, falx cerebelli
12 Medulla oblongata
13 Central canal

14 Cerebellomedullary cistern
15 Dens of the axis (odontoid process)
16 Spinal cord
17 Superior sagittal sinus
18 Anterior cerebral artery
19 Anterior commissure
20 Frontal sinus
21 Crista galli
22 Optic chiasma
23 Pituitary gland (hypophysis)
24 Superior nasal concha
25 Middle nasal concha and sphenoid sinus
26 Inferior nasal concha

27 Pharyngeal opening of auditory tube
28 Superior longitudinal muscle of
   tongue
29 Vertical muscle of the tongue
30 Uvula
31 Genioglossus
32 Pharynx
33 Epiglottis
34 Geniohyoid
35 Mylohyoid
36 Hyoid bone
37 Vocal fold and sinus of larynx
38 Esophagus

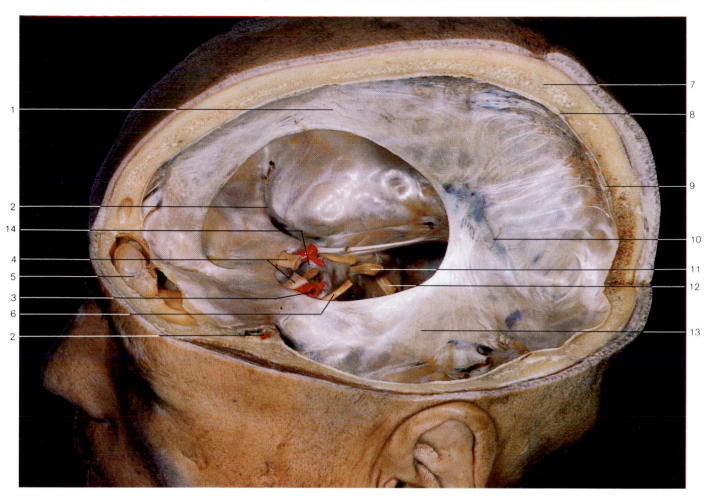

Dura mater and venous sinuses of the dura mater. The brain has been removed (oblique lateral aspect).

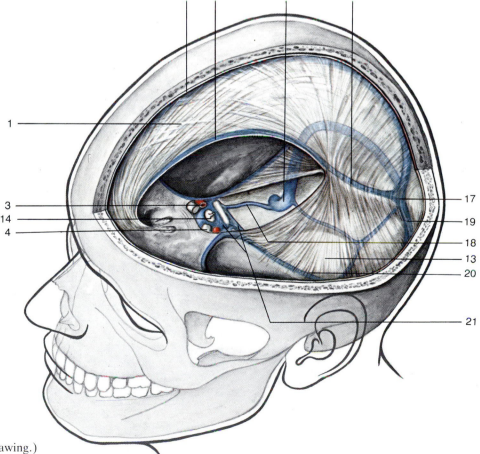

1 Falx cerebri
2 Position of middle meningeal
   artery and vein
3 Internal carotid artery
4 Optic nerves
5 Frontal sinus
6 Oculomotor nerve
7 Diploe
8 Dura mater
9 Superior sagittal sinus
10 Straight sinus
11 Trigeminal nerve
12 Facial and vestibulocochlear nerve
13 Tentorium cerebelli
14 Pituitary gland (hypophysis)
15 Inferior sagittal sinus
16 Sigmoid sinus
17 Confluence of sinuses
18 Inferior petrosal sinus
19 Transverse sinus
20 Superior petrosal sinus
21 Cavernous and intercavernous sinuses

Dura mater and **venous sinuses**
(left lateral aspect). (Semischematic drawing.)

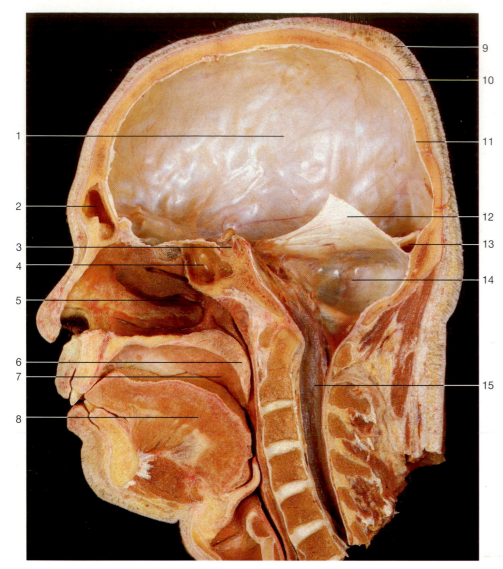

1. **Cranial cavity** with dura mater containing mainly the right cerebral hemisphere
2. Frontal sinus
3. Hypophysial fossa with pituitary gland
4. Sphenoidal sinus
5. **Nasal cavity**
6. Soft palate
7. **Oral cavity**
8. Tongue
9. Skin
10. Calvaria
11. Dura mater
12. Tentorium cerebelli
13. Confluence of sinuses
14. **Infratentorial space** containing cerebellum and part of the brain stem
15. Vertebral canal
16. Frontal branch of middle meningeal artery and veins
17. Middle meningeal artery
18. Diploe
19. Parietal branch of middle meningeal artery and vein
20. Occipital pole of left hemisphere covered with dura mater

Median section through the head. Right half. **Demonstration of dura mater covering the cranial cavity.** Brain completely removed (lateral aspect).

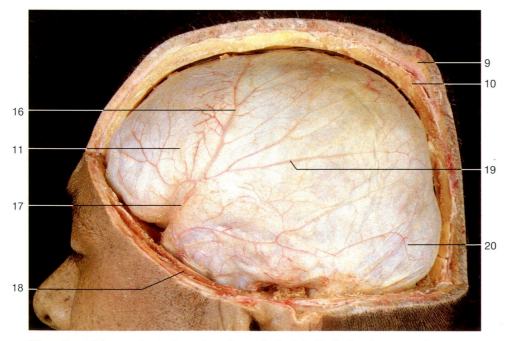

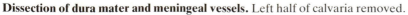

Dissection of dura mater and meningeal vessels. Left half of calvaria removed.

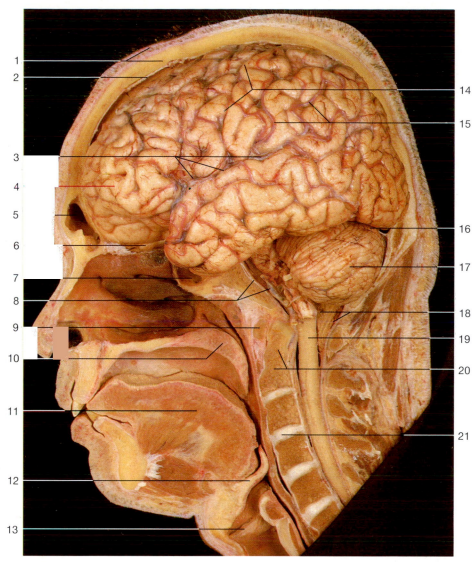

1	Calvaria and skin of the scalp
2	Dura mater (divided)
3	Position of lateral sulcus
4	Frontal lobe with pia mater
5	Frontal sinus
6	Olfactory bulb
7	Sphenoidal sinus
8	Clivus, basilar artery
9	Atlas, anterior arch (divided)
10	Soft palate
11	Tongue
12	Epiglottis
13	Vocal fold
14	Position of central sulcus
15	Superior cerebral veins
16	Tentorium (divided)
17	Cerebellum
18	Cerebellomedullary cistern
19	Position of foramen magnum, spinal cord
20	Dens of axis
21	Intervertebral disc

Dissection of the brain with pia mater in situ. The facial part of the head is cut in half. The brain is shown in its entirety.

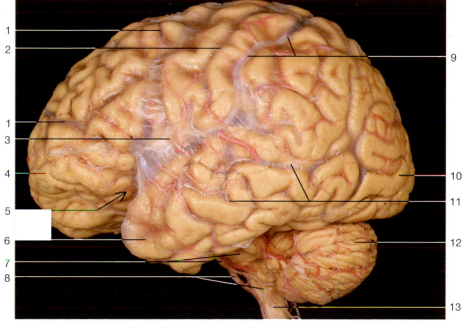

1	Superior cerebral veins
2	Position of central sulcus
3	Position of lateral sulcus, cistern of lateral cerebral fossa
4	Frontal pole
5	Lateral sulcus (arrow)
6	Temporal pole
7	Pons, basilar artery
8	Vertebral arteries
9	Superior anastomotic vein
10	Occipital pole
11	Inferior cerebral veins
12	Hemisphere of cerebellum
13	Medulla oblongata

Brain with pia mater. Frontal pole to the left (lateral aspect).

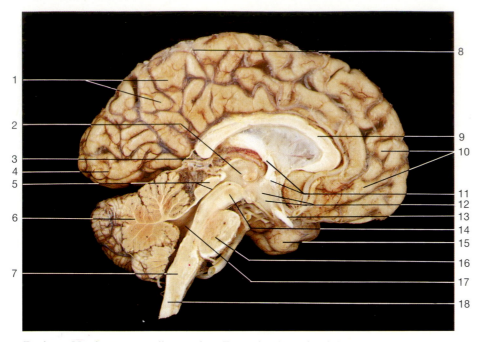

1 Parietal lobe
2 Thalamus, third ventricle and
   intermediate mass
3 Great cerebral vein
4 Occipital lobe
5 Colliculi of the midbrain
   and aqueduct
6 Cerebellum
7 Medulla oblongata
8 Central sulcus
9 Corpus callosum
10 Frontal lobe
11 Fornix and anterior commissure
12 Hypothalamus
13 Optic chiasma
14 Midbrain
15 Temporal lobe
16 Pons
17 Fourth ventricle
18 Spinal cord
19 Inferior concha,
   nasal cavity
20 Alveolar process of maxilla
21 Apex of tongue
22 Dens of axis
23 Oral part of pharynx
24 Alveolar process of mandible
25 Epiglottis

Brain and brain stem, median section. Frontal pole to the right.

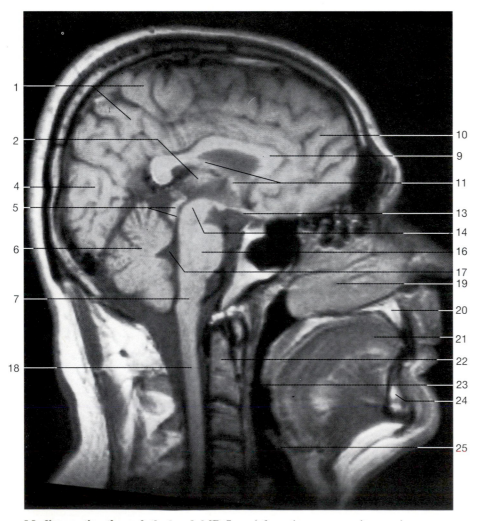

Median section through the head. MR-Scan (cf. section on opposite page).

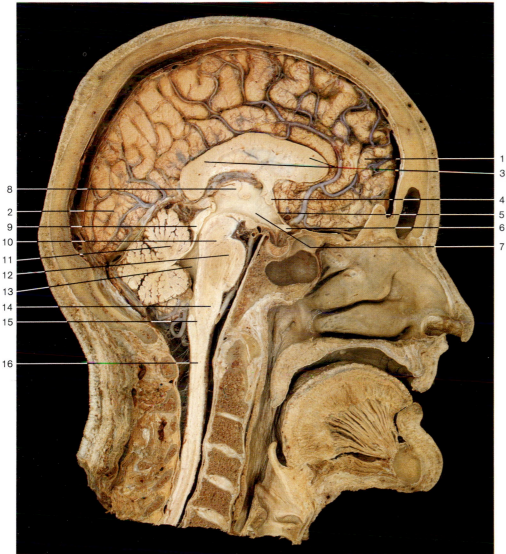

1	Frontal lobe of cerebrum
2	Occipital lobe of cerebrum
3	Corpus callosum
4	Anterior commissure
5	Lamina terminalis
6	Optic chiasma
7	Hypothalamus
8	Thalamus, third ventricle
9	Colliculi of the midbrain
10	Midbrain (inferior portion)
11	Cerebellum
12	Pons
13	Fourth ventricle
14	Medulla oblongata
15	Central canal
16	Spinal cord

Median section through the head. Regions of the brain. Falx cerebri removed.

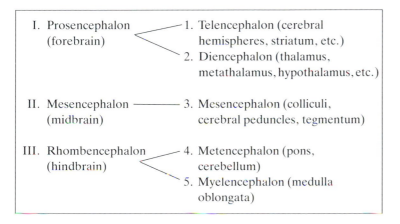

I. Prosencephalon (forebrain)	1. Telencephalon (cerebral hemispheres, striatum, etc.)
	2. Diencephalon (thalamus, metathalamus, hypothalamus, etc.)
II. Mesencephalon (midbrain)	3. Mesencephalon (colliculi, cerebral peduncles, tegmentum)
III. Rhombencephalon (hindbrain)	4. Metencephalon (pons, cerebellum)
	5. Myelencephalon (medulla oblongata)

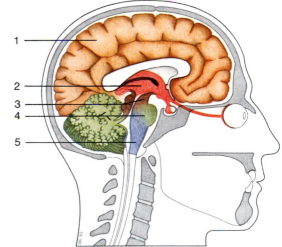

Main divisions of the brain. (Semidiagrammatic scheme) (O.).
I–III = primary brain vesicles (cf. table);
I–5 = secondary brain vesicles.
Midbrain, pons and medulla oblongata are collectively termed the **brain stem.**

The Cerebral Arteries und Veins

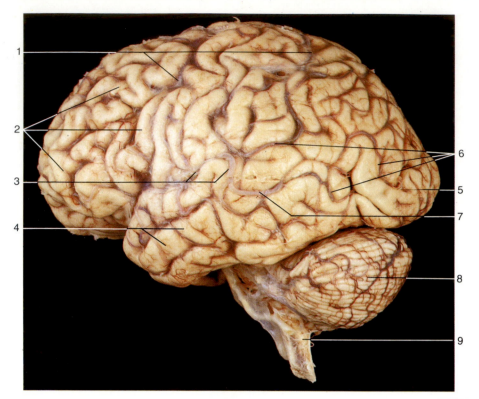

1 Superior cerebral veins, parietal lobe
2 Frontal lobe
3 Superficial middle cerebral vein
4 Temporal lobe
5 Occipital lobe
6 Inferior cerebral veins and transverse occipital sulcus
7 Inferior anastomotic vein
8 Cerebellum
9 Medulla oblongata

Brain with pia mater. Cerebral veins (bluish). In the lateral sulcus the cistern of the lateral fossa is recognizable. Frontal lobe to the left.

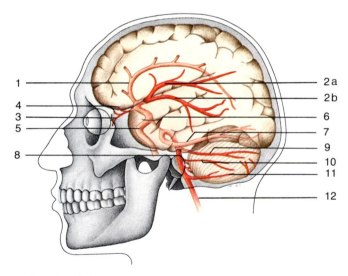

Arteries of the brain. Main branches of internal carotid and vertebral artery (lateral aspect) (O.).

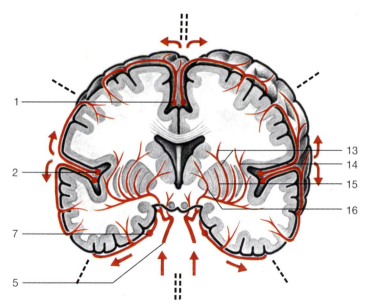

Arteries of the brain. Coronal section. Areas supplied by cortical and central arteries (O.). Dotted lines indicate arterial supply areas; arrows = direction of blood flow.

1 Anterior cerebral artery
2 Middle cerebral artery
  a Parietal branches
  b Temporal branches
3 Ophthalmic artery
4 Anterior and posterior ethmoidal arteries

5 Internal carotid artery
6 Posterior communicating artery
7 Posterior cerebral artery
8 Basilar artery
9 Superior cerebellar artery
10 Anterior inferior cerebellar artery

11 Posterior inferior cerebellar artery
12 Vertebral artery
13 Posterior striate branches
14 Insular artery
15 Pallidostriate artery
16 Thalamic artery

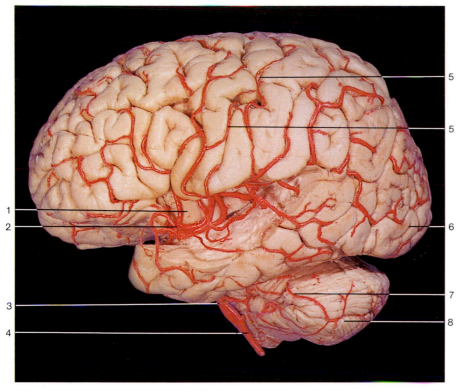

Cerebral arteries. Lateral aspect of the left hemisphere. The upper part of the temporal lobe has been removed to display the insula and cerebral arteries.

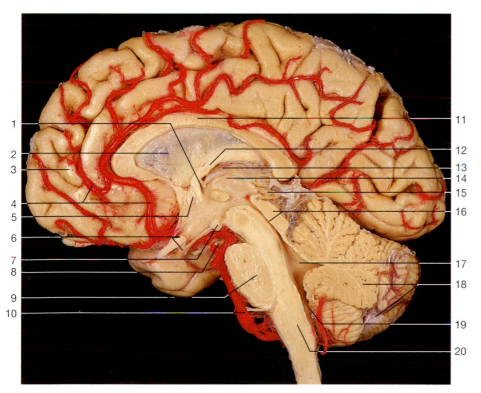

Median section through the brain and brain stem. Cerebral arteries injected with red resin.

The brain is supplied by a great number of arteries. The superficial arteries approach the brain via the pia mater supplying only the cortex (cortical arteries). The subcortical structures (striatum, thalamus, etc.) are supplied by perforating branches (central arteries) which penetrate the brain at its base. They extend as far as the subcortical white matter which therefore is a kind of "watershed" between the two zones of supply.

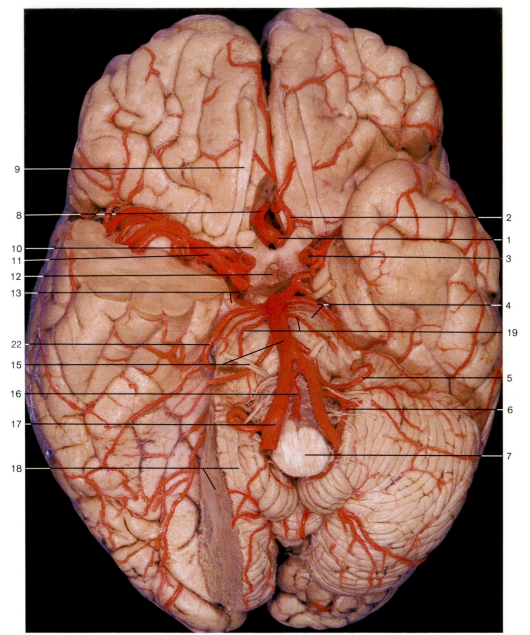

1 Anterior communicating artery
2 Left anterior cerebral artery
3 Internal carotid artery
4 Pons, left superior cerebellar artery
5 Anterior inferior cerebellar artery
6 Posterior inferior cerebellar artery
7 Medulla oblongata
8 Right anterior cerebral artery
9 Olfactory tract
10 Optic nerve
11 Middle cerebral artery
12 Infundibulum
13 Oculomotor nerve, posterior communicating artery
14 Posterior cerebral artery
15 Basilar artery and abducens nerve (n. VI)
16 Anterior spinal artery
17 Vertebral artery
18 Cerebellum
19 Labyrinthine arteries
20 Ophthalmic artery
21 Posterior spinal artery
22 Right superior cerebellar artery

Arteries of the brain (inferior aspect). Frontal pole above; right temporal lobe and cerebellum partly removed.

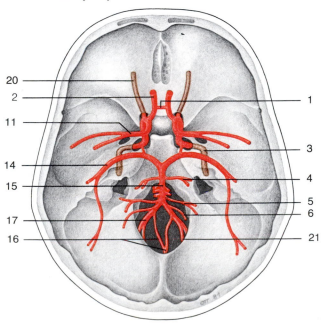

Circulus arteriosus cerebri (superior aspect). (Schematic drawing) (O.).

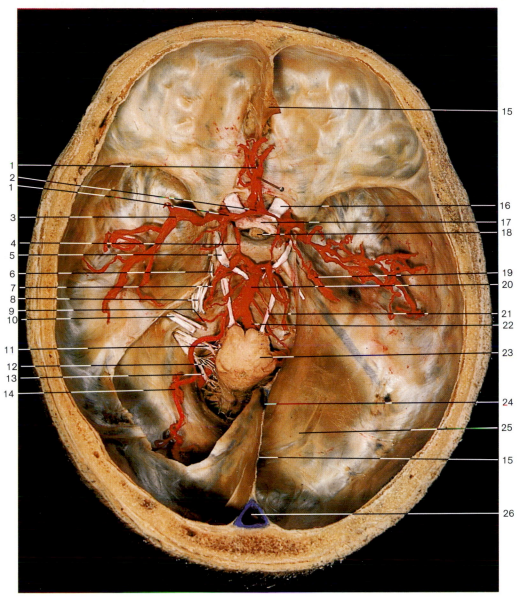

1	Anterior cerebral artery
2	Anterior communicating artery
3	Middle cerebral artery
4	Posterior communicating artery
5	Oculomotor nerve
6	Trochlear nerve
7	Posterior cerebral artery
8	Trigeminal nerve
9	Internal auditory artery
10	Facial nerve, vestibulocochlear nerve
11	Glossopharyngeal nerve, vagus nerve
12	Hypoglossal nerve
13	Accessory nerve
14	Anterior inferior cerebellar artery
15	Falx cerebri
16	Optic nerve
17	Optic chiasma
18	Infundibulum and pituitary gland
19	Anterior choroidal artery, choroid plexus
20	Basilar artery
21	Abducens nerve
22	Vertebral arteries
23	Medulla oblongata
24	Inferior sagittal sinus
25	Tentorium cerebelli
26	Superior sagittal sinus and confluence of sinuses
27	Posterior inferior cerebellar artery
28	Internal carotid artery

Base of the cranial cavity (internal aspect). Left tentorium has been cut.

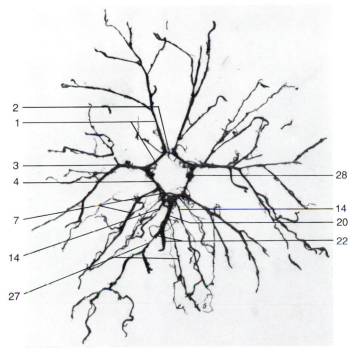

Circulus arteriosus cerebri (isolated from the brain and projected on cardboard).

The Lobes of the Brain

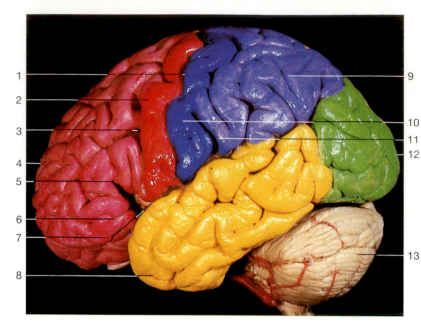

1 Central sulcus
2 Precentral gyrus
3 Precentral sulcus
4 Frontal lobe
5 Anterior ascending ramus of lateral sulcus
6 Anterior horizontal ramus of lateral sulcus
7 Lateral sulcus
8 Temporal lobe
9 Parietal lobe
10 Postcentral gyrus
11 Postcentral sulcus
12 Occipital lobe
13 Cerebellum
14 Superior frontal sulcus
15 Middle frontal gyrus
16 Lunate sulcus
17 Longitudinal fissure
18 Arachnoid granulations

Brain, left hemisphere (lateral aspect, frontal pole to the left).

Pink	= Frontal lobe
Blue	= Parietal lobe
Green	= Occipital lobe
Yellow	= Temporal lobe
Dark red	= Precentral gyrus
Dark blue	= Postcentral gyrus

Brain (superior aspect). Right hemisphere with pia mater.

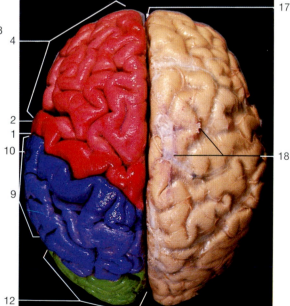

Brain (superior aspect). Lobes of the left hemisphere indicated by color; right hemisphere is covered with pia mater.

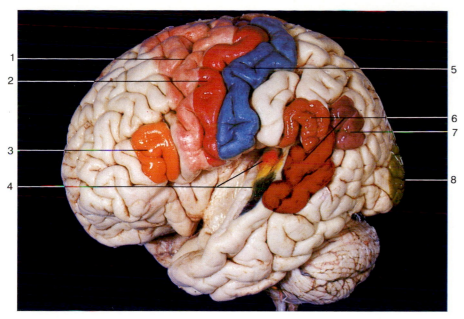

Brain, left hemisphere (lateral aspect). **Main cortical areas** are colored.
The lateral sulcus has been opened to display the insula and the inner surface of
the temporal lobe.

1 Premotor area
2 Somatomotor area
3 Motor speech area of Broca
4 Acoustic area
  (red: high tone; blue: low tone)
5 Somatosensory area
6 Sensory speech area of Wernicke
7 Reading comprehension area
8 Visuosensory area

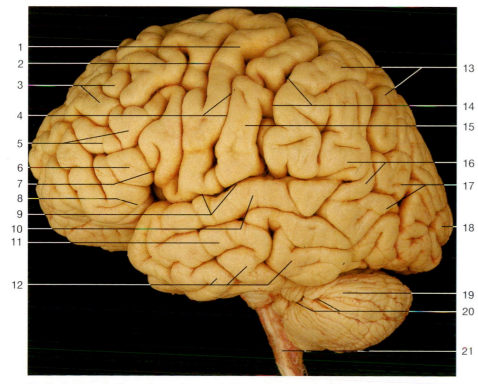

Brain, left hemisphere (lateral aspect). Frontal pole to the left.

1 Precentral gyrus
2 Precentral sulcus
3 Superior frontal gyrus
4 **Central sulcus**
5 Middle frontal gyrus
6 Inferior frontal gyrus
7 Ascending ramus ⎫
8 Horizontal ramus ⎬ of lateral
9 Posterior ramus ⎭ sulcus
10 Superior temporal gyrus
11 Middle temporal gyrus
12 Inferior temporal gyrus
13 Superior parietal lobule
14 Postcentral sulcus
15 Postcentral gyrus
16 Supramarginal gyrus
17 Angular gyrus
18 **Occipital lobe**
19 **Cerebellum**
20 Horizontal fissure of cerebellum
21 Medulla oblongata

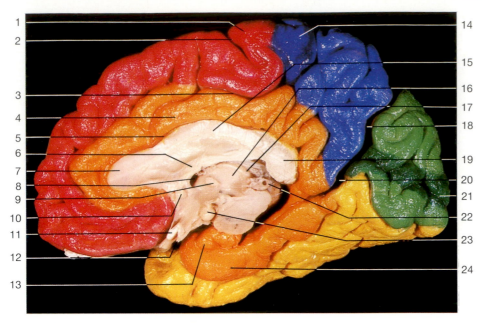

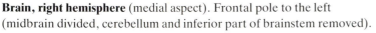

Brain, right hemisphere (medial aspect). Frontal pole to the left (midbrain divided, cerebellum and inferior part of brainstem removed).

1 Precentral gyrus
2 Precentral sulcus
3 Cingulate sulcus
4 Cingulate gyrus
5 Sulcus of corpus callosum
6 Fornix
7 Genu of corpus callosum
8 Interventricular foramen
9 Intermediate mass
10 Anterior commissure
11 Optic chiasma
12 Infundibulum
13 Uncus hippocampi
14 Postcentral gyrus
15 Body of corpus callosum
16 Third ventricle, thalamus
17 Stria medullaris
18 Parietooccipital sulcus
19 Splenium of corpus callosum
20 Communication of calcarine and parietooccipital sulcus
21 Occipital pole
22 Pineal body
23 Mamillary body
24 Parahippocampal gyrus
25 Olfactory bulb
26 Olfactory tract
27 Gyrus rectus
28 Optic nerve
29 Infundibulum, optic chiasma
30 Optic tract
31 Oculomotor nerve
32 Crus cerebri
33 Red nucleus
34 Cerebral aqueduct
35 Corpus callosum
36 Longitudinal fissure
37 Orbital gyri
38 Lateral root of olfactory tract
39 Medial root of olfactory tract
40 Olfactory tubercle, anterior perforated substance
41 Tuber cinereum
42 Interpeduncular fossa
43 Substantia nigra
44 Colliculi of the midbrain
45 Lateral occipitotemporal gyrus
46 Medial occipitotemporal gyrus

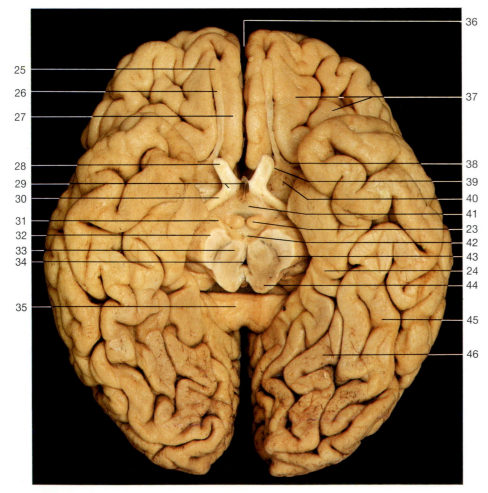

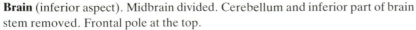

Brain (inferior aspect). Midbrain divided. Cerebellum and inferior part of brain stem removed. Frontal pole at the top.

Pink	= Frontal lobe
Blue	= Parietal lobe
Green	= Occipital lobe
Yellow	= Temporal lobe
Dark red	= Precentral lobe
Dark blue	= Postcentral lobe
Orange	= Limbic cortex (cingulate and parahippocampal gyri)

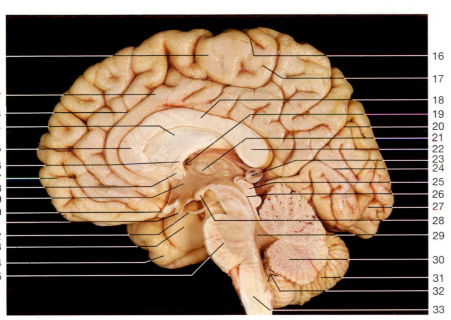

Brain (sagittal section). Frontal pole to the left.

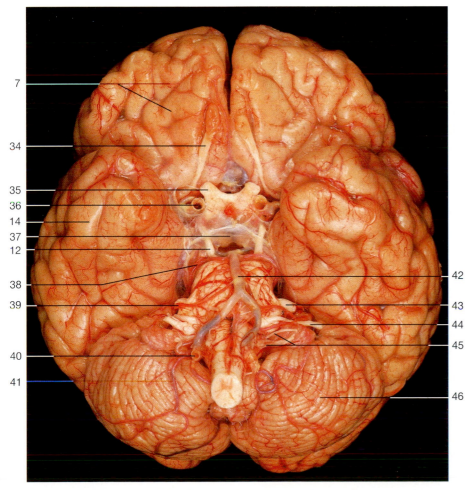

Brain, with pia mater and blood vessels (inferior aspect).

1 Precentral gyrus
2 Cingulate gyrus
3 Cingulate sulcus
4 Septum pellucidum
5 Genu of corpus callosum
6 Fornix
7 **Frontal lobe**
8 Anterior commissure
9 **Hypothalamus**
10 Optic chiasma
11 Infundibulum
12 Oculomotor nerve
13 Uncus
14 **Temporal lobe**
15 Pons
16 Central sulcus
17 Postcentral gyrus
18 Body of corpus callosum
19 Interventricular foramen (arrow)
20 Parietooccipital sulcus
21 Intermediate mass
22 Splenium of corpus callosum
23 Pineal body
24 Calcarine sulcus
25 Colliculi of midbrain
26 Cerebral aqueduct
27 **Occipital lobe**
28 Mamillary body
29 Fourth ventricle
30 Vermis of cerebellum
31 Right hemisphere of cerebellum
32 Median aperture of Magendi (arrow)
33 Medulla oblongata
34 Olfactory tract
35 Optic nerve
36 **Internal carotid artery**
37 Interpeduncular cistern
38 Superior cerebellar artery
39 Anterior inferior cerebellar artery
40 **Vertebral artery**
41 Posterior inferior cerebellar artery
42 **Basilar artery**
43 Trigeminal nerve (n. V)
44 Facial nerve (n. VII)
45 Accessory nerve (n. XI), hypoglossal nerve (n. XII)
46 Cerebellum

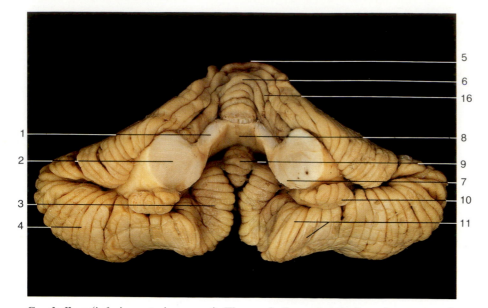

1 Superior cerebellar peduncle
2 Middle cerebellar peduncle
3 Cerebellar tonsil
4 Inferior semilunar lobule
5 Vermis
6 Central lobule of vermis
7 Inferior cerebellar peduncle
8 Superior medullary velum
9 Nodule of vermis
10 Flocculus
11 Biventral lobule
12 Fissura prima
13 Culmen ⎫
14 Declive ⎬ of vermis
15 Folium of the vermis
16 Ala of central lobule
17 Quadrangular lobule
18 Lobulus simplex
19 Superior semilunar lobule
20 Horizontal cerebellar fissure
21 Inferior semilunar lobule
22 Tuber of vermis
23 Pyramid of vermis
24 Uvula of vermis
25 Biventral lobule

Cerebellum (inferior anterior aspect). The cerebellar peduncles have been severed.

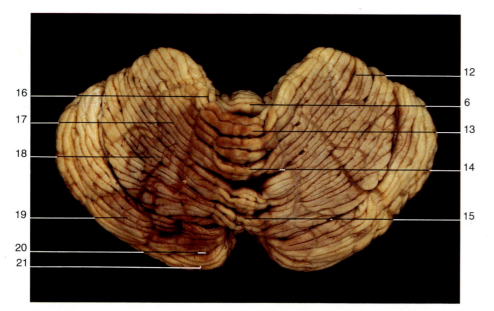

Cerebellum (superior aspect).

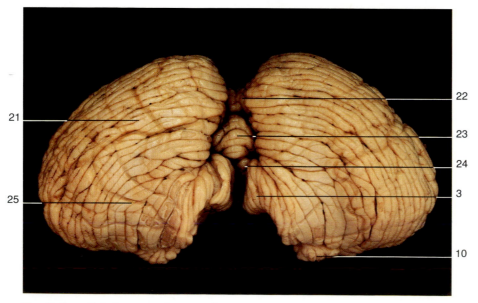

Cerebellum (inferior posterior aspect).

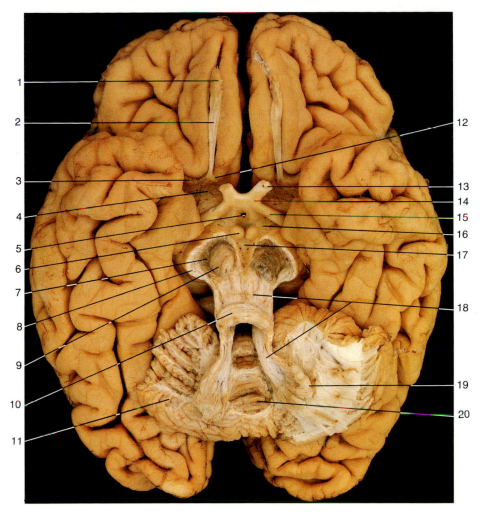

1	Olfactory bulb
2	Olfactory tract
3	Lateral olfactory stria
4	Anterior perforated substance
5	Infundibulum (divided)
6	Mamillary body
7	Substantia nigra
8	Crus cerebri
9	Red nucleus
10	Decussation of superior cerebellar peduncle
11	Cerebellar hemisphere
12	Medial olfactory stria
13	Optic nerve
14	Optic chiasma
15	Optic tract
16	Posterior perforated substance
17	Interpeduncular fossa
18	Superior cerebellar peduncle, cerebellorubral tract
19	Dentate nucleus
20	Vermis of the cerebellum
21	Cerebellar hemisphere
22	Vermis (central lobule)
23	Cerebellar lingula
24	Ala of central lobule
25	Superior cerebellar peduncle
26	Fastigium
27	Fourth ventricle
28	Middle cerebellar peduncle
29	Nodule of vermis
30	Flocculus of cerebellum
31	Cerebellar tonsil
32	Culmen of vermis
33	Declive of vermis
34	Tuber of vermis
35	Inferior semilunar lobule
36	Pyramis of vermis
37	Uvula of vermis

Brain and cerebellum (inferior aspect). Parts of the cerebellum have been removed to display the dentate nucleus and the main pathway to the midbrain (cerebellorubral tract).

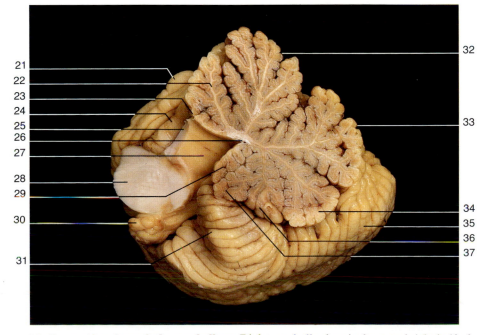

Median section through the cerebellum. Right cerebellar hemisphere and right half of vermis.

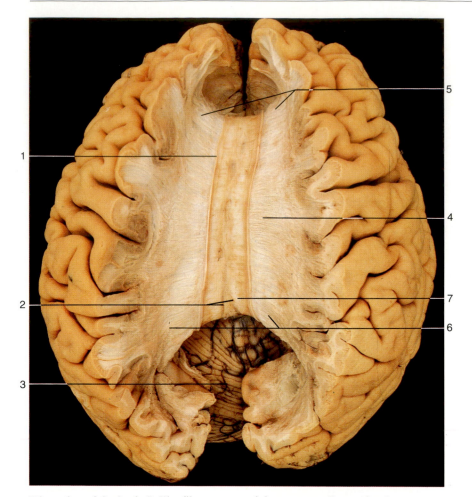

1 Lateral longitudinal stria
  of indusium griseum
2 Medial longitudinal stria
  of indusium griseum
3 Cerebellum
4 Radiating fibers of the corpus callosum
5 Forceps minor of corpus callosum
6 Forceps major of corpus callosum
7 Splenium of corpus callosum

Dissection of the brain I. The fiber system of the corpus callosum has been displayed by removing the cortex lying above it (frontal pole at top).

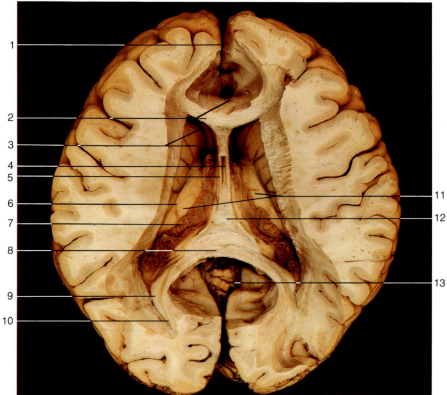

1 Longitudinal cerebral fissure
2 Genu of corpus callosum
3 Head of caudate nucleus and
  anterior horn of lateral ventricle
4 Cavum of septum pellucidum
5 Septum pellucidum
6 Stria terminalis
7 Choroid plexus of lateral ventricle
8 Splenium of corpus callosum
9 Calcar avis
10 Posterior horn of lateral ventricle
11 Thalamus, Lamina affixa
12 Commissure of fornix
13 Vermis of cerebellum

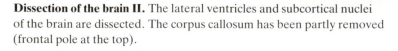

Dissection of the brain II. The lateral ventricles and subcortical nuclei of the brain are dissected. The corpus callosum has been partly removed (frontal pole at the top).

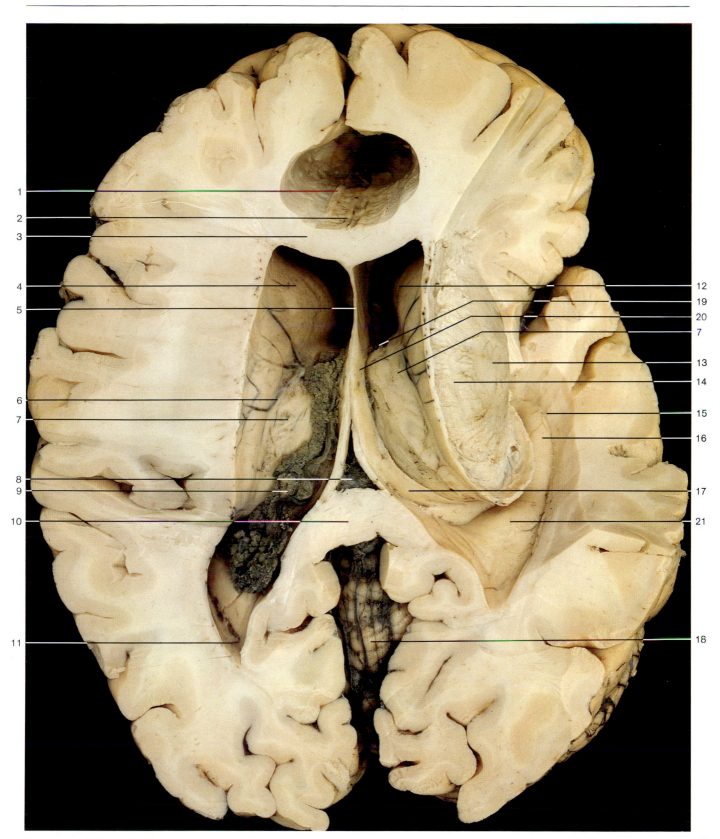

Dissection of the brain III. Superior view of lateral ventricle and subcortical nuclei of the brain. Corpus callosum partly removed. At right, the entire lateral ventricle has been opened, the insula with claustrum, extreme and external capsules have been removed, exposing the lentiform nucleus and the internal capsule.

1	Lateral longitudinal stria	8	Choroid plexus of third ventricle
2	Medial longitudinal stria	9	Choroid plexus of lateral ventricle
3	Genu of corpus callosum	10	Splenium of corpus callosum
4	Head of caudate nucleus	11	Posterior horn of lateral ventricle
5	Septum pellucidum	12	Anterior horn of lateral ventricle, head of
6	Stria terminalis		caudate nucleus
7	Thalamus, Lamina affixa	13	Putamen of lentiform nucleus

14 Internal capsule
15 Inferior horn of lateral ventricle
16 Pes hippocampi
17 Crus of fornix
18 Vermis of cerebellum with pia mater
19 Interventricular foramen
20 Right column of fornix
21 Collateral eminence

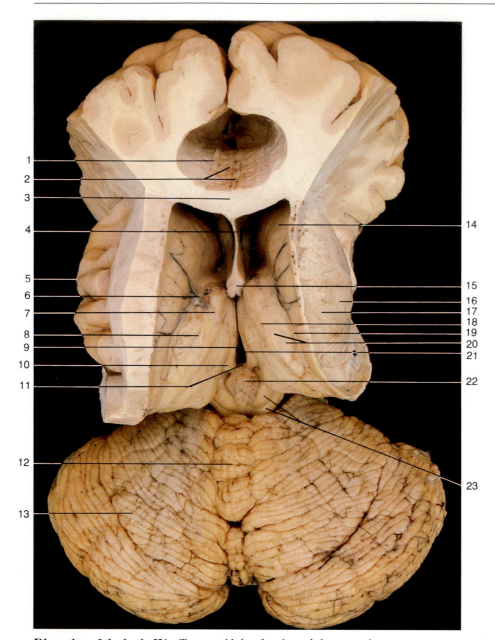

1 Lateral longitudinal stria
2 Medial longitudinal stria
3 Corpus callosum
4 Septum pellucidum
5 Insular gyri
6 Thalamostriate vein
7 Anterior tubercle of thalamus
8 Thalamus
9 Medullary stria of thalamus
10 Habenular trigone
11 Habenular commissure
12 Vermis of the cerebellum
13 Left hemisphere of cerebellum
14 Head of caudate nucleus
15 Columns of fornix
16 Putamen of lentiform nucleus
17 Internal capsule
18 Taenia of choroid plexus
19 Stria terminalis, thalamostriate vein
20 Lamina affixa
21 Third ventricle
22 Pineal body
23 Superior and inferior colliculus
   of midbrain

Dissection of the brain IVa. Temporal lobe, fornix and the posterior corpus callosum have been removed (this part of the specimen is depicted below). Frontal pole at top, superior aspect.

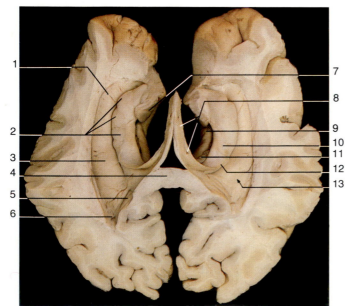

1 Inferior horn of lateral ventricle
2 Hippocampal digitations
3 Collateral eminence
4 Splenium of corpus callosum
5 Calcar avis
6 Posterior horn of lateral ventricle
7 Uncus of parahippocampal gyrus
8 Body and crus of fornix
9 Parahippocampal gyrus
10 Pes hippocampi
11 Dentate gyrus
12 Hippocampal fimbria
13 Lateral ventricle

Dissection of the brain IVb. Depicted is the portion of the brain removed from the specimen above. **Temporal lobe and limbic system.** Superior aspect, Columns of fornix are served.

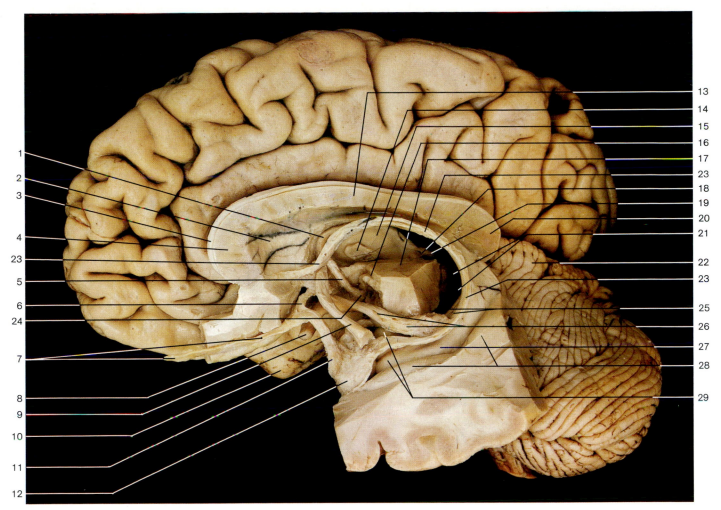

Dissection of the limbic system. Lateral aspect, left side (corpus callosum has been cut in the median plane, the left thalamus and the left hemisphere have been partly removed).

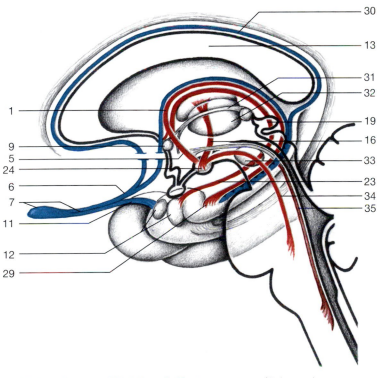

Main pathways of **limbic and olfactory system.** (Schematic drawing) (O.). Blue = afferent pathways; red = efferent pathways.

1	Body of fornix	25	Fimbria of hippocampus, pes hippocampi
2	Septum pellucidum		
3	Lateral longitudinal stria	26	Left optic tract, lateral geniculate body
4	Genu of corpus callosum		
5	Column of fornix	27	Lateral ventricle, parahippocampal gyrus
6	Medial olfactory stria		
7	Olfactory bulb and olfactory tract	28	Collateral eminence
8	Optic nerve	29	Hippocampal digitations
9	Anterior commissure, left half	30	Supracallosal gyrus (longitudinal stria)
10	Right temporal lobe	31	Stria medullaris thalami
11	Lateral olfactory stria	32	Thalamus
12	Amygdala	33	Red nucleus
13	Body of corpus callosum	34	Mamillotegmental tract
14	Interthalamic adhesion	35	Dorsal longitudinal fasciculus (Schütz)
15	Third ventricle and right thalamus		
16	Mamillothalamic tract		
17	Part of the thalamus		
18	Habenular commissure		
19	Pineal body		
20	Splenium of corpus callosum		
21	Colliculi of midbrain		
22	Vermis of cerebellum		
23	Stria terminalis		
24	Mamillary body		

The Hypothalamus

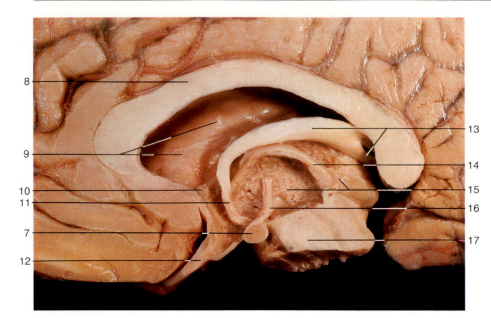

1 Paraventricular nucleus ⎫
2 Preoptic nucleus ⎪
3 Ventromedial nucleus ⎬ Hypothalamic
4 Supraoptic nucleus ⎪ nuclei
5 Posterior nucleus ⎪
6 Dorsomedial nucleus ⎭
7 Mamillary body
8 Corpus callosum
9 Lateral ventricle
10 Anterior commissure
11 Column of fornix
12 Optic chiasma
13 Crus of fornix
14 Medullary stria of thalamus
15 Thalamus and interthalamic adhesion
16 Mamillothalamic tract of Vicq d'Azyr
17 Cerebral peduncle
18 Pineal body
19 Tectum of midbrain
20 Lamina terminalis

Median section through the diencephalon. Medial part of the thalamus and septum pellucidum have been removed to show the fornix and mamillothalamic tract.

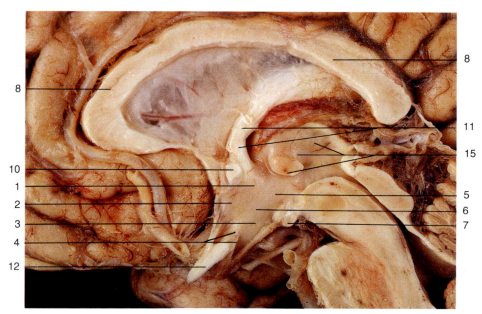

Median section through the diencephalon and midbrain; location of hypothalamic nuclei.

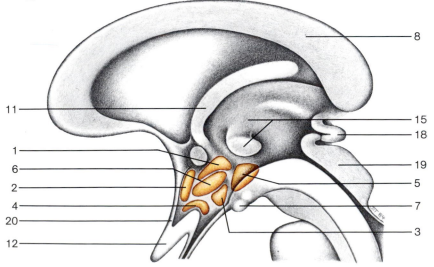

Position of main hypothalamic nuclei. (Schematic diagram) (O.).

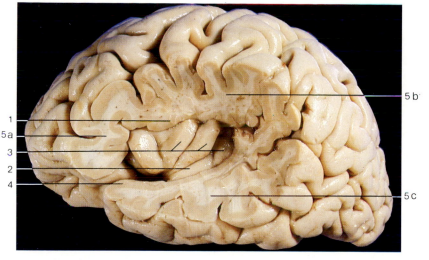

1   Circular sulcus of insula
2   Long gyrus of insula
3   Short gyri of insula
4   Limen insulae
5   Opercula (cut)
   a Frontal operculum
   b Frontoparietal operculum
   c Temporal operculum
6   Corona radiata
7   Lentiform nucleus
8   Anterior commissure
9   Olfactory tract
10 Cerebral arcuate fibers
11 Optic radiation
12 Cerebral peduncle
13 Trigeminal nerve
14 Flocculus of cerebellum
15 Pyramidal tract
16 Decussation of pyramidal tract
17 Internal capsule
18 Optic tract
19 Optic nerve
20 Infundibulum
21 Temporal lobe (right side)
22 Mamillary bodies
23 Oculomotor nerve
24 Transverse fibers of pons

Insula (Reili). The opercula of the frontal, parietal and temporal lobes have been removed to display the insular gyri. Left hemisphere.

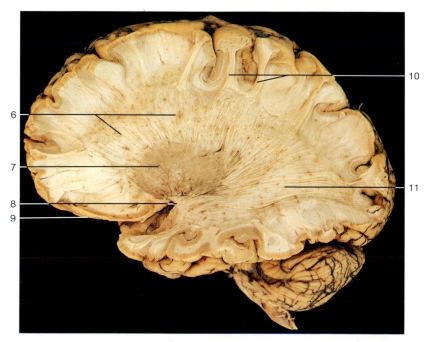

Dissection of the corona radiata, left hemisphere (frontal pole on the left).

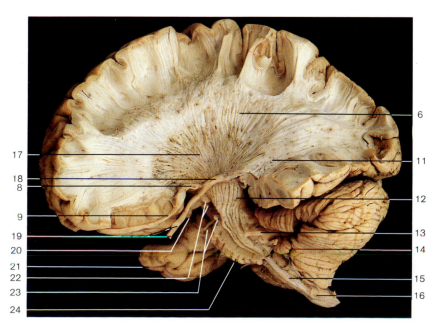

◁ **Corona radiata and internal capsule,** left hemisphere. Lentiform nucleus removed (frontal pole to the left).

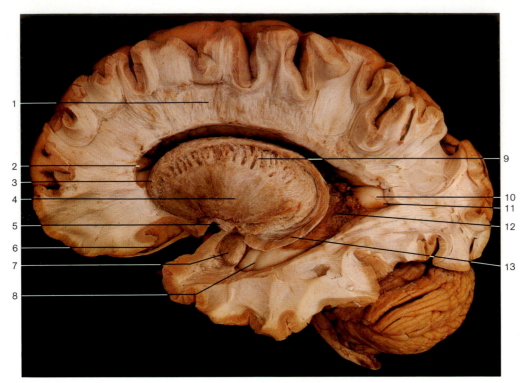

1　Corona radiata
2　Anterior horn of lateral ventricle
3　Head of caudate nucleus
4　Putamen
5　Anterior commissure
6　Olfactory tract
7　Amygdala
8　Hippocampal digitations
9　Internal capsule
10　Calcar avis
11　Posterior horn of lateral ventricle
12　Choroid plexus of lateral ventricle
13　Caudal extremity of caudate nucleus
14　Thalamus
15　Cerebral arcuate fibers
16　Globus pallidus (remnants)

Dissection of the subcortical nuclei and internal capsule, left hemisphere (lateral aspect). Frontal pole to the left. The lateral ventricle has been opened, and the insular gyri and claustrum have been removed, revealing the lentiform nucleus and the internal capsule.

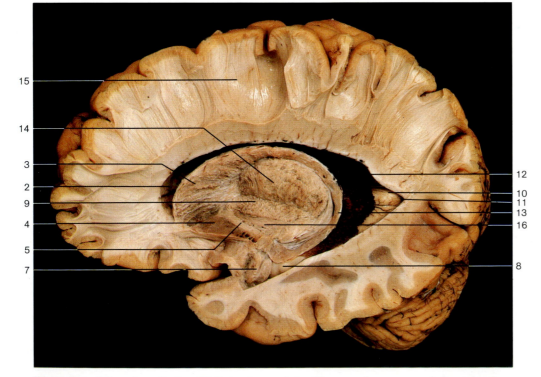

Dissection of the subcortical nuclei (lateral aspect, lentiform nucleus removed, frontal pole to the left).

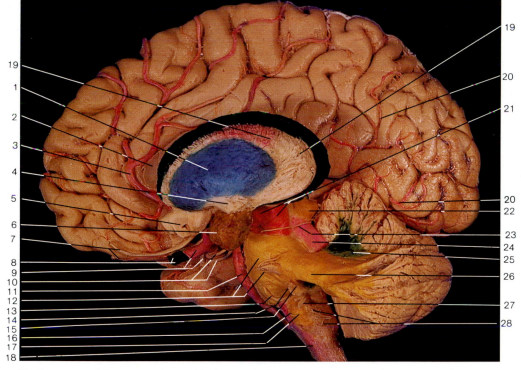

1 Putamen
2 Genu of corpus callosum
3 Anterior cerebral artery
4 Anterior commissure
5 Subcallosal area
6 Amygdala
7 Olfactory tract
8 Optic nerve
9 Internal carotid artery, infundibulum
10 Oculomotor nerve (right and left nerve)
11 Basilar artery
12 Pons and trigeminal nerve
13 Abducens nerve
14 Facial nerve
15 Vestibulocochlear nerve
16 Hypoglossal nerve
17 Olive
18 Pyramidal tract
19 Internal capsule
20 Posterior cerebral artery
21 Cerebral peduncle
22 Colliculi of midbrain
23 Trochlear nerve
24 Superior cerebellar peduncle
25 Inferior cerebellar peduncle
26 Middle cerebellar peduncle
27 Glossopharyngeal nerve
28 Vagus and accessory nerves
29 Corpus callosum
30 Lateral ventricle (anterior horn)
31 Caudate nucleus
32 Internal capsule (anterior limb)
33 Insula
34 Claustrum
35 Thalamus
36 Superior and inferior colliculus of midbrain
37 Cerebellum
38 Middle peduncle of cerebellum (efferent tracts)
39 Medulla oblongata (afferent tracts)
40 Putamen of lentiform nucleus
41 Globus pallidus of lentiform nucleus
42 Genu and posterior limb of internal capsule

Brain stem and the connections with the cerebellum. Internal capsule (lateral aspect). Red = pyramidal tract; yellow = middle cerebellar peduncle; green = inferior cerebellar peduncle; pink = superior cerebellar peduncle.

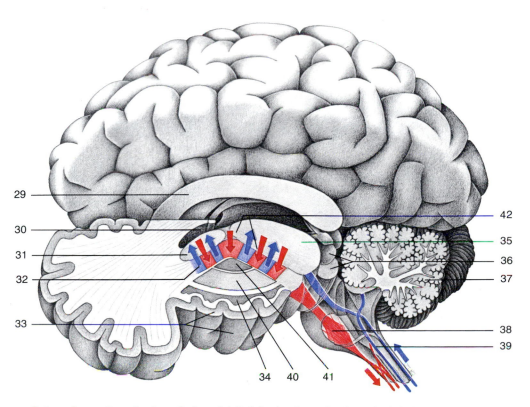

Internal capsule and subcortical nuclei (left brain, frontal pole to the left, horizontal section, semischematic drawing) (O.). Blue = afferent tracts; red = efferent tracts.

107

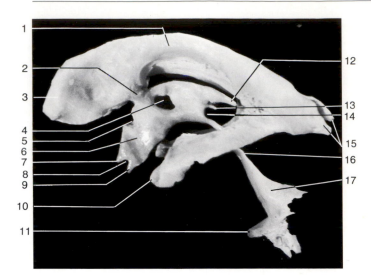

1   Central part of the lateral ventricle
2   Interventricular foramen of Monro
3   Anterior horn of the lateral ventricle
4   Site of interthalamic adhesion
5   Notch for anterior commissure
6   Third ventricle
7   Optic recess
8   Notch for optic chiasma
9   Infundibular recess
10 Inferior horn of lateral ventricle with indentation
    of amygdaloid body
11 Lateral recess and lateral aperture of Luschka
12 Suprapineal recess
13 Pineal recess
14 Notch for posterior commissure
15 Posterior horns of lateral ventricle
16 Aqueduct
17 Fourth ventricle
18 Median aperture of Magendie
19 Cerebellomedullary cistern

Cast of ventricular cavities of the brain (lateral aspect), frontal pole to the left.

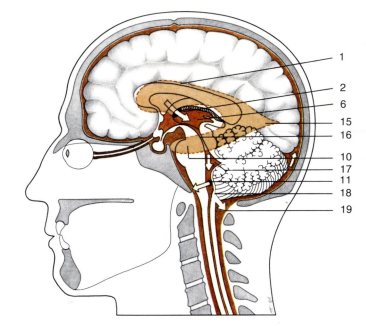

Position of ventricular cavities. (Schematic diagram) (O.). The direction of flow of cerebrospinal fluid is indicated by arrows. Dotted line = outline of right lateral ventricle.

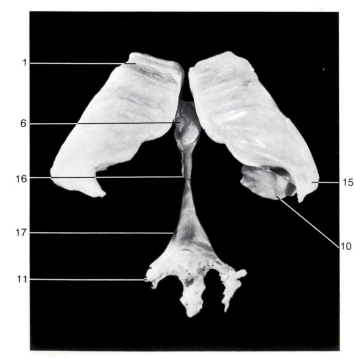

Cast of ventricular cavities (posterior aspect).

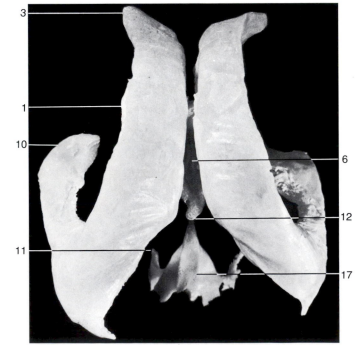

Cast of ventricular cavities (superior aspect). Frontal pole at top.

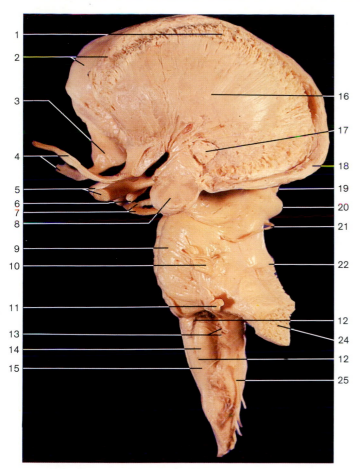

1 Internal capsule
2 Head of the caudate nucleus
3 Olfactory trigone
4 Olfactory tracts
5 Optic nerves
6 Infundibulum
7 Oculomotor nerve
8 Amygdaloid body
9 Pons
10 Trigeminal nerve
11 Facial and vestibulocochlear nerves
12 Hypoglossal nerve
13 Glossopharyngeal and vagus nerves
14 Olive
15 Medulla oblongata
16 Lentiform nucleus
17 Anterior commissure
18 Tail of caudate nucleus
19 Superior colliculus
20 Inferior colliculus
21 Trochlear nerve
22 Superior cerebellar peduncle
23 Inferior cerebellar peduncle
24 Middle cerebellar peduncle
25 Accessory nerve (n. XI)
26 Columns of fornix (divided)
27 Lamina affixa
28 Third ventricle
29 Pulvinar of thalamus
30 Inferior brachium
31 Frenulum veli
32 Superior medullary velum
33 Facial colliculus
34 Striae medullares, rhomboid fossa
35 Hypoglossal triangle
36 Stria terminalis, thalamostriate vein
37 Habenular trigone
38 Choroid plexus of lateral ventricle
39 Pineal body
40 Lateral geniculate body
41 Cerebral peduncle
42 Choroid plexus of fourth ventricle
43 Clava
44 Dorsal root of cervical nerve
45 Cuneate tubercle

Brain stem (left lateral aspect). Cerebellar peduncles have been severed, cerebellum and cerebral cortex have been removed.

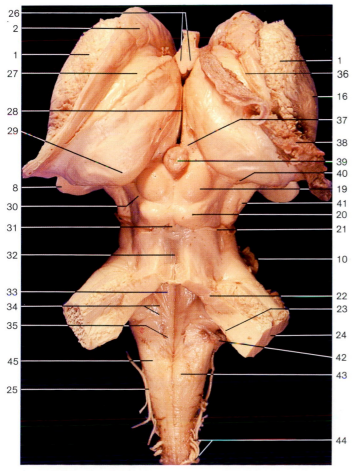

Brain stem (dorsal aspect). Cerebellum removed.

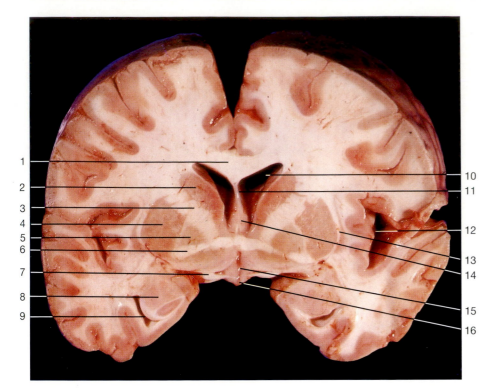

1	Corpus callosum
2	Head of **caudate nucleus**
3	**Internal capsule**
4	**Putamen**
5	**Globus pallidus**
6	Anterior commissure
7	Optic tract
8	Amygdaloid body
9	Inferior horn of lateral ventricle
10	**Lateral ventricle**
11	Septum pellucidum
12	Insula
13	External capsule
14	Column of fornix
15	Optic recess
16	Infundibulum
17	**Thalamus**
18	Claustrum
19	Lenticular ansa
20	**Third ventricle, hypothalamus**
21	Basilar artery, pons
22	Cortex of temporal lobe
23	Inferior colliculus
24	Superior colliculus
25	Aqueduct
26	Red nucleus
27	Substantia nigra
28	Cerebral peduncle
29	Trochlear nerve (n. IV)
30	Gray matter
31	Nucleus of oculomotor nerve (nucleus of Edinger-Westphal)
32	Fibers of oculomotor nerve (n. III)
33	Vermis of cerebellum
34	Fourth ventricle
35	Reticular formation
36	Pons, transverse pontine fibers
37	Emboliform nucleus
38	Dentate nucleus
39	Middle cerebellar peduncle
40	Choroid plexus
41	Hypoglossal nucleus at rhomboid fossa
42	Medial longitudinal fasciculus
43	Trigeminal nerve (n. V.)
44	Inferior olivary nucleus
45	Corticospinal fibers, arcuate fibers
46	Fourth ventricle with choroid plexus
47	Vestibular nuclei
48	Nucleus and tractus solitarius
49	Inferior cerebellar peduncle (restiform body)
50	Reticular formation
51	Medial lemniscus
52	Cuneate nucleus of Burdach
53	Central canal
54	**Pyramidal tract**
55	Flocculus of cerebellum
56	Cerebellar hemisphere with pia mater
57	"Arbor vitae" of cerebellum
58	Nucleus gracilis of Goll
59	Lateral recess of choroid plexus of IVth ventricle
60	Posterior inferior cerebellar artery

Coronal section through the brain at the level of the anterior commissure. Section 1.

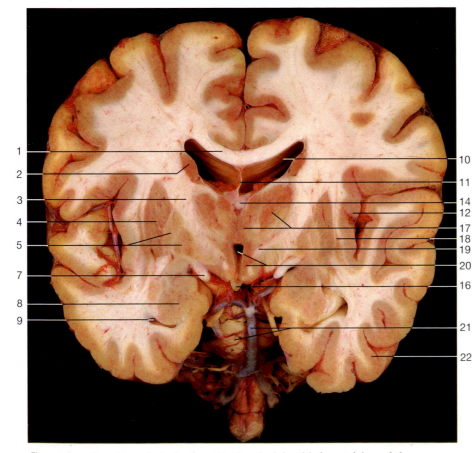

Coronal section through the brain at the level of the third ventricle and the interthalamic adhesion. Section 2.

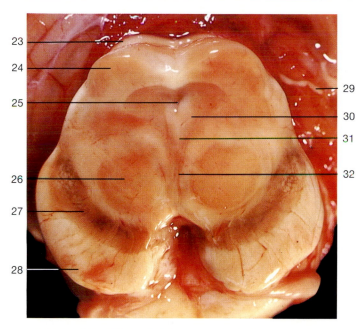

23
24
25
26
27
28

29
30
31
32

Cross-section of the midbrain (mesencephalon) at the level of the superior colliculus (superior aspect). Section 3.

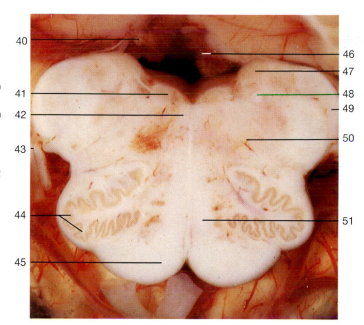

40
41
42
43
44
45

46
47
48
49
50
51

Cross-section of the rhombencephalon at the level of the olive (inferior aspect). Section 5.

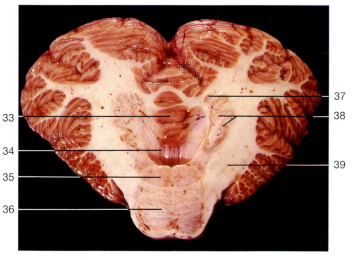

33
34
35
36

37
38
39

Cross-section through the rhombencephalon at the level of pons (inferior aspect). Section 4.

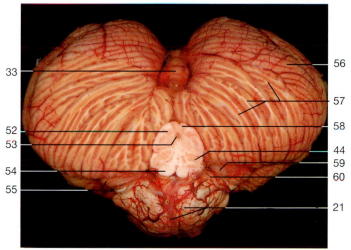

33
52
53
54
55

56
57
58
44
59
60
21

Cross-section through medulla oblongata and cerebellum (inferior aspect). Section 6.

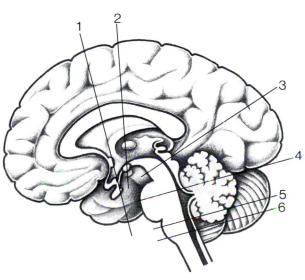

1
2
3
4
5
6

Drawing indicating the levels of brain sections (O.).

111

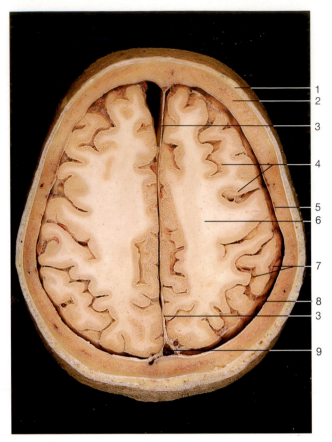

Horizontal section through the head.
Section 1.

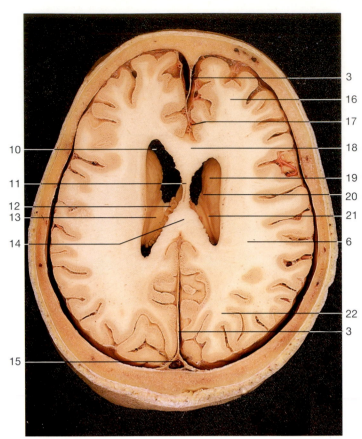

Horizontal section through the head.
Section 2.

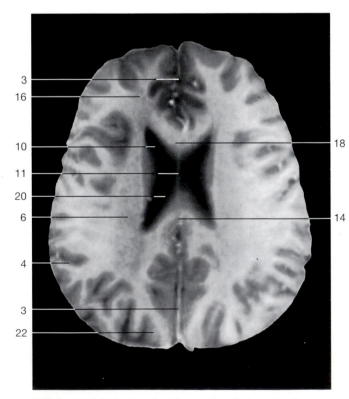

MR-Scan of the human head at the level of section 2.

1 Skin of scalp
2 Calvaria (diploe of the skull)
3 **Falx cerebri**
4 Gray matter of brain (cortex)
5 Dura mater
6 **White matter of brain**
7 Pia mater with vessels
8 Subarachnoidal space
9 Superior sagittal sinus
10 Anterior horn of lateral ventricle
11 **Septum pellucidum**
12 Choroid plexus
13 Thalamus
14 Splenium of corpus callosum
15 Confluence of sinuses
16 Frontal lobe
17 Anterior cerebral artery
18 Genu of corpus callosum
19 Caudate nucleus
20 **Central part of lateral ventricle**
21 Stria terminalis
22 Occipital lobe

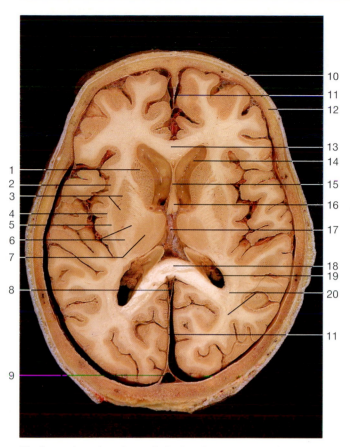

1 Caudate nucleus
2 Insula
3 Lentiform nucleus
4 Claustrum
5 External capsule
6 Internal capsule
7 Thalamus
8 Straight sinus (sinus rectus)
9 Superior sagittal sinus, confluence of sinuses
10 Skin of scalp
11 Falx cerebri
12 Calvaria (diploe of skull)
13 Genu of corpus callosum
14 Anterior horn of lateral ventricle
15 Septum pellucidum
16 Column of fornix
17 Choroid plexus of third ventricle
18 Splenium of corpus callosum
19 Entrance to inferior horn of lateral ventricle with choroid plexus
20 Optic radiation
21 Third ventricle

Horizontal section through the head at the level of third ventricle of internal capsule and neighbouring nuclei. Section 3.

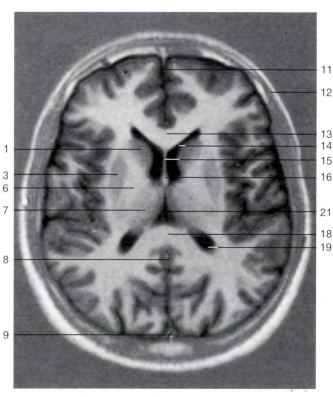

MR-Scan at the corresponding level to the above figure. Section 3.

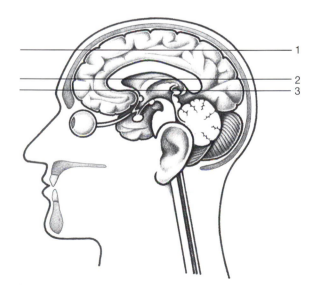

Sagittal section through the head. Levels of sections. (Schematic drawing) (O.).

113

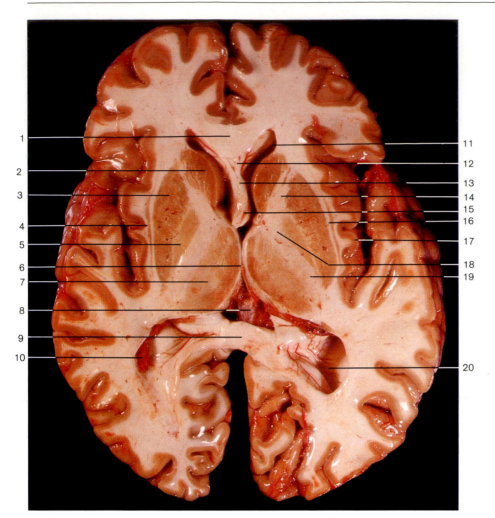

1	Genu of corpus callosum
2	Head of caudate nucleus
3	Putamen
4	Claustrum
5	Globus pallidus
6	Third ventricle
7	Thalamus
8	Pineal body
9	Splenium of corpus callosum
10	Choroid plexus of the lateral ventricle
11	Anterior horn of lateral ventricle
12	Cavity of septum pellucidum
13	Septum pellucidum
14	Anterior limb of internal capsule
15	Column of fornix
16	External capsule
17	Insula
18	Genu of internal capsule
19	Posterior limb of internal capsule
20	Posterior horn of lateral ventricle
21	Anterior commissure
22	Optic radiation
23	Falx cerebri
24	Maxillary sinus
25	Position of auditory tube
26	Tympanic cavity
27	External acoustic meatus
28	Medulla oblongata
29	Fourth ventricle
30	Cerebellum (left hemisphere)
31	Temporomandibular joint
32	Tympanic membrane
33	Base of cochlea
34	Mastoid air cells
35	Sigmoid sinus
36	Vermis of cerebellum
37	Intermediate mass

Horizontal section through the brain, showing the subcortical nuclei and internal capsule. Section 1.

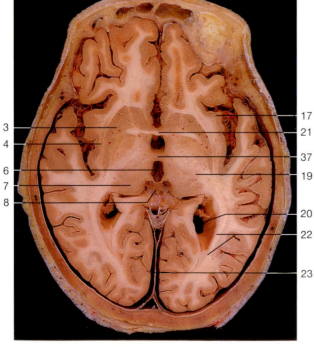

Horizontal section through the head. Section 2.

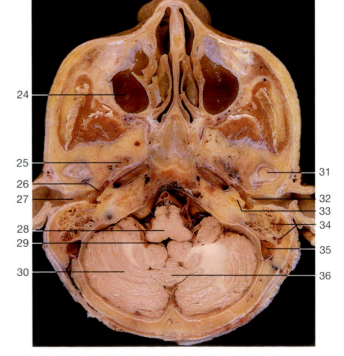

Horizontal section through the head. Section 4.

114

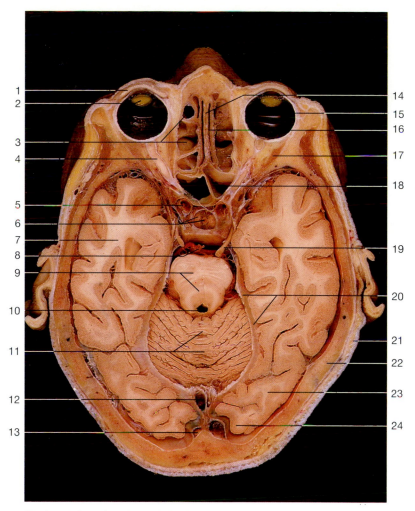

1 Upper lid, tarsal plate
2 Lens
3 Ethmoidal sinus
4 **Optic nerve**
5 Internal carotid artery
6 Infundibulum, **pituitary gland**
7 Temporal lobe
8 Basilar artery
9 Pons, cross section of brain stem
10 **Cerebral aqueduct,** beginning of fourth ventricle
11 Vermis of cerebellum
12 Straight sinus
13 Transverse sinus
14 Nasal septum
15 **Eyeball** (sclera)
16 Nasal cavity
17 Lateral rectus
18 Sphenoidal sinus
19 Oculomotor nerve (n. III)
20 **Tentorium of cerebellum**
21 Skin of scalp
22 Calvaria
23 Occipital lobe
24 Striate cortex (visual cortex)

Horizontal section through the head. Section 3.

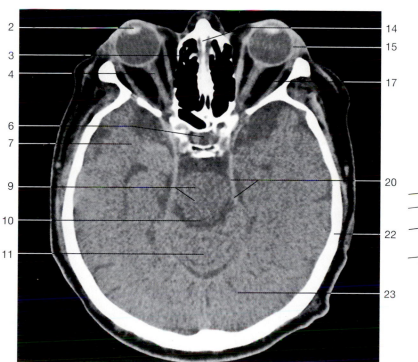

Horizontal section through the head. CT-Scan, Section 3.

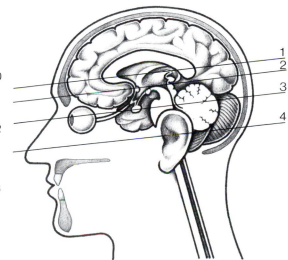

Sagittal section through the head.
Levels of sections. (Schematic drawing) (O.).

115

The Auditory and Vestibular Apparatus

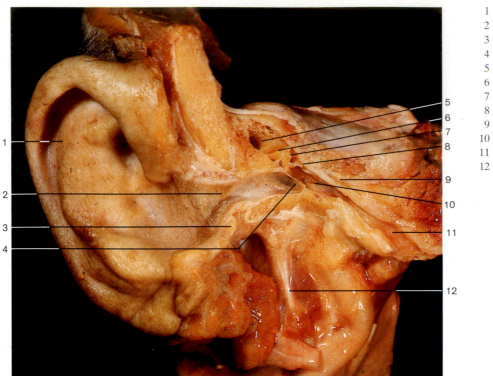

1 Auricle or pinna
2 External acoustic meatus
3 Cartilage of the external acoustic meatus
4 Tympanic membrane
5 Mastoid antrum
6 Incus
7 Head of malleus
8 Stapes
9 Tensor tympani
10 Tympanic cavity
11 Auditory tube
12 Styloid process

Longitudinal section through the right external acoustic meatus and middle ear, showing auditory ossicles and auditory tube.

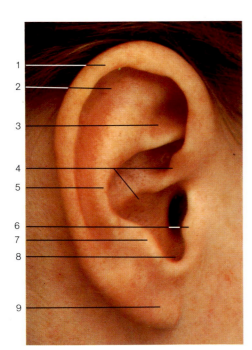

Right auricle (lateral aspect).

1 Helix
2 Scaphoid fossa
3 Triangular fossa
4 Concha
5 Antihelix
6 Tragus
7 Antitragus
8 Intertragic notch
9 Lobule

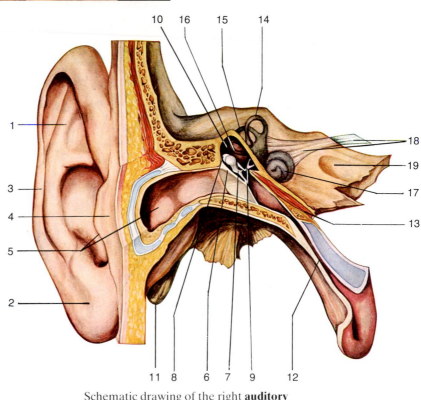

Schematic drawing of the right auditory and vestibular apparatus (anterior aspect).

Outer Ear
1 Auricle
2 Lobule of auricle
3 Helix
4 Tragus
5 External acoustic meatus

Middle Ear
6 Tympanic membrane
7 Malleus
8 Incus
9 Stapes

10 Tympanic cavity
11 Mastoid process
12 Auditory tube
13 Tensor tympani

Inner Ear
14 Anterior semicircular duct
15 Posterior semicircular duct
16 Lateral semicircular duct
17 Cochlea
18 Vestibulocochlear nerve
19 Petrous part of the temporal bone

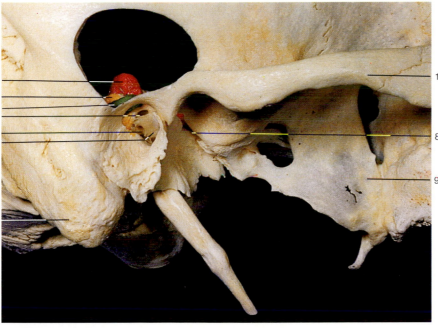

1 Anterior semicircular canal
2 Posterior semicircular canal
3 Lateral or horizontal semicircular canal
4 Fenestra vestibuli
5 Fenestra cochleae
6 Tympanic cavity
7 Mastoid process
8 Petrotympanic fissure (Chorda tympani = red probe)
9 Lateral pterygoid plate
10 Mastoid air cells
11 Facial canal
12 Foramen ovale
13 Carotid canal
14 Tympanic ring
15 Petromastoid part of temporal bone
16 Squamous part of temporal bone
17 Squamomastoid suture
18 Zygomatic process
19 Incisure of tympanic ring
20 Promontory
21 Apex of cochlea (cupula)
22 Spiral canal of cochlea at base of cochlea
23 Epitympanic recess
24 Auditory ossicles, tympanic cavity
25 Hypotympanic recess

Right temporal bone (lateral aspect). Petrosquamous portion has been partly removed to display the semicircular canals.

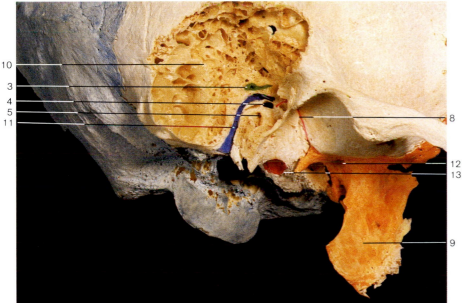

Right temporal bone (lateral aspect). Mastoid process has been opened to show the mastoid air cells and their connection with the tympanic cavity.

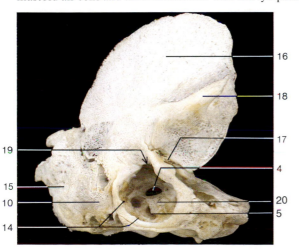

Right temporal bone of the newborn (lateral aspect).

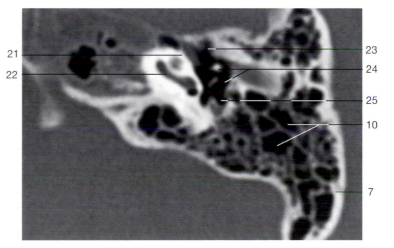

Frontal section through petrous part. MR-Scan.

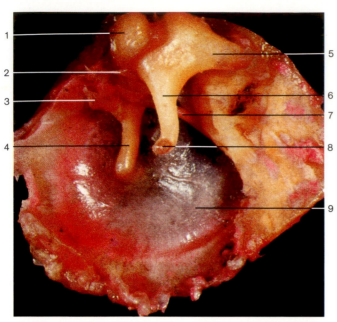

1 Head of malleus
2 Anterior ligament of malleus
3 Tendon of tensor tympani
4 Handle of malleus
5 Short crus of incus
6 Long crus of incus
7 Chorda tympani
8 Lenticular process
9 Tympanic membrane

Tympanic membrane with malleus and incus (internal aspect).

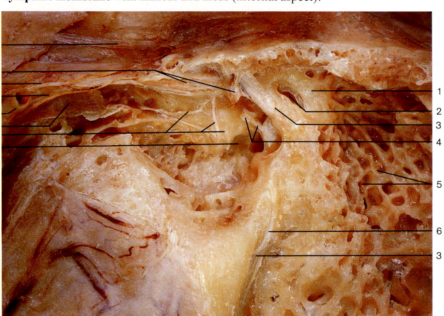

1 Tympanic antrum
2 Lateral semicircular canal
3 Facial canal
4 Stapes with tendon of stapedius
5 Mastoid air cells
6 Chorda tympani (intracranial part)
7 Greater petrosal nerve
8 Tensor tympani, processus cochleariformis
9 Lesser petrosal nerve
10 Anterior tympanic artery
11 Middle meningeal artery
12 Auditory tube
13 Promontory with tympanic plexus
14 Fenestra cochleae

Tympanic cavity, medial wall. External auditory meatus and lateral wall of tympanic cavity together with incus. Malleus and tympanic membrane have been removed; mastoid air cells are opened.

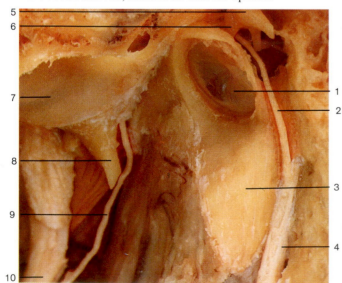

1 Tympanic membrane
2 Chorda tympani (intracranial part)
3 Floor of the external acoustic meatus
4 Facial nerve, facial canal
5 Incus
6 Head of malleus
7 Mandibular fossa
8 Spine of sphenoid
9 Chorda tympani (extracranial part)
10 Styloid process

Tympanic membrane (lateral aspect). External acoustic meatus and facial canal have been opened to expose the chorda tympani (magn. ~1.5×).

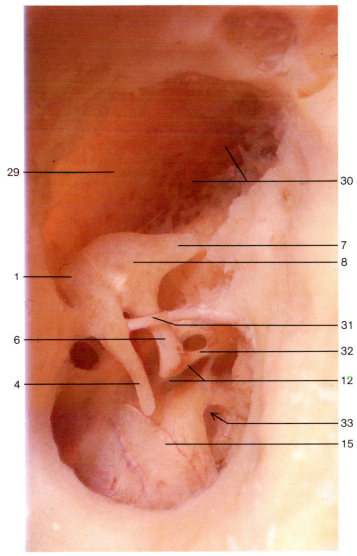

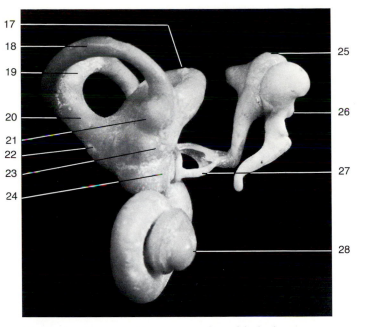

Chain of auditory ossicles in connection with the inner ear (anterior-lateral aspect, left side).

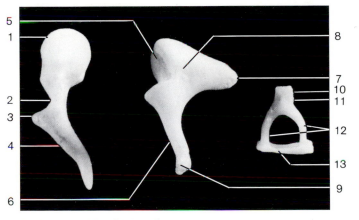

Tympanic cavity with malleus, incus and stapes (lateral aspect, left side). Tympanic membrane removed, mastoid antrum opened.

Auditory ossicles (isolated).

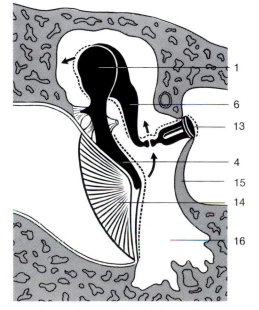

Position and movements of the auditory ossicles. (Schematic diagram.)

Malleus
1 Head
2 Neck
3 Lateral process
4 Handle

Incus
5 Articular facet for malleus
6 Long crus
7 Short crus
8 Body
9 Lenticular process

Stapes
10 Head
11 Neck
12 Anterior and posterior crura
13 Base

Walls of tympanic cavity
14 Tympanic membrane
15 Promontory
16 Hypotympanic recess of tympanic cavity

Internal ear (labyrinth)
17 Lateral semicircular duct
18 Anterior semicircular duct
19 Posterior semicircular duct
20 Common crus
21 Ampulla
22 Beginning of endolymphatic duct
23 Utricular prominence
24 Saccular prominence
25 Incus
26 Malleus
27 Stapes
28 Cochlea

Tympanic cavity
29 Epitympanic recess
30 Mastoid antrum
31 Chorda tympani
32 Tendon of stapedius muscle
33 Round window (fenestra cochleae)

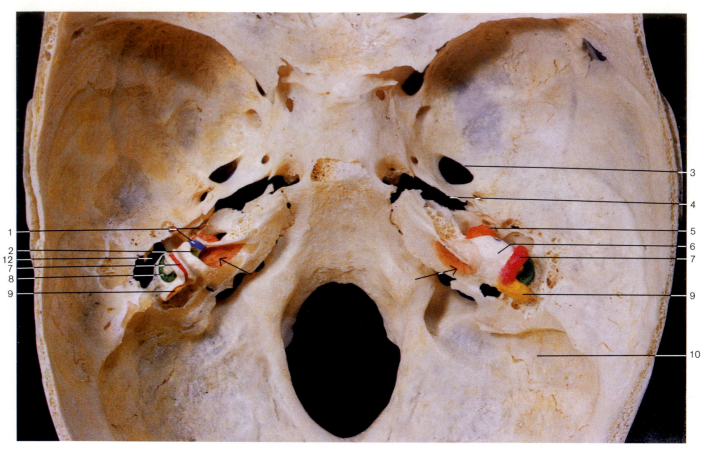

Bony labyrinth, petrous part of the temporal bone (from above). At left: semicircular canals opened, at right closed. Arrows: internal acoustic meatus.

1 Facial canal and semicanal of auditory tube	9 Posterior semicircular canal	17 Fenestra vestibuli
2 Superior vestibular area	10 Groove for sigmoid sinus	18 Promontory
3 Foramen ovale	11 Sigmoid sinus	19 Zygomatic process
4 Foramen lacerum	12 Tympanic cavity	20 Fenestra cochleae
5 Cochlea	13 Auditory tube	21 Mastoid process
6 Vestibule	14 Mastoid air cells	
7 Anterior semicircular canal	15 Facial and vestibulocochlear nerves	
8 Lateral semicircular canal	16 Temporal fossa	

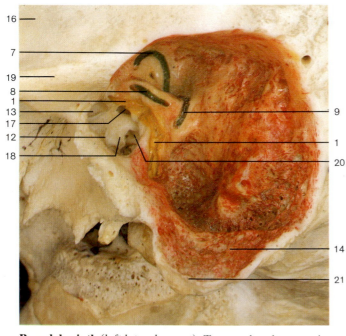

Bony labyrinth (left lateral aspect). Temporal and tympanic bone partly removed, semicircular canals opened.

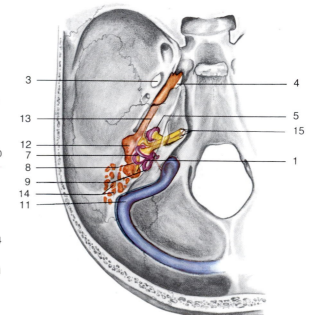

Internal ear. Diagram showing the position of the membranous labyrinth and the tympanic cavity.

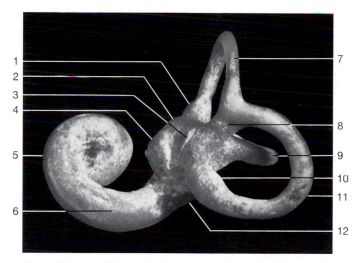

1 Ampulla (anterior semicircular canal)	16 External acoustic meatus
2 Elliptical recess	17 Mastoid air cells
3 Aqueduct of the vestibule	18 Tympanic cavity, fenestra cochleae (probe)
4 Spherical recess	19 External acoustic meatus
5 Cochlea	20 Facial canal
6 Base of cochlea	21 Base of cochlea, canalis musculotubarius
7 Anterior semicircular canal	22 Malleus and incus
8 Crus commune or common limb	23 Stapes
9 Lateral semicircular canal	24 Tympanic membrane
10 Posterior bony ampulla	25 Tympanic cavity
11 Posterior semicircular canal (posterior canal)	26 Aqueduct of cochlea
12 Fenestra cochleae	27 Saccus endolymphaticus
13 Bony ampulla	28 Ductus endolymphaticus
14 Fenestra vestibuli	29 Macula of utricle
15 Cupula of cochlea	30 Macula of saccule

Cast of the right labyrinth (postero-medial aspect).

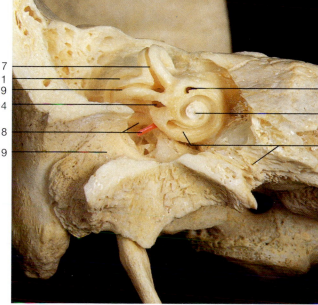

Cast of the right labyrinth (lateral aspect).

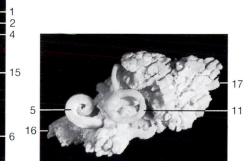

Cast of the labyrinth and mastoid cells.
Life size (posterior aspect).

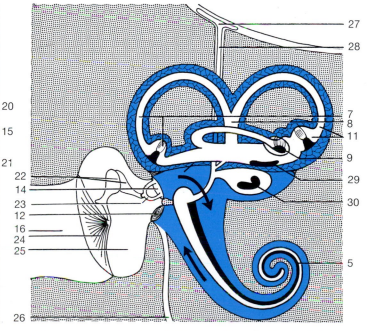

Dissection of bony labyrinth in situ. Semicircular canals and cochlear duct opened.

Schematic diagram of the **auditory and vestibular apparatus.**
Arrows: direction of sound waves; blue = perilymphatic ducts.

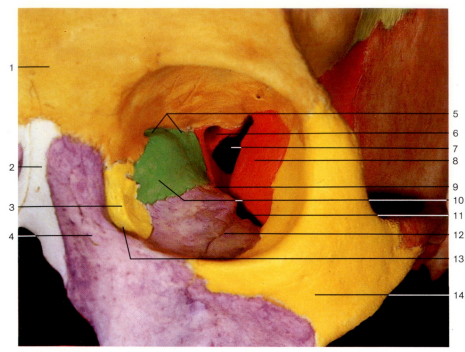

1 Frontal bone
2 Nasal bone
3 Lacrimal bone
4 Maxilla, frontal process
5 Ethmoidal foramina
6 Lesser wing of sphenoid bone and optic canal
7 Superior orbital fissure
8 Greater wing of sphenoid bone
9 Orbital process of palatine bone
10 Orbital plate of ethmoid bone
11 Inferior orbital fissure
12 Infraorbital sulcus
13 Nasolacrimal canal
14 Zygomatic bone
15 Frontal sinus
16 Superior rectus
17 Orbital fatty tissue
18 Optic nerve
19 Tenon's space
20 Inferior rectus
21 Periorbita and maxilla
22 Maxillary sinus
23 Levator palpebrae superioris
24 Superior conjunctival fornix
25 Superior tarsal plate
26 Inferior tarsal plate
27 Inferior conjunctival fornix
28 Inferior oblique
29 Lateral rectus
30 Medial rectus
31 Superior oblique
32 Nasal septum
33 Middle nasal concha
34 Inferior nasal concha
35 Sclera
36 Ophthalmic artery
37 Cornea
38 Lens

Bones of the left orbit (indicated by different colors).

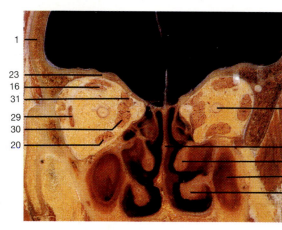

Frontal section through the posterior part of the orbit.

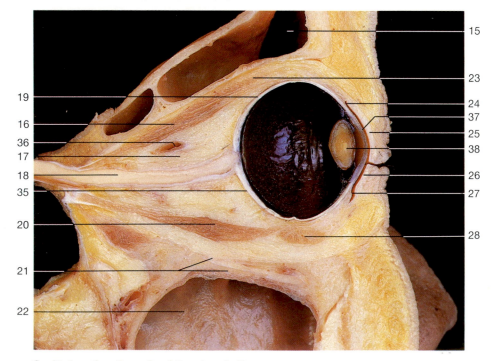

Sagittal section through orbit and eyeball.

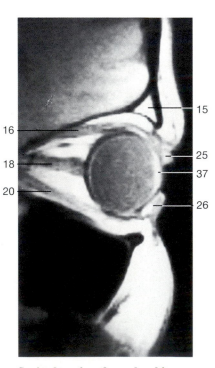

Sagittal section through orbit and eyeball. MR-Scan.

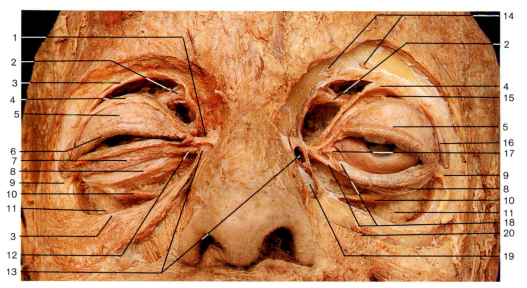

Eyelids and lacrimal apparatus. On the left side the lacrimal sac has been opened. Orbital septum removed.

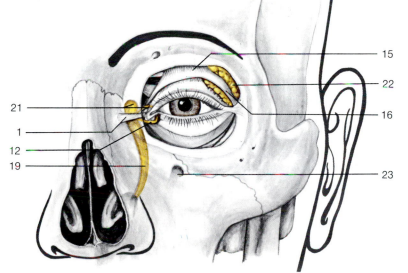

Lacrimal apparatus of left eye (anterior aspect).

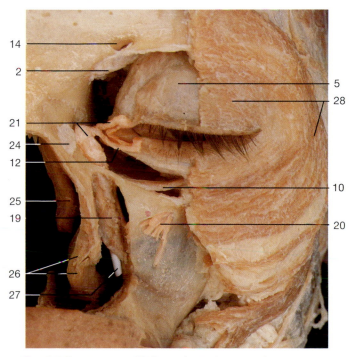

Lacrimal apparatus of left eye (anterior aspect).

1 **Medial palpebral ligament**
2 Tendon of superior oblique
3 Orbital septum (severed)
4 Aponeurosis of levator palpebrae superioris
5 Superior tarsal plate
6 Margin of lid
7 Inferior tarsal plate
8 Inferior tarsal muscle
9 Lateral palpebral ligament
10 Inferior oblique
11 Orbital fat
12 **Inferior lacrimal canaliculus**
13 Lacrimal sac, left side fenestrated
14 Supraorbital foramen
15 Levator palpebrae superioris
16 Lateral fixation of aponeurosis of levator palpebrae
17 Semilunar fold of conjunctiva
18 Lacrimal punctum and inferior lacrimal canaliculus
19 **Nasolacrimal duct**
20 Infraorbital nerve
21 **Lacrimal sac, superior lacrimal canaliculus**
22 Lacrimal gland
23 Infraorbital foramen
24 Medial palpebral ligament (divided)
25 Middle nasal concha
26 **Inferior nasal concha**
27 Opening of nasolacrimal duct (probe)
28 Orbicularis oculi

The Eyeball

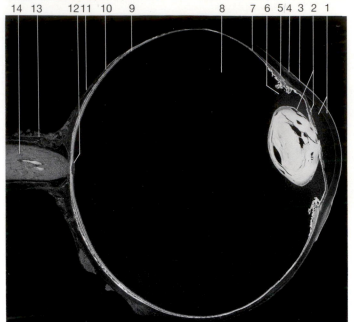

Horizontal section through the human eye (2×).

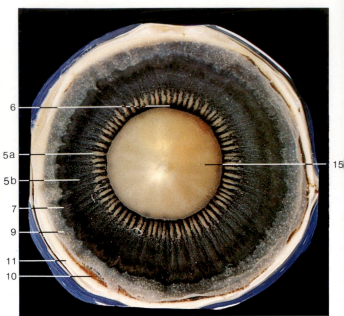

Anterior segment of the eyeball (posterior aspect) (the opacity of the lens is an artifact).

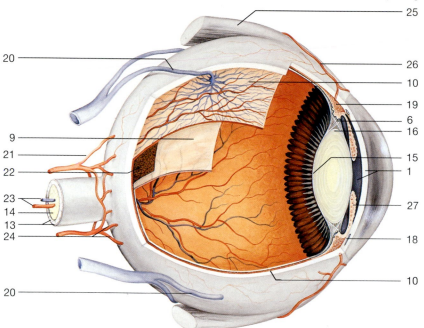

Organization of the eyeball. Demonstration of vascular tunic of bulb. (Schematic drawing.)

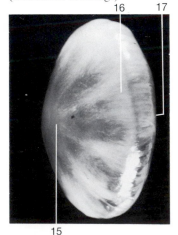

Equatorial aspect of the lens, anterior pole to the right.

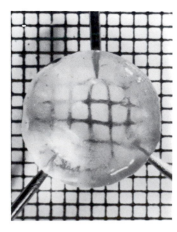

Frontal aspect of the lens. (Note the magnification effect.)

1   Cornea and anterior chamber
2   Iris, lens
3   Transitional zone between corneal and conjunctival epithelium
4   Conjunctiva of the eyeball
5   Ciliary body
    a Ciliary processes (pars plicata)
    b Ciliary ring (pars plana)
6   Zonular fibers
7   Ora serrata
8   Vitreous body
9   Retina
10 Choroid
11 Sclera
12 Optic disc
13 Dura mater and subarachnoid space
14 Optic nerve
15 Lens (posterior pole)
16 Equator of lens
17 Lens (anterior pole)
18 Canal of Schlemm
19 Ciliary muscle
20 Vena vorticosa
21 Long posterior ciliary artery
22 Retinal pigmented epithelium
23 Central retinal artery and vein
24 Short posterior ciliary arteries
25 External ocular muscle
26 Anterior ciliary artery
27 Iris

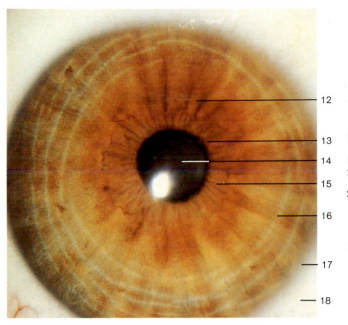

Anterior segment of the eye. (Courtesy of Dr. G. O. H. NAUMANN, Eye Dept., University of Erlangen.)

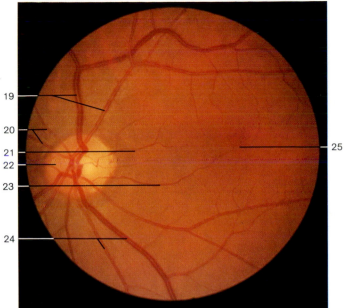

Fundus of a normal left eye. (Courtesy of Dr. G. O. H. NAUMANN, Eye Dept., University of Erlangen.)

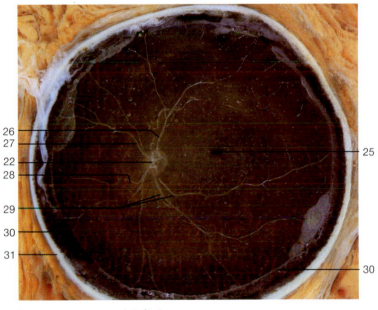

Posterior segment of the left eye.

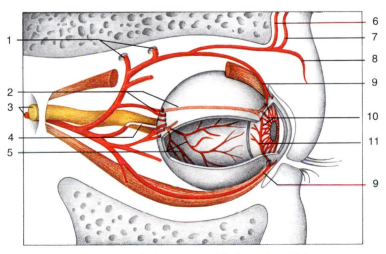

Diagram of the ophthalmic artery and its branches (O.).

1 Posterior and anterior ethmoidal arteries
2 Long and short posterior ciliary arteries
3 Optic nerve and ophthalmic artery
4 Central retinal artery
5 Retinal arteries
6 Supratrochlear artery
7 Supraorbital artery
8 Dorsal nasal artery
9 Anterior ciliary artery
10 Iridial arteries
11 Circulus arteriosus major of iris
12 Iridial fold
13 Pupillary margin of iris
14 Anterior pole of lens
15 Lesser circle of iris
16 Greater circle of iris
17 Margin of cornea or limbus
18 Sclera
19 Superior temporal artery and vein of retina
20 Superior nasal artery and vein of retina
21 Superior macular artery
22 **Optic disc**
23 Inferior macular artery
24 Inferior temporal artery and vein
25 Fovea centralis, macula lutea
26 Superior temporal artery ⎫
27 Superior nasal artery   ⎬ of retina
28 Inferior nasal artery   ⎪
29 Inferior temporal artery ⎭
30 Retina
31 Sclera

The Extraocular Muscles

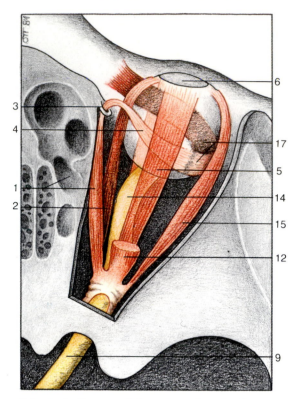

Schematic diagram of the extraocular muscles.
Right orbit (from above) (O.).
Levator palpebrae superior has been severed.

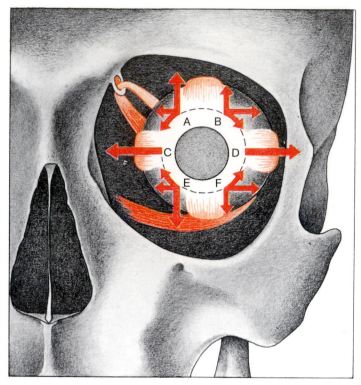

The action of the extraocular muscles.
Left orbit (anterior aspect).

A Superior rectus	C Medial rectus	E Inferior rectus
B Inferior oblique	D Lateral rectus	F Superior oblique

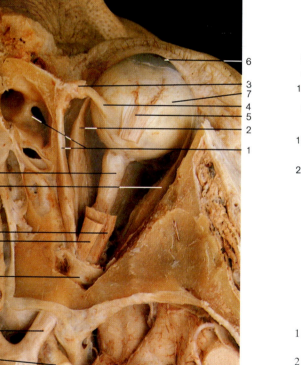

Right orbit with eyeball and extraocular muscles
(from above). The roof of the orbit has been
removed, the superior rectus and the levator
palpebrae superior have been severed.

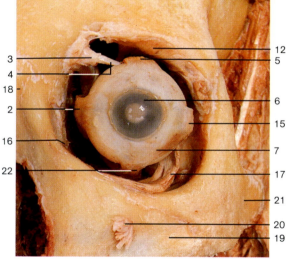

Left orbit with eyeball and extraocular muscles
(anterior aspect). Lids, conjunctiva and lacrimal
apparatus have been removed.

1 Superior oblique muscle and ethmoid air cells	12 Levator palpebrae superioris
2 Medial rectus	13 Superior rectus
3 Trochlea	14 Optic nerve (extracranial part)
4 Tendon of superior oblique	15 Lateral rectus
5 Superior rectus	16 Nasolacrimal duct
6 Cornea	17 Inferior oblique
7 Eyeball	18 Nasal bone
8 Optic chiasma	19 Maxilla
9 Optic nerve (intracranial part)	20 Infraorbital foramen and nerves
10 Internal carotid artery	21 Zygomatic bone
11 Common annular tendon	22 Inferior rectus

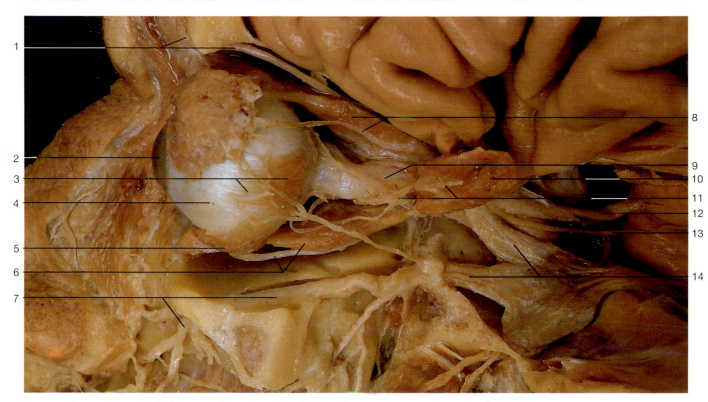

Extraocular muscles and their nerves (lateral aspect of left eye). Lateral rectus divided and reflected.

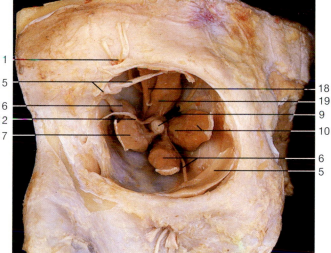

Left orbit with extraocular muscles (anterior aspect). Eyeball removed.

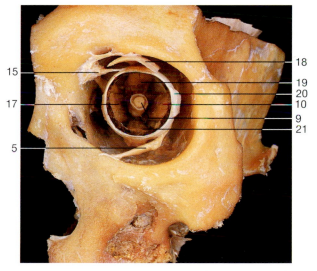

Left orbit with extraocular muscles (anterior aspect). Eyeball removed with the exception of a small ring of sclera.

1   Supraorbital nerve
2   Cornea
3   Insertion of lateral rectus
4   Eyeball
5   **Inferior oblique**
6   Inferior rectus, inferior branch of oculomotor nerve
7   Infraorbital nerve
8   Superior rectus, lacrimal nerve
9   Optic nerve
10 **Lateral rectus**
11 Ciliary ganglion, abducens nerve (n. VI)
12 Oculomotor nerve (n. III)

13 Trochlear nerve (n. IV)
14 Ophthalmic nerve (n. V$_1$), maxillary nerve (n. V$_2$)
15 Trochlea, tendon of superior oblique
16 **Superior oblique**
17 **Medial rectus**
18 Levator palpebrae superioris
19 **Superior rectus**
20 Ring of sclera (cornea and posterior portion of the eyeball removed)
21 **Inferior rectus**

The Visual Pathway

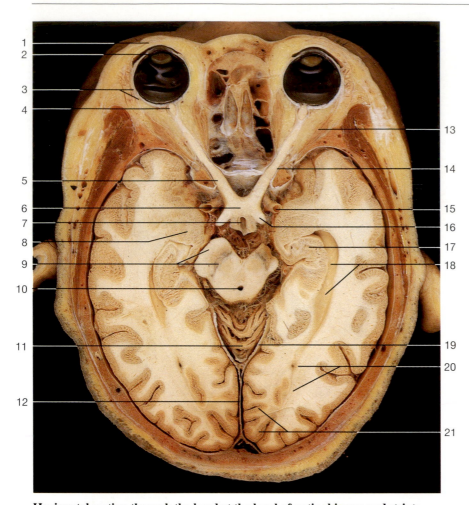

1	Upper lid
2	Cornea
3	**Eyeball** (sclera, retina)
4	Head of optic nerve
5	Optic nerve
6	**Optic chiasma**
7	Infundibular recess of hypothalamus
8	Amygdaloid body
9	Substantia nigra, crus cerebri
10	Cerebral aqueduct
11	Vermis of cerebellum
12	Falx cerebri
13	Lateral rectus
14	Optic canal
15	Internal carotid artery
16	**Optic tract**
17	Hippocampus
18	Inferior horn of lateral ventricle
19	Tentorium cerebelli
20	Optic radiation
21	**Striate cortex** (visual cortex)

Horizontal section through the head at the level of optic chiasma and striate cortex (superior aspect). Note the relationship of hypothalamic infundibulum to optic chiasma.

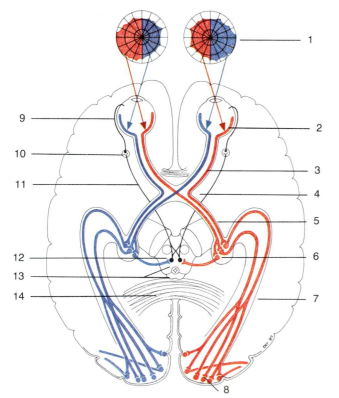

◁

1	Visual fields
2	Retina
3	Optic nerve
4	Optic chiasma
5	Optic tract
6	Lateral geniculate body
7	Optic radiation
8	Visual cortex
9	Ciliary nerves (long and short)
10	Ciliary ganglion
11	Oculomotor nerve
12	Accessory oculomotor nucleus
13	Colliculi of midbrain
14	Corpus callosum

Diagram of the visual pathway and path of the light reflex (O.).

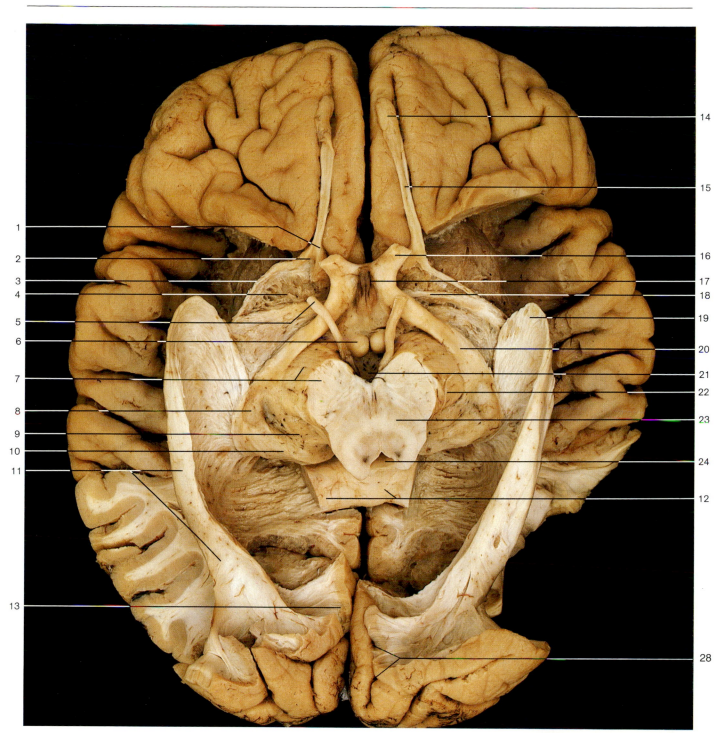

Dissection of the visual pathway (inferior aspect). Frontal pole at top, midbrain divided.

1 Medial olfactory stria
2 Olfactory trigone
3 Lateral olfactory stria
4 Anterior perforated substance
5 Oculomotor nerve
6 Mamillary body
7 Cerebral peduncle
8 Lateral geniculate body
9 Medial geniculate body
10 Pulvinar of the thalamus
11 Optic radiation
12 Splenium of the corpus callosum, commissural fibers
13 Cuneus
14 Olfactory bulb

15 Olfactory tract
16 Optic nerve
17 Infundibulum
18 Anterior commissure
19 Genu of optic radiation
20 Optic tract
21 Interpeduncular fossa and posterior perforated substance
22 Trochlear nerve
23 Substantia nigra
24 Cerebral aqueduct
25 Visual cortex
26 Line of Gennari
27 Gyrus of striate cortex
28 Calcarine sulcus

Frontal section of the striate cortex at the level of the striate area in the occipital lobe.

129

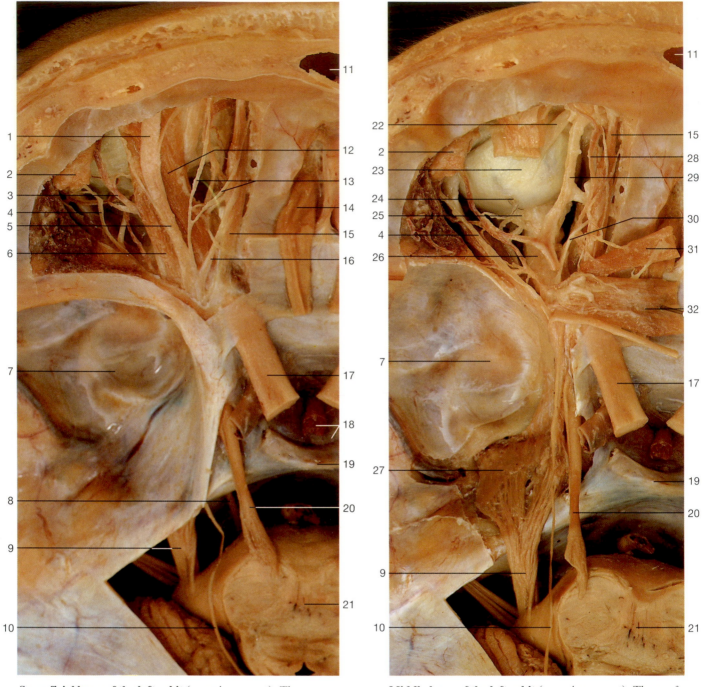

Superficial layer of the left orbit (superior aspect). The roof of the orbit has been removed, the left tentorium fenestrated.

Middle layer of the left orbit (superior aspect). The roof of the orbit has been removed and the superior extraocular muscles have been divided and reflected.

1	Lateral branch of frontal nerve
2	Lacrimal gland
3	Lacrimal vein
4	Lacrimal nerve
5	**Frontal nerve**
6	Superior rectus
7	Middle cranial fossa
8	**Abducens nerve** (n. VI)
9	Trigeminal nerve (n. V)
10	**Trochlear nerve** (intracranial part) (n. IV)
11	Frontal sinus
12	Levator palpebrae superioris
13	Branches of supratrochlear nerve
14	Olfactory bulb
15	Superior oblique
16	**Trochlear nerve** (intraorbital part) (n. IV)
17	**Optic nerve** (intracranial part)
18	Pituitary gland, infundibulum
19	Dorsum sellae
20	**Oculomotor nerve** (n. III)
21	Midbrain
22	Tendon of superior oblique
23	Eyeball
24	Vena vorticosa
25	Short ciliary nerves
26	Optic nerve (extracranial part)
27	**Trigeminal ganglion**

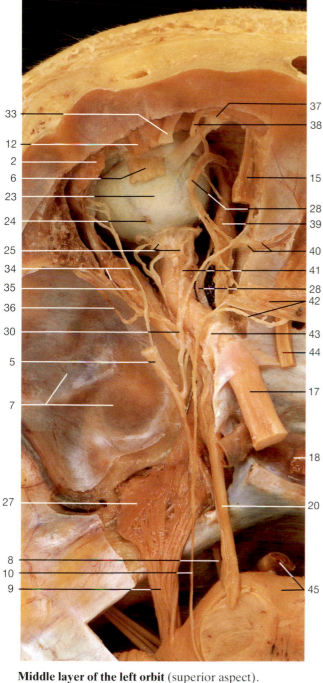

Middle layer of the left orbit (superior aspect). The roof of the orbit and the superior extraocular muscles have been removed.

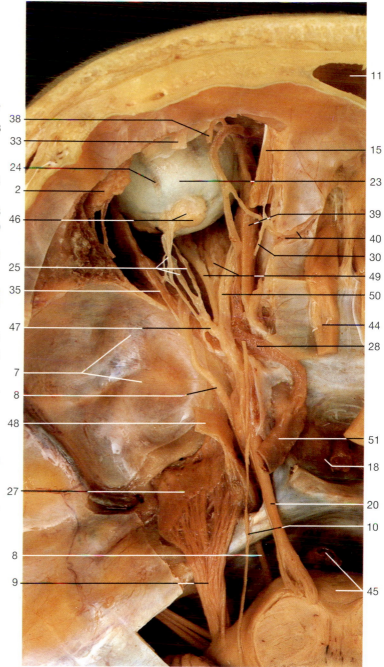

Deeper layer of the left orbit (superior aspect). The optic nerve has now been removed.

28	**Ophthalmic artery**	
29	Superior ophthalmic vein	
30	**Nasociliary nerve**	
31	Levator palpebrae superioris (reflected)	
32	Superior rectus (reflected)	
33	Lateral branch of supraorbital nerve	
34	Lacrimal nerve and artery	
35	Lateral rectus	
36	Meningolacrimal artery (anastomosing with middle meningeal artery)	

37	Trochlea
38	Medial branch of supraorbital nerve
39	Medial rectus
40	Anterior ethmoidal artery and nerve
41	Long ciliary nerve
42	Superior oblique, trochlear nerve
43	Common tendinous ring
44	Olfactory tract
45	Basilar artery, pons
46	Optic nerve, external sheath of optic nerve (divided)

47	**Ciliary ganglion**
48	Ophthalmic nerve (divided, reflected)
49	Inferior branch of oculomotor nerve, inferior rectus
50	Superior branch of oculomotor nerve
51	Internal carotid artery

131

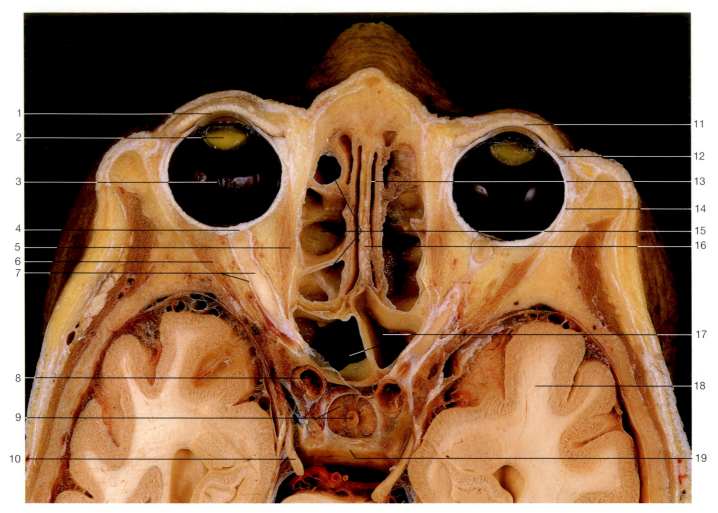

Horizontal section through the nasal cavity, the orbits and temporal lobes of the brain at the level of pituitary gland.

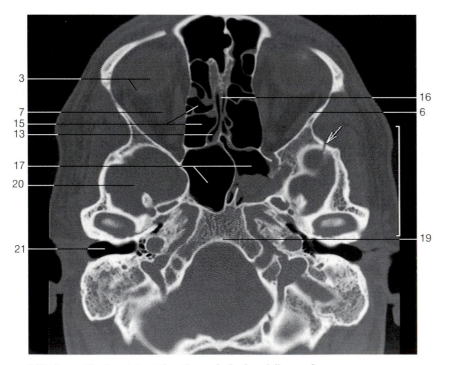

1 Cornea
2 Lens
3 Vitreous body, eyeball
4 Head of optic nerve
5 Medial rectus
6 Lateral rectus
7 Optic nerve with dural sheath
8 Internal carotid artery
9 Pituitary gland, infundibulum
10 Oculomotor nerve
11 Superior tarsal plate of eye lid
12 Fornix of conjunctiva
13 Nasal cavity
14 Sclera
15 Ethmoidal sinus
16 Nasal septum
17 Sphenoidal sinus
18 Temporal lobe
19 Clivus
20 Middle cranial fossa
21 External acoustic meatus

MR-Scan. Horizontal section through the head (bar = 2 cm; arrow: fracture).

1 Crista galli
2 Pituitary gland, sella turcica
3 Sphenoidal air sinus (relatively large)
4 Tubal elevation
5 Pharyngeal opening of the auditory tube
6 Pharyngeal recess
7 Atlas (anterior arch)
8 Soft palate
9 Frontal sinus
10 Perpendicular plate of ethmoid
11 Cartilage of nasal septum
12 Vomer
13 Hard palate
14 Nasal branch of anterior ethmoidal artery and anterior ethmoidal nerve
15 Nasopharynx
16 Nasal septum
17 Olfactory nerves
18 Septal artery
19 Crest of nasal septum
20 Incisive canal
21 Anterior ethmoidal artery
22 Olfactory bulb
23 Olfactory tract
24 Internal carotid artery
25 Posterior nasal and septal arteries
26 Nasopalatine nerve
27 Choana (arrow)
28 Tongue

Nasal septum, covered by a mucous membrane.

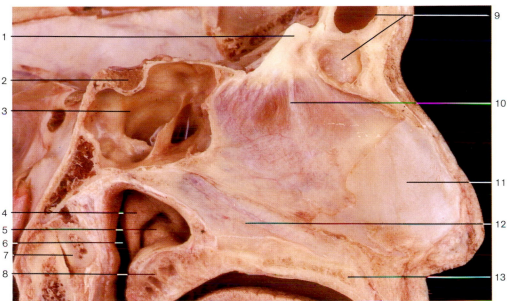

Nasal septum. Mucous membrane removed.

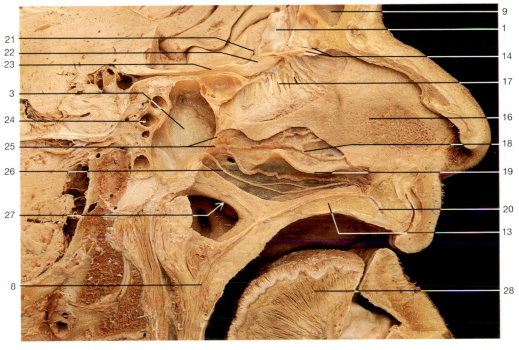

Nasal septum. Dissection of nerves and vessels.

133

The Nasal Cavity and Paranasal Sinuses

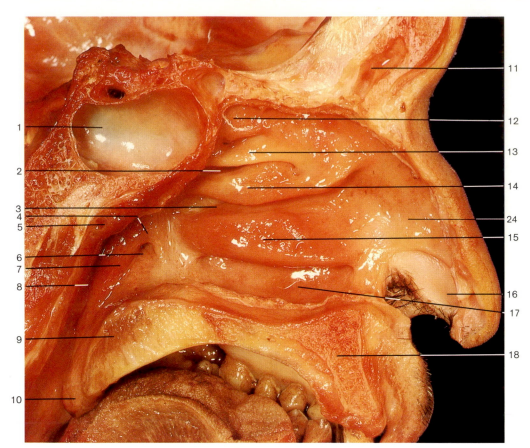

1   Sphenoidal sinus
2   Superior meatus
3   Middle meatus
4   Tubal elevation
5   Pharyngeal tonsil
6   Pharyngeal orifice
    of auditory tube
7   Salpingopharyngeal fold
8   Pharyngeal recess
9   Soft palate
10 Uvula
11 Frontal sinus
12 Sphenoethmoidal recess
13 Superior nasal concha
14 Middle nasal concha
15 Inferior nasal concha
16 Vestibule
17 Inferior meatus
18 Hard palate
19 Opening of sphenoidal sinus
20 Opening of maxillary sinus
21 Palatine tonsil
22 Openings of ethmoidal
    air cells
23 Opening of frontal sinus
24 Atrium
25 Opening of nasolacrimal
    duct
26 Ethmoidal air cells
27 Maxillary sinus
28 Nasal septum

Lateral wall of the nasal cavity (septum removed).

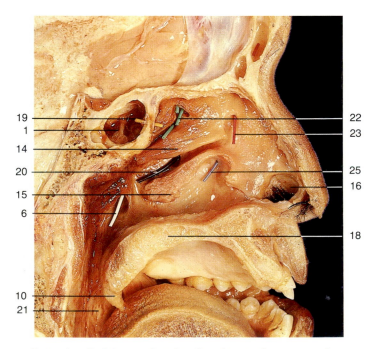

Lateral wall of the nasal cavity. Openings to the paranasal sinuses (indicated by probes). Inferior and middle nasal conchae partly removed.

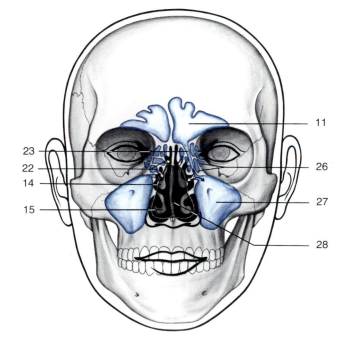

Schematic diagram showing the position of paranasal sinuses (K.-B.) (openings indicated by arrows).

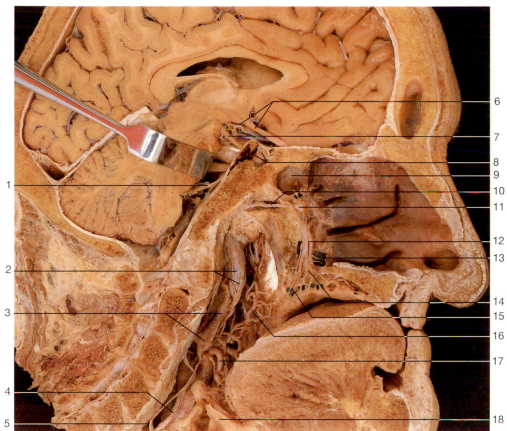

1 Facial nerve
2 Internal carotid artery, internal carotid plexus
3 **Superior cervical ganglion**
4 Vagus nerve
5 Sympathetic trunk
6 Optic nerve, ophthalmic artery
7 Oculomotor nerve
8 Internal carotid artery, cavernous sinus
9 Sphenoidal sinus
10 Nerve of the pterygoid canal
11 **Pterygopalatine ganglion**
12 Descending palatine artery
13 Lateral inferior posterior nasal branches, lateral posterior nasal and septal arteries
14 Greater palatine nerves and artery
15 Lesser palatine nerves and arteries
16 Branches of ascending pharyngeal artery
17 Lingual artery
18 Epiglottis
19 Tentorium, trochlear nerve
20 Trigeminal nerve, motor root
21 Vagus, glossopharyngeal and accessory nerves
22 Lingual nerve with chorda tympani
23 Branch of greater palatine artery, hard palate
24 Inferior alveolar nerve
25 Hyoid bone, epiglottis

Nerves of the lateral wall of nasal cavity I. Sagittal section through the head. Mucous membranes partly removed, pterygoid canal opened.

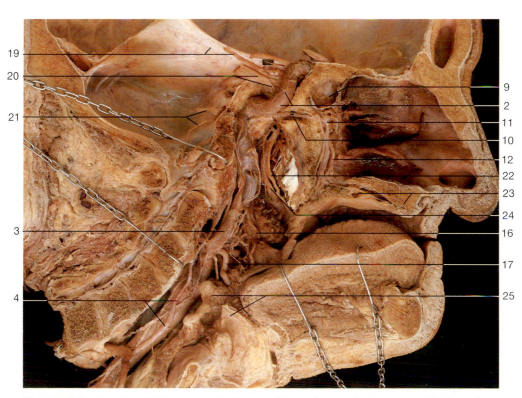

Nerves of the lateral wall of nasal cavity II. Carotid canal opened, mucous membranes of pharynx and nasal cavity partly removed.

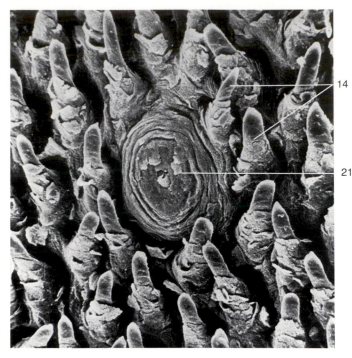

Surface of the tongue, showing filiform and fungiform papillae (scanning electron micrograph).

1 Hard palate
2 Superior longitudinal muscle of tongue
3 Median fibrous septum
4 Inferior longitudinal muscle of tongue
5 Sublingual gland
6 Mandible
7 Geniohyoid
8 Mylohyoid
9 Platysma
10 Vertical and transverse muscles
11 Buccinator
12 Genioglossus
13 Anterior belly of digastric muscle
14 Filiform papillae
15 Foramen cecum
16 Root of tongue, lingual tonsil
17 Palatine tonsil
18 Vallecula of epiglottis
19 Vestibule of larynx
20 Median sulcus of tongue
21 Fungiform papillae
22 Foliate papillae
23 Circumvallate papilla
24 Sulcus terminalis
25 Epiglottis
26 Greater cornu of hyoid bone

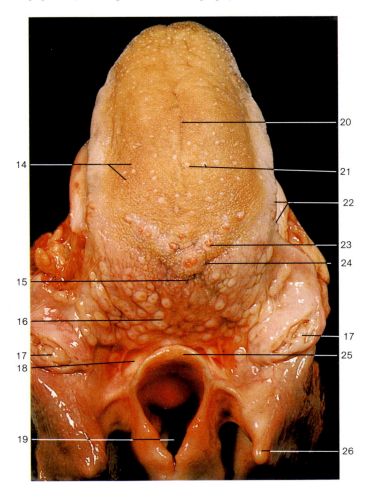

Dorsal surface of the tongue and laryngeal inlet.

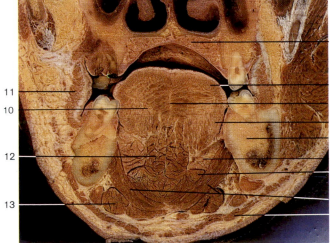

Coronal section through the oral cavity.

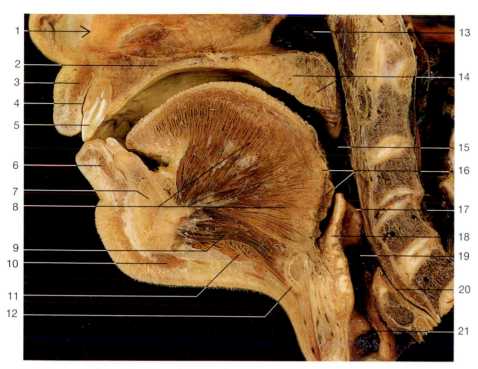

1	Nasal cavity
2	Hard palate
3	Upper lip
4	Vestibule of oral cavity
5	First incisor
6	Orbicularis oris
7	Mandible
8	Genioglossus
9	Geniohyoid muscle
10	Anterior belly of digastric muscle
11	Mylohyoid muscle
12	Hyoid bone
13	Nasopharynx
14	Soft palate and uvula
15	Oropharynx
16	Lingual tonsil
17	Laryngopharynx
18	Epiglottis
19	Aryepiglottic fold
20	Laryngopharynx continuous with esophagus
21	Larynx

Median sagittal section through the oral cavity and pharynx.

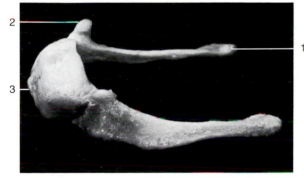 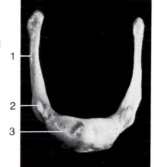

1	Greater cornu	⎫
2	Lesser cornu	⎬ of hyoid bone
3	Body	⎭

Hyoid bone (oblique lateral aspect).   **Hyoid bone** (anterior aspect).

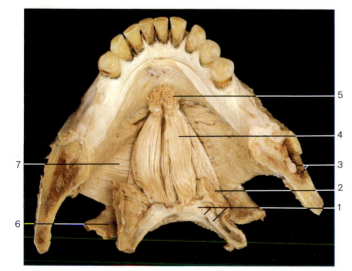

Muscles of the floor of the oral cavity (superior aspect).

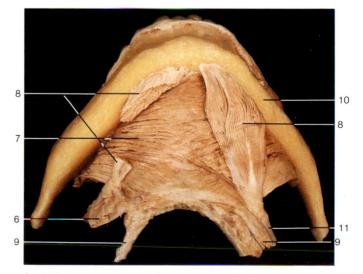

Oral diaphragm, muscles (inferior aspect). Cut on the base.

1 Lesser cornu and body of hyoid bone
2 Hyoglossus muscle (divided)
3 Ramus of mandible, inferior alveolar nerve
4 Geniohyoid muscle
5 Genioglossus muscle (divided)
6 Stylohyoid muscle (divided)

7 Mylohyoid muscle
8 Anterior belly of digastric muscle
9 Hyoid bone
10 Mandible
11 Intermediate tendon of digastric muscle

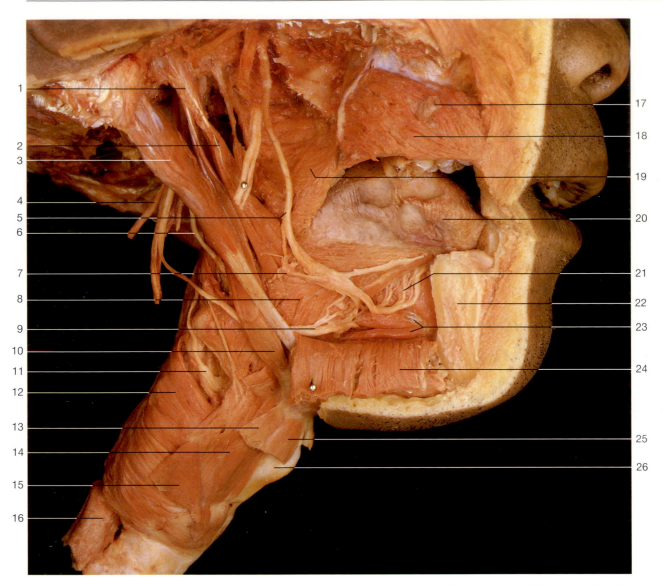

Parapharyngeal and sublingual regions. Innervation of the tongue. Lateral part of face and mandible removed, oral cavity opened.

1 Styloid process	14 Thyrohyoid muscle
2 Styloglossus muscle	15 Sternothyroid muscle
3 Digastric muscle (posterior belly)	16 Esophagus
4 Vagus nerve (n. X)	17 Parotid duct (divided)
5 **Lingual nerve** (n. V₃)	18 Buccinator
6 **Glossopharyngeal nerve** (n. IX)	19 Superior constrictor of pharynx
7 Submandibular ganglion	20 Tongue
8 Hyoglossus muscle	21 Terminal branches of lingual nerve
9 **Hypoglossal nerve** (n. XII)	22 Mandible (divided)
10 Stylohyoid muscle	23 Genioglossus, geniohyoideus
11 Superior laryngeal nerve (branch of vagus nerve, not visible)	24 Mylohyoid muscle (divided and reflected)
12 Middle constrictor of pharynx	25 Sternohyoid muscle (divided)
13 Omohyoid muscle (divided)	26 Thyroid cartilage

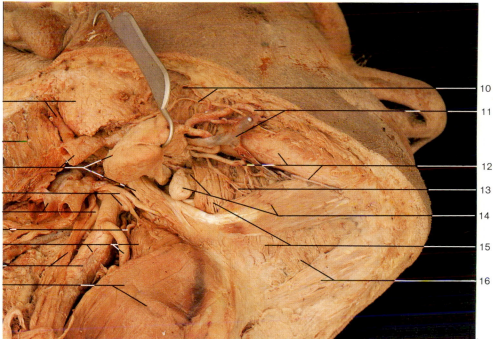

Submandibular triangle, superficial dissection. Right side (inferior aspect).
Submandibular gland has been reflected.

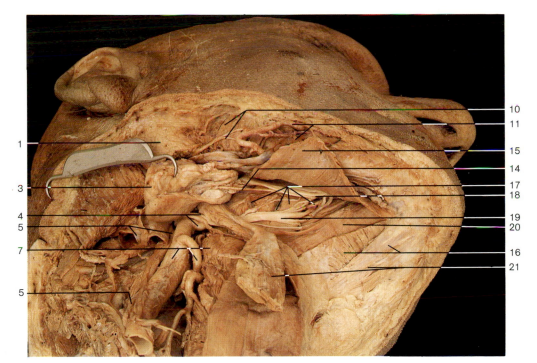

Submandibular triangle, deep dissection. Right side. Mylohyoid has been severed and
reflected to display the lingual and hypoglossal nerves.

1 Parotid gland and retromandibular vein
2 Sternocleidomastoid
3 Retromandibular vein, submandibular gland, stylohyoid muscle
4 Hypoglossal nerve, lingual artery
5 Vagus nerve, internal jugular vein
6 Superior laryngeal artery
7 External carotid artery, thyrohyoid muscle,
   superior thyroid artery
8 Common carotid artery, superior root of ansa cervicalis
9 Omohyoid, sternohyoid
10 Masseter, marginal mandibular branch of facial nerve

11 Facial artery and vein
12 Mandible, submental artery and vein
13 Mylohyoid nerve
14 Submandibular duct, sublingual gland, anterior belly
   of digastric muscle
15 Mylohyoid (right side)
16 Mylohyoid (left side) and right digastric muscle
17 Hyoglossus muscle, lingual artery
18 Lingual nerve
19 Hypoglossal nerve
20 Geniohyoid muscle
21 Anterior belly of digastric muscle (reflected)

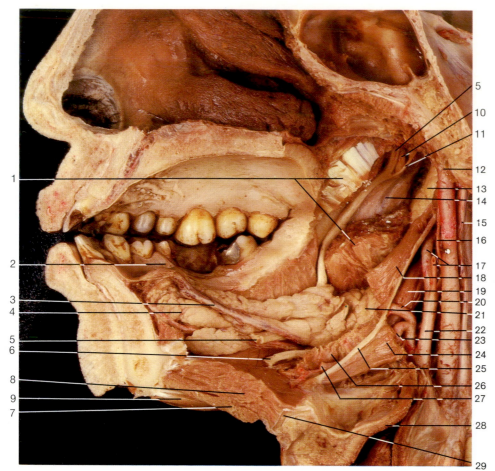

Oral cavity (internal aspect). Tongue and pharyngeal wall removed.

1 Medial pterygoid muscle
2 Sublingual papilla
3 Submandibular duct
4 Sublingual gland
5 Lingual nerve
6 Hypoglossal nerve
7 Mylohyoid
8 Geniohyoid
9 Anterior belly of digastric muscle
10 Inferior alveolar nerve
11 Chorda tympani
12 Internal carotid artery
13 Parotid gland
14 Sphenomandibular ligament
15 Vagus nerve
16 Glossopharyngeal nerve
17 Superficial temporal artery, ascending pharyngeal artery
18 Styloglossus
19 Posterior belly of digastric muscle
20 Facial artery
21 Submandibular gland
22 External carotid artery
23 Lingual artery
24 Middle pharyngeal constrictor muscle
25 Stylohyoid ligament
26 Hyoglossus
27 Deep lingual artery
28 Epiglottis
29 Hyoid bone
30 Hiatus semilunaris
31 Opening of nasolacrimal duct
32 Opening of auditory tube
33 Levator veli palatini
34 Tensor veli palatini
35 Submandibular ganglion

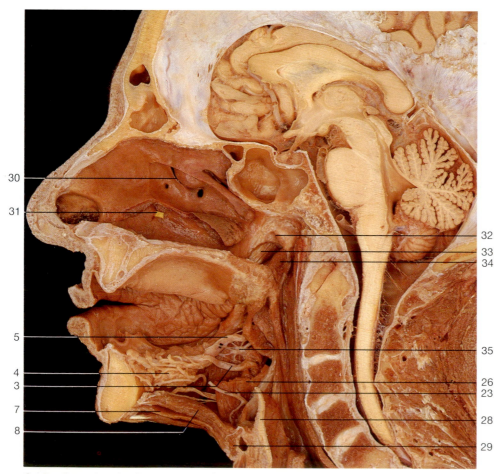

Oral and nasal cavity (internal aspect). Tongue removed.

Chapter III
Neck

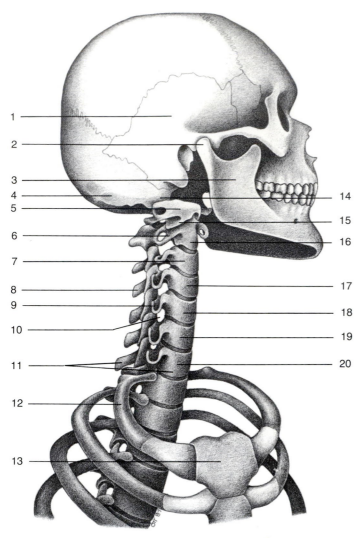

1 Temporal bone
2 Temporomandibular joint
3 Mandible
4 Occipital bone
5 Atlas
6 Axis
7 Third cervical vertebra
8 Spinous process of fourth cervical vertrebra
9 Transverse process of fifth cervical vertebra
   with groove for spinal nerve
10 Intervertebral foramen
11 Vertebra prominens (C₇)
12 First rib
13 Sternum (manubrium sterni)
14 Atlantooccipital joint
15 Lateral atlantoaxial joint
16 Body of axis
17 Body of fourth cervical vertebra
18 Body of fifth cervical vertebra
19 Body of sixth cervical vertebra
20 Body of seventh cervical vertebra

Cervical spine (oblique lateral aspect) (O.).

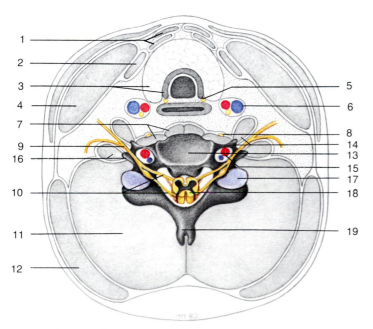

1 Infrahyoid muscles
2 Omohyoid muscle
3 Thyroid gland and trachea
4 Sternocleidomastoid muscle
5 Recurrent laryngeal nerve
6 Internal jugular vein, common carotid artery and vagus
7 Longus colli and longus capitis muscles
8 Prevertebral muscles and sympathetic trunk
9 Spinal nerve
10 Ventral and dorsal root of spinal nerve
11 True muscles of the neck
12 Trapezius
13 Body of cervical vertebra
14 Anterior tubercle of transverse process,
    origin of scalenus anterior
15 Vertebral artery, vertebrarterial foramen
16 Posterior tubercle of transverse process,
    origin of scalenus medius and posterior
17 Superior facet of articular process
18 Spinal cord
19 Spinous process

Cervical vertebra and the **organization of the neck.**
(Schematic drawing) (O.).

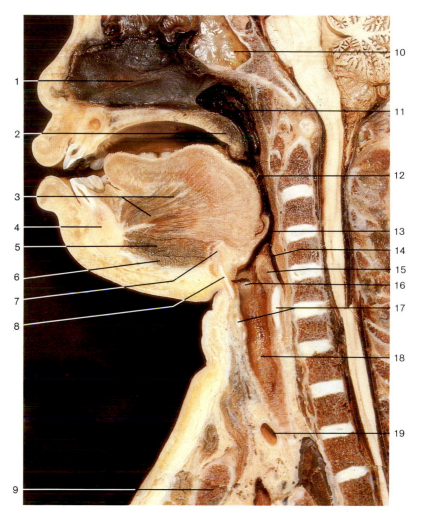

1 Nasal septum
2 Uvula
3 Genioglossus
4 Mandible
5 Geniohyoid
6 Mylohyoid
7 Hyoid bone
8 Thyroid cartilage
9 Manubrium sterni
10 Sphenoidal air cells
11 Nasopharynx
12 Oropharynx
13 Epiglottis
14 Laryngopharynx
15 Arytenoid muscle
16 Vocal fold
17 Cricoid cartilage
18 Trachea
19 Left brachiocephalic vein
20 Thymus
21 Esophagus
22 Occipital lobe
23 Cerebellum, 4th ventricle
24 Medulla oblongata
25 Dens of axis
26 Intervertebral discs
   of cervical vertebral column

Median section through adult head and neck. Note the low position of the adult larynx when compared with that of the neonate (cf. with figure below).

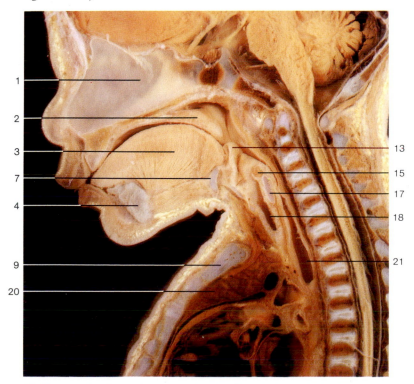

Median section through neonate head and neck. Note the high position of the larynx permitting the epiglottis nearly to reach the uvula (cf. with the figure above).

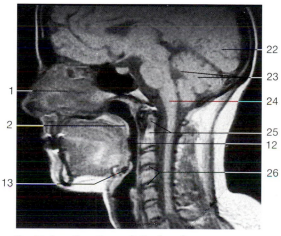

Sagittal section through the head. MR-Scan.

143

Muscles of the Neck

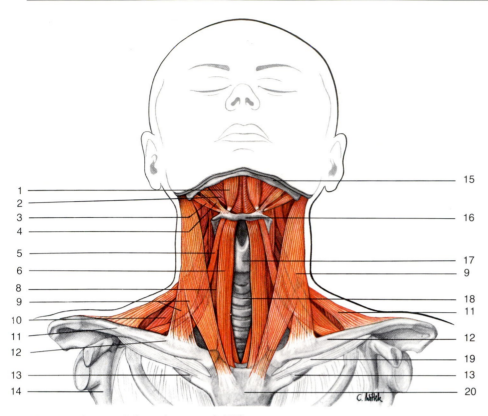

Muscles of the neck (anterior aspect) (W.).

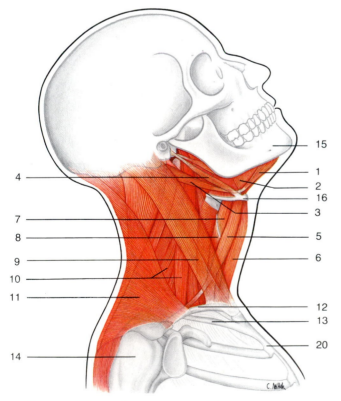

Muscles of the neck (lateral aspect) (W.).

1	Anterior belly of digastric	⎫
2	Mylohyoid	⎬ Suprahyoid muscles
3	Posterior belly of digastric	⎪
4	Stylohyoid	⎭
5	Omohyoid	⎫
6	Sternohyoid	⎬ Infrahyoid muscles
7	Thyrohyoid	⎪
8	Sternothyroid	⎭
9	Sternocleidomastoid	
10	Scalene muscles	
11	Trapezius	
12	Clavicle	
13	First rib	
14	Scapula	
15	Mandible	
16	Hyoid bone	
17	Larynx (thyroid cartilage)	
18	Trachea	
19	Subclavius	
20	Manubrium sterni	

144

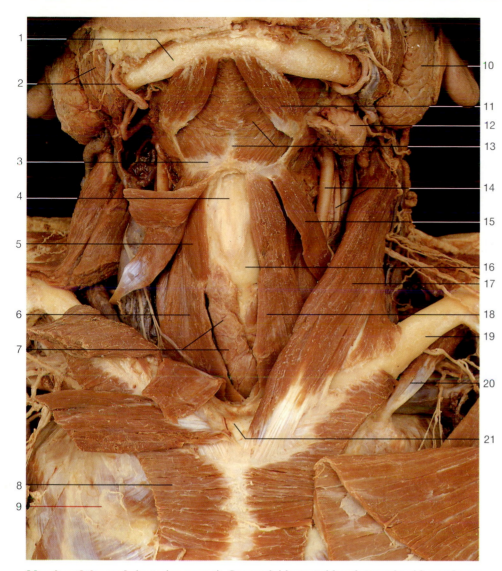

1	Mandible
2	Masseter, facial artery
3	Hyoid bone
4	Median thyrohyoid ligament
5	Thyrohyoid muscle
6	Sternothyroid muscle
7	Thyroid gland (pyramidal lobe)
8	Pectoralis major muscle
9	Second rib
10	Parotid gland
11	Anterior belly of digastric muscle
12	Submandibular gland (divided)
13	Mylohyoid muscle, mylohyoid raphe
14	External carotid artery, vagus nerve
15	Omohyoid muscle
16	Thyroid cartilage
17	Sternocleidomastoid muscle
18	Sternohyoid muscle
19	Clavicle
20	Subclavius
21	Jugular fossa or suprasternal notch

Muscles of the neck (anterior aspect). Sternocleidomastoid and sternohyoid muscle on the right have been divided and reflected.

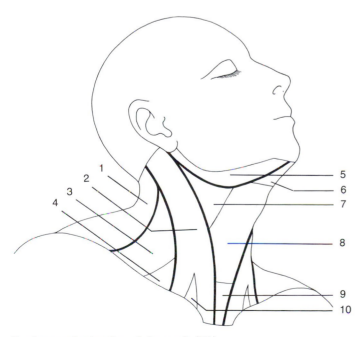

Regions and triangles of the neck (W.).

1	Trapezius
2	Sternocleidomastoid
3	Occipital triangle } Posterior triangle
4	Omoclavicular triangle
5	Submandibular triangle } Anterior triangle
6	Submental triangle
7	Carotid triangle
8	Muscular triangle
9	Jugular fossa
10	Lesser supraclavicular fossa

145

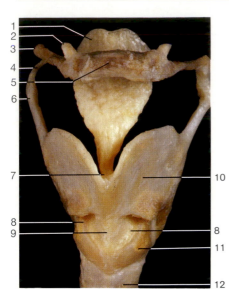

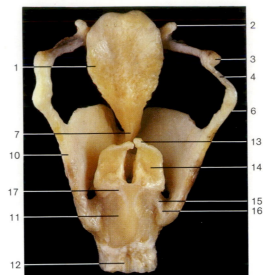

1 Epiglottis
2 Lesser cornu of hyoid bone
3 Greater cornu of hyoid bone
4 Lateral thyrohyoid ligament
5 Body of hyoid bone
6 Superior cornu of thyroid cartilage
7 Thyroepiglottic ligament
8 Conus elasticus
9 Cricothyroid ligament
10 Thyroid cartilage
11 Cricoid cartilage
12 Trachea
13 Corniculate cartilage
14 Arytenoid cartilage
15 Posterior cricoarytenoid ligament
16 Cricothyroid joint
17 Cricoarytenoid joint

Cartilages of the larynx and the hyoid bone (anterior aspect).

Cartilages of the larynx and the hyoid bone (posterior aspect).

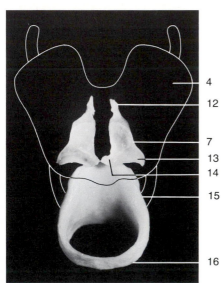

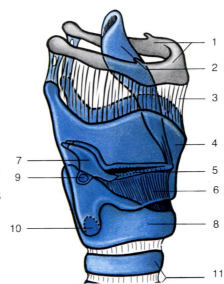

1 Hyoid bone
2 Epiglottis
3 Thyrohyoid membrane
4 Thyroid cartilage
5 Vocal ligament
6 Conus elasticus
7 Arytenoid cartilage
8 Cricoid cartilage
9 Cricoarytenoid joint
10 Cricothyroid joint
11 Tracheal cartilages
12 Corniculate cartilage
13 Muscular process of arytenoid cartilage
14 Vocal process of arytenoid cartilage
15 Lamina of cricoid cartilage
16 Arch of cricoid cartilage

Cartilages of the larynx (anterior aspect). Thyroid cartilage is indicated by the outline.

Cartilages and ligaments of the larynx (lateral aspect). (Schematic drawing) (W.).

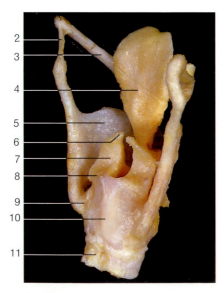

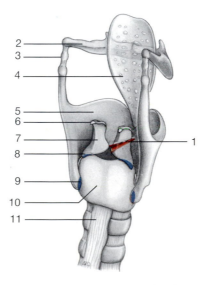

1 Vocal ligament
2 Lateral thyrohyoid ligament
3 Greater cornu of hyoid bone
4 Epiglottis
5 Thyroid cartilage
6 Corniculate cartilage
7 Arytenoid cartilage
8 Cricoarytenoid joint
9 Cricothyroid joint
10 Cricoid cartilage
11 Trachea

Cartilages of the larynx (oblique-posterior aspect).

Cartilages of the larynx (oblique-posterior aspect) (W.).

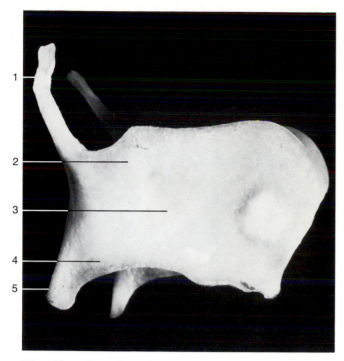

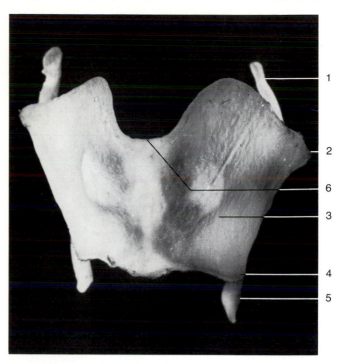

Thyroid cartilage (lateral aspect).

Thyroid cartilage (anterior aspect).

1 Superior cornu
2 Superior thyroid tubercle
3 Lamina of thyroid cartilage

4 Inferior thyroid tubercle
5 Inferior cornu
6 Superior thyroid notch

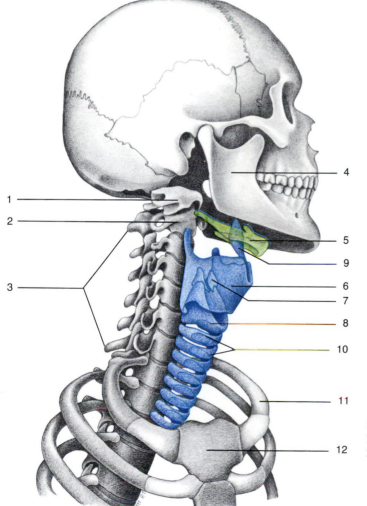

1 Atlas
2 Axis
3 Cervical vertebrac (C_2-C_7)
4 Mandible
5 Hyoid bone
6 Thyroid cartilage
7 Arytenoid cartilage
8 Cricoid cartilage
9 Epiglottis
10 Tracheal cartilages
11 First rib
12 Manubrium sterni

Position of the larynx in the neck (oblique lateral aspect).
(Schematic drawing) (O.).

147

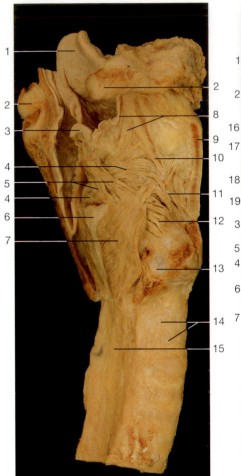

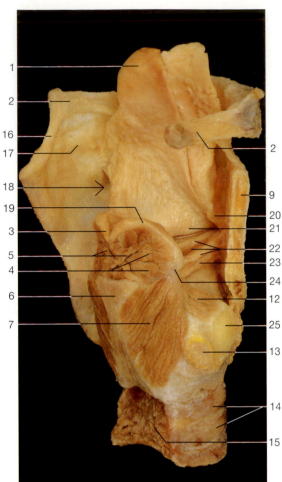

1 Epiglottis
2 Greater horn of hyoid bone
3 Corniculate cartilage
4 Transverse arytenoid muscle
5 Oblique arytenoid muscle
6 Lamina of cricoid cartilage
7 **Posterior cricoarytenoid muscle**
8 Aryepiglottic fold and muscle
9 Lamina of thyroid cartilage
10 Thyroepiglottic muscle
11 Thyroarytenoid muscle
12 **Lateral cricoarytenoid muscle**
13 Articular facet of thyroid cartilage
14 Cartilages of trachea
15 Membranous part of trachea
16 Lateral thyrohyoid ligament
17 Thyrohyoid membrane
18 Position of piriform recess
19 Arytenoid cartilage
20 Stem of epiglottis
21 Vestibular fold
22 Vocal folds, fissure of glottis
23 **Vocalis muscle**
24 Cricoarytenoid articulation
25 Arch of cricoid cartilage
26 Cricothyroid muscle
27 Cricoid cartilage
28 Piriform recess
29 Superior horn of thyroid cartilage
30 Vocal ligament

Laryngeal muscles I (lateral aspect). Thyroid cartilage and thyroarytenoid muscle partly removed.

Laryngeal muscles II (lateral aspect). Half of thyroid cartilage removed.

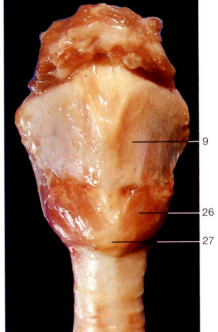

Laryngeal muscles, larynx (anterior aspect).

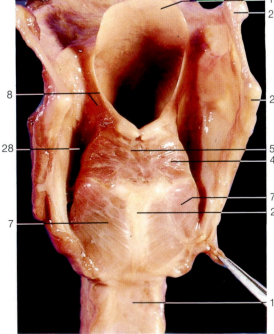

Laryngeal muscles, larynx (posterior aspect).

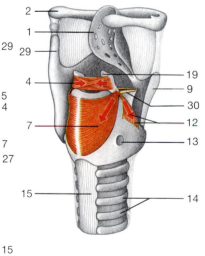

Action of internal muscles of the larynx. (Schematic drawing) (O.).

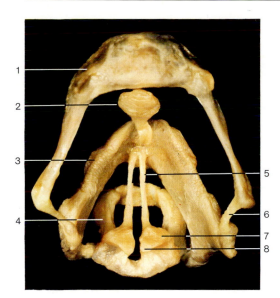

Laryngeal cartilages and ligaments (superior aspect).

△

1 Hyoid bone
2 Epiglottis
3 Thyroid cartilage
4 Cricoid cartilage
5 Vocal ligament
6 Thyrohyoid ligament
7 Arytenoid cartilage
8 Corniculate cartilage
9 Vocal fold
10 Vestibular fold
11 Aryepiglottic fold
12 Interarytenoid notch

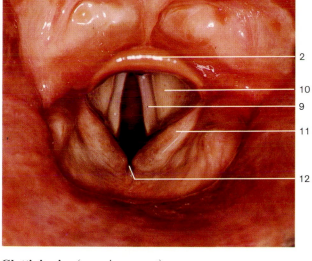

Glottis in vivo (superior aspect).

1 Root of the tongue
2 Thyroarytenoid muscle, lateral part
3 Thyroid cartilage
4 Vocal fold
5 Lateral cricoarytenoid muscle
6 Cricothyroid muscle
7 Arch of cricoid cartilage
7' Lamina of cricoid cartilage
8 Thyroid gland
9 Epiglottis
▽

10 Vestibular fold
11 Thyrohyoid muscle
12 Ventricle
13 Vocal ligament
14 Vocalis muscle
15 Fissure of glottis
16 Trachea
17 Superior cornu of thyroid cartilage
18 Arytenoid muscle

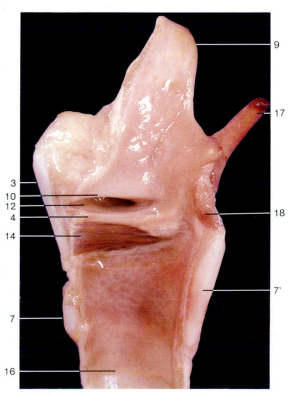

Sagittal section through the larynx.

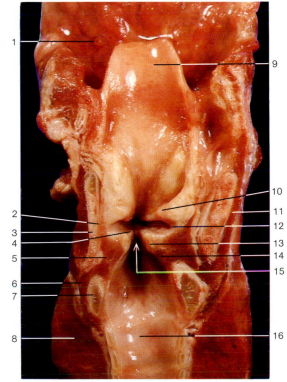

Coronal section through larynx and trachea.

Innervation of the Larynx

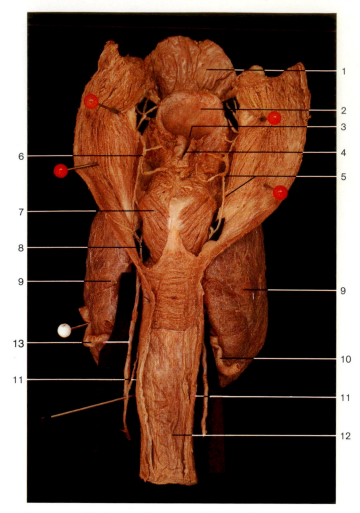

1 Tongue
2 Epiglottis
3 Inlet to the larynx
4 Interarytenoid notch
5 Piriform recess
6 Internal branch of superior laryngeal nerve
7 Posterior cricoarytenoid muscle
8 Inferior laryngeal nerve
9 Thyroid gland
10 Inferior thyroid artery
11 Esophagus
12 Mucous membrane of esophagus
13 Recurrent laryngeal nerve

Larynx and its innervation (posterior aspect).
Pharynx exposed posteriorly.

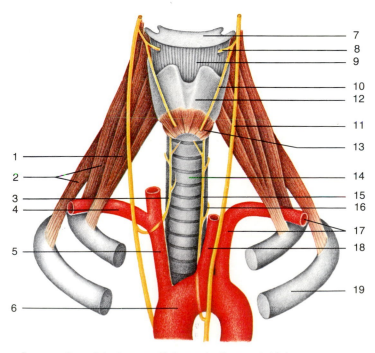

1 Scalenus anterior
2 Scalenus medius and posterior
3 Right recurrent laryngeal nerve
4 Right subclavian artery
5 Brachiocephalic trunk
6 Ascending aorta
7 Hyoid bone
8 Internal branch of superior laryngeal nerve
9 Thyrohyoid membrane
10 External branch of superior laryngeal nerve
11 Vagus
12 Thyroid cartilage
13 Cricothyroid muscle
14 Trachea
15 Left recurrent laryngeal nerve
16 Esophagus
17 Left subclavian artery
18 Left common carotid artery
19 Second rib

Innervation of the larynx. (Schematic diagram) (O.).

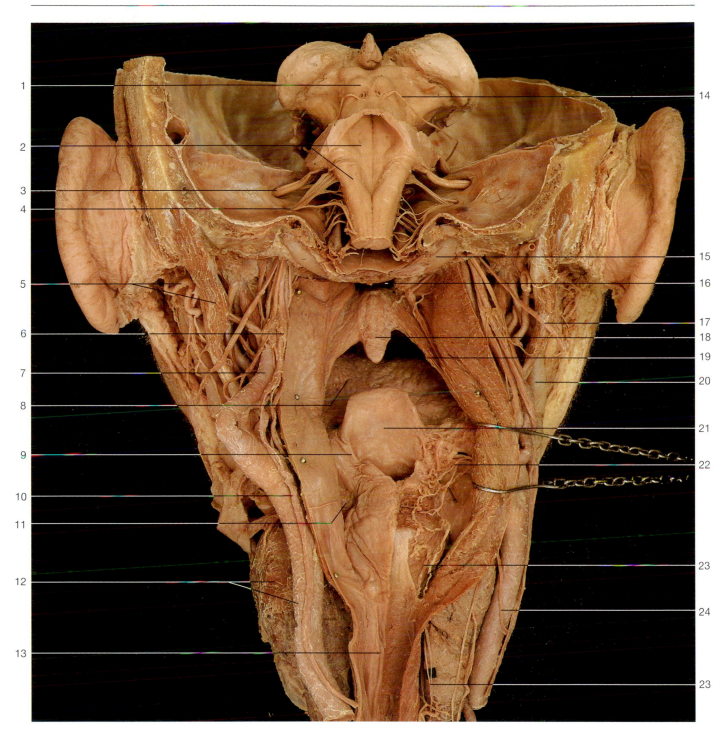

Larynx and oral cavity (posterior aspect). Mucous membrane on the right half of pharynx has been removed.

1	Midbrain (inferior colliculus)	13	Esophagus
2	Rhomboid fossa, medulla oblongata	14	Trochlear nerve
3	Vestibulocochlear and facial nerve	15	Occipital condyle
4	Glossopharyngeal, vagus and accessory nerve	16	**Nasal cavity** (choane)
5	Occipital artery, posterior belly of digastric muscle	17	Accessory nerve
6	Superior cervical ganglion	18	**Uvula,** soft palate
7	**Internal carotid artery**	19	Palatopharyngeal muscle
8	Tongue, **oral cavity**	20	External carotid artery
9	Aryepiglottic fold	21	Epiglottis
10	Vagus nerve	22	**Superior laryngeal nerve**
11	**Piriform recess**	23	**Inferior laryngeal nerve**
12	Thyroid gland, common carotid artery	24	Ansa cervicalis

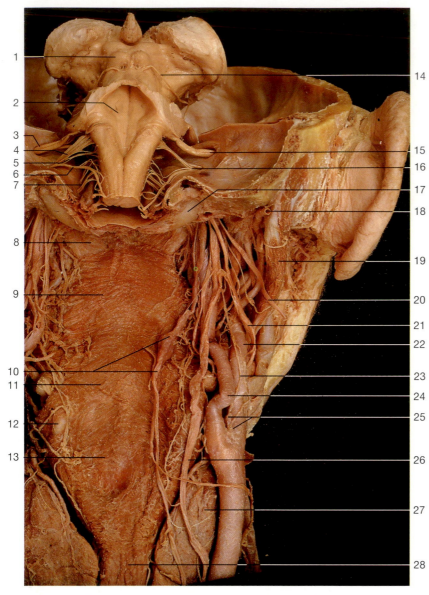

1 Inferior colliculus of midbrain
2 Facial colliculus in floor of rhomboid fossa
3 Vestibulocochlear and facial nerve
4 Glossopharyngeal nerve
5 Vagus nerve
6 Accessory nerve
7 Hypoglossal nerve
8 Pharyngobasilar fascia
9 Superior constrictor of pharynx
10 Sympathetic trunk, superior cervical ganglion (medially displaced)
11 Middle constrictor of pharynx
12 Greater cornu of hyoid bone
13 Inferior constrictor of pharynx
14 Trochlear nerve
15 Internal acoustic meatus with facial and vestibulocochlear nerve
16 Jugular foramen with glossopharyngeal, vagus and assessory nerve
17 Occipital condyle
18 Occipital artery
19 Posterior belly of digastric muscle
20 Accessory nerve (extracranial part)
21 Hypoglossal nerve (extracranial part)
22 External carotid artery
23 Carotid sinus nerve
24 Internal carotid artery
25 Carotid sinus, carotid body
26 Vagus nerve
27 Thyroid gland
28 Esophagus
29 Choanae
30 Medial pterygoid plate
31 Foramen lacerum
32 **Pharyngeal tubercle**
33 Hard palate
34 Greater and lesser palatine foramen
35 Pterygoid hamulus
36 Lateral pterygoid plate
37 Pterygoid canal
38 Foramen ovale
39 Mandibular fossa
40 Carotid canal
41 Styloid process, stylomastoid foramen

Pharynx and parapharyngeal nerves in connection with brain stem (posterior aspect).

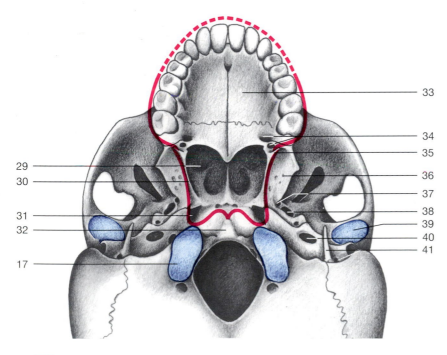

Inferior aspect of the skull. Red line = outline of superior constrictor in continuation with buccinator and orbicularis oris. (Semischematic drawing) (O.).

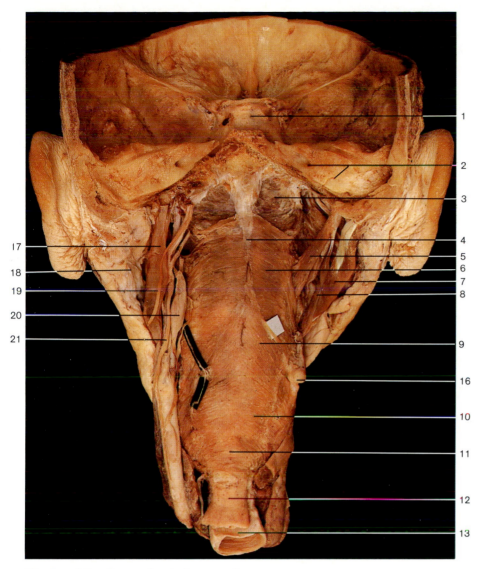

1	Sella turcica
2	Internal acoustic meatus and petrous part of temporal bone
3	Pharyngobasilar fascia
4	Fibrous raphe of pharynx
5	Stylopharyngeus
6	Superior constrictor of pharynx
7	Posterior belly of digastric muscle
8	Stylohyoid
9	Middle constrictor of pharynx
10	Inferior constrictor of pharynx
11	Muscle-free area (Kilian's triangle)
12	Esophagus
13	Trachea
14	Thyroid and parathyroid glands
15	Medial pterygoid
16	Greater cornu of hyoid bone
17	Internal jugular vein
18	Parotid gland
19	Accessory nerve
20	Superior ganglion of sympathetic trunk
21	Vagus nerve

Muscles of the pharynx (posterior aspect).

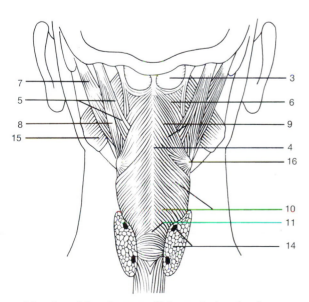

Muscles of the pharynx. (Schematic drawing.)

The **pharynx** is fixed to the base of the skull and is continuous with the esophagus below the level of the larynx. Although part of the digestive system, the pharynx does not show the arrangement of layers characteristic of the gastrointestinal tract. In contrast to the esophagus and intestine, the layer of circular pharyngeal muscles (constrictors) is located externally and the longitudinal muscle layer internally. Therefore, between esophagus and pharynx, muscle-free areas (e.g. Laimer's triangle) are occasionally found where diverticula or herniae can develop. The oropharynx opens anteriorly into the oral cavity and its muscular wall becomes continuous with buccinator in the cheek.

153

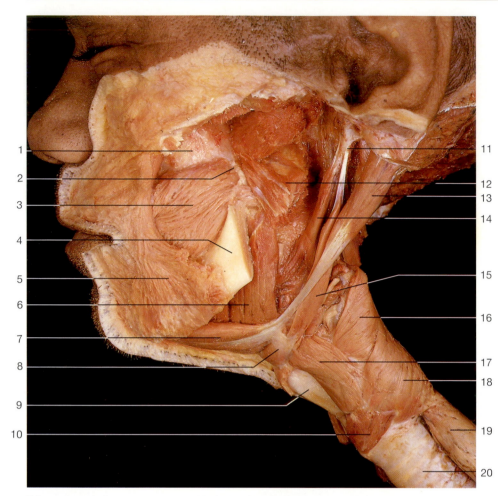

Dissection of pharynx, supra- and infrahyoid muscles I. Mandible partly removed (lateral aspect).

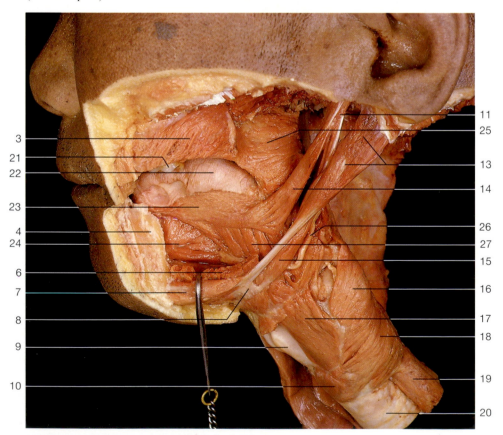

Dissection of pharynx, supra- and infrahyoid muscles II. Oral cavity opened (lateral aspect).

154

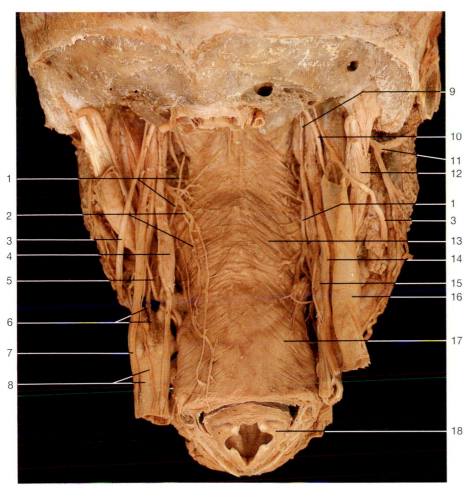

Parapharyngeal nerves and vessels. Dorsal aspect of the pharynx.

1. Ascending pharyngeal artery
2. Pharyngeal plexus
3. Accessory nerve
4. Superior cervical ganglion of sympathetic trunk
5. Superior laryngeal nerve
6. Carotid body and carotid sinus nerve
7. Left vagus
8. Common carotid artery and cardiac branch of vagus nerve
9. Glossopharyngeal nerve
10. Hypoglossal nerve
11. Facial nerve
12. Posterior belly of digastric
13. Middle constrictor of pharynx
14. Right vagus
15. Sympathetic trunk
16. Internal jugular vein
17. Inferior constrictor of pharynx
18. Larynx
19. Buccinator
20. Pterygomandibular raphe
21. **Tensor veli palatini**
22. Uvula of palate
23. Pharynx
24. Styloid process with stylopharyngeus and stylohyoid
25. Internal carotid artery, internal jugular vein
26. Dens of axis
27. Atlas
28. Spinal cord
29. Orbicularis oris
30. Masseter
31. Mandible
32. Mandibular canal
33. Medial and lateral pterygoid muscle
34. External carotid artery
35. Parotid gland
36. Vertebral artery
37. Dura mater
38. Splenius capitis

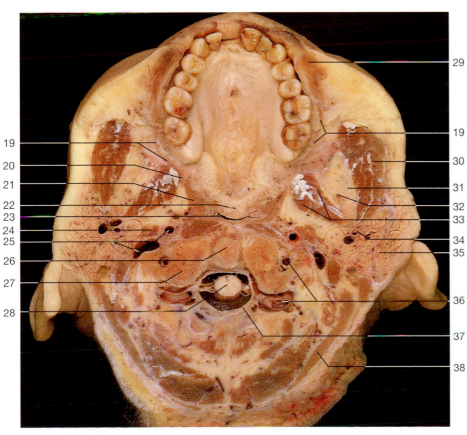

Cross-section of head and neck at the level of atlas (from below).

155

Arteries of the Head and Neck

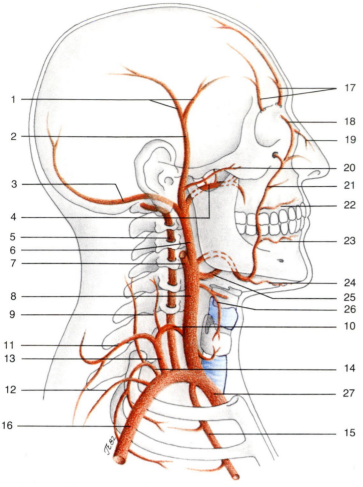

1 Frontal and parietal branches of superficial temporal artery
2 Superficial temporal artery
3 Occipital artery
4 Maxillary artery
5 Vertebral artery
6 External carotid artery
7 Internal carotid artery
8 Common carotid artery (divided)
9 Ascending cervical artery
10 Inferior thyroid artery
11 Transverse cervical artery with 2 branches, superficial cervical artery and descending scapular artery
12 Suprascapular artery
13 Thyrocervical trunk
14 Costocervical trunk with 2 branches – deep cervical artery and superior intercostal artery
15 Internal thoracic artery
16 Subclavian artery
17 Supraorbital and supratrochlear arteries
18 Angular artery
19 Dorsal nasal artery
20 Transverse facial artery
21 Facial artery
22 Superior labial artery
23 Inferior labial artery
24 Submental artery
25 Lingual artery
26 Superior thyroid artery
27 Brachiocephalic trunk

Arteries of head and neck. Diagram of the main branches of external carotid and subclavian artery (Tr.).

to page 157 ▷

1 Galea aponeurotica
2 Frontal branch } of superficial
3 Parietal branch } temporal artery
4 Superior auricular muscle
5 **Superficial temporal artery and vein**
6 Middle temporal artery
7 Auriculotemporal nerve
8 Parotid plexus of facial nerve
9 Facial nerve
10 **External carotid artery** within the retromandibular fossa
11 Posterior belly of digastric muscle
12 Sternocleidomastoid artery
13 Sympathetic trunk, superior cervical ganglion
14 Sternocleidomastoid (divided and reflected)
15 Clavicle (divided)
16 Transverse cervical artery
17 Ascending cervical artery, phrenic nerve
18 Anterior scalene muscle
19 Suprascapular artery
20 Dorsal scapular artery

21 Brachial plexus, **axillary artery**
22 Thoracoacromial artery
23 Lateral thoracic artery
24 Median nerve (displaced), pectoralis minor (reflected)
25 Frontal belly of occipitofrontalis muscle
26 Orbital part of orbicularis oculi
27 **Angular artery** and vein
28 **Facial artery**
29 Superior labial artery
30 Zygomaticus major
31 Inferior labial artery
32 Parotid duct
33 Fatty tissue of cheek
34 **Maxillary artery**
35 Masseter
36 Facial artery, mandible
37 Submental artery
38 Anterior belly of digastric muscle

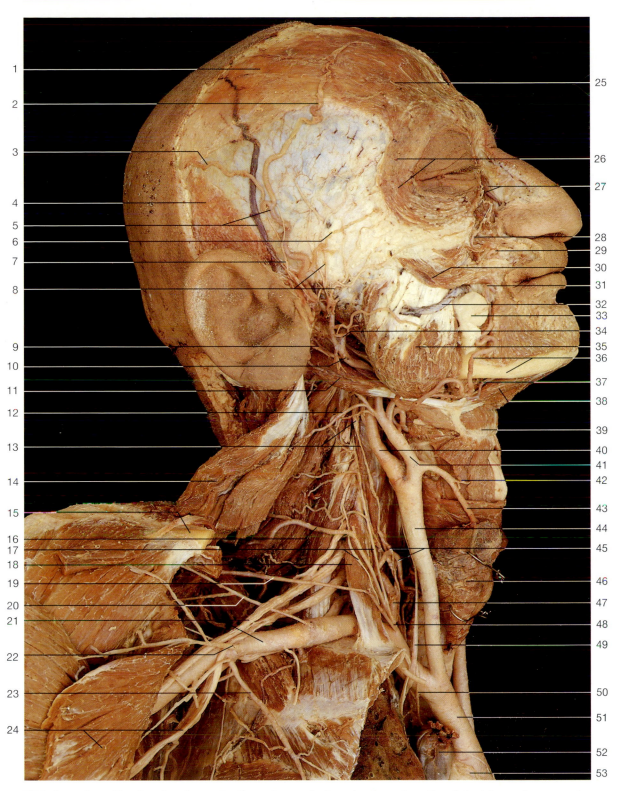

Main branches of head and neck arteries (lateral aspect). Anterior thoracic wall and clavicle partly removed; pectoralis muscles have been reflected to display the subclavian and axillary arteries.

39	Hyoid bone	46	Thyroid gland (right lobe)
40	**Internal carotid artery**	**47**	**Vertebral artery**
41	**External carotid artery**	**48**	**Thyrocervical trunk**
42	Superior laryngeal artery	49	Vagus nerve
43	Superior thyroid artery	50	Ansa subclavia of sympathetic trunk
44	**Common carotid artery**	**51**	**Brachiocephalic trunk**
45	Thyroid ansa of sympathetic trunk, **inferior thyroid artery**	52	Superior vena cava (divided)
		53	Aortic arch

157

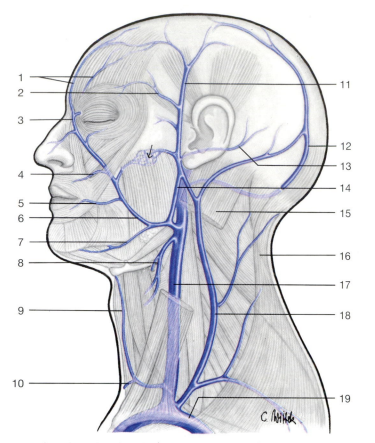

1 Supraorbital veins
2 Middle temporal vein
3 Angular vein
4 Superior labial vein
5 Inferior labial vein
6 **Facial vein**
7 Submental vein
8 Superior thyroid vein
9 Anterior jugular vein
10 Jugular venous arch
11 Superficial temporal vein
12 Occipital vein
13 Posterior auricular vein
14 Retromandibular vein
15 Sternocleidomastoid
16 Trapezius
17 **Internal jugular vein**
18 External jugular vein
19 Subclavian vein
20 Submental nodes
21 **Thoracic duct**
22 Retroauricular nodes
23 Parotid nodes
24 Occipital nodes
25 Submandibular nodes
26 Jugulo-digastric nodes ⎤ deep cervical
27 Jugulo-omohyoid nodes ⎦ nodes
28 Jugular trunk
29 Subclavian trunk
30 Infraclavicular nodes

Veins of head and neck. (Schematic diagram) (W.). Sternocleidomastoid has been partly removed to expose the internal jugular vein.
Arrow: Pterygoid plexus.

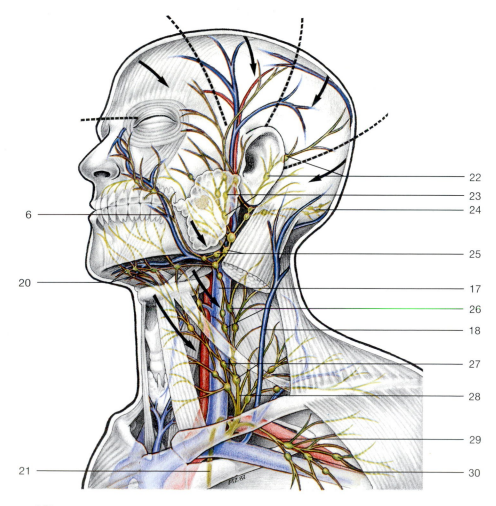

Lymph nodes and veins of head and neck (A.). Dotted lines = border between irrigation areas; arrows = direction of lymph flow.

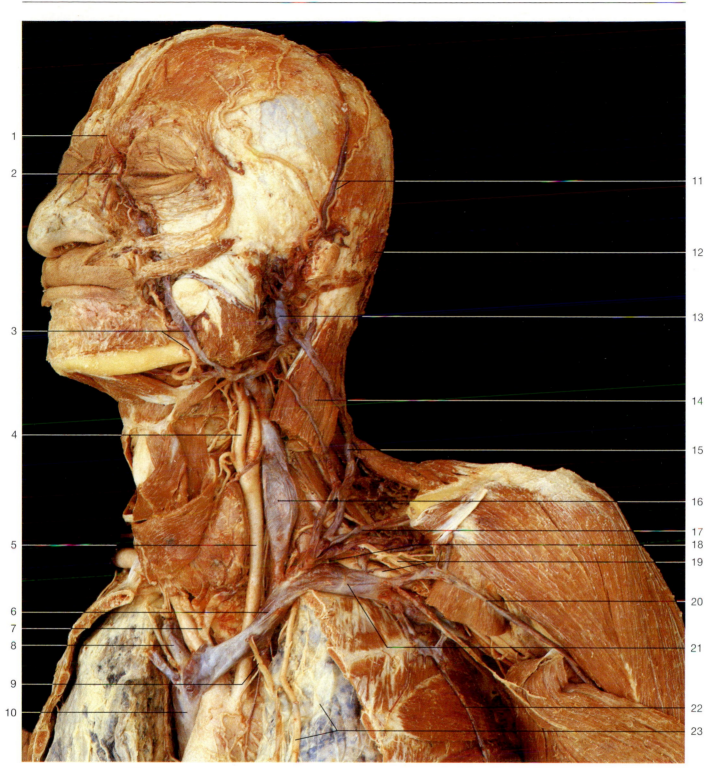

Dissection of veins of head and neck (oblique-lateral aspect). Sternocleidomastoid divided, anterior thoracic wall and clavicle removed.

1	Supraorbital vein	10	**Superior vena cava**
2	**Angular vein**	11	**Superficial temporal vein** and artery
3	**Facial** artery and **vein**	12	Occipital vein
4	External carotid artery	13	**Retromandibular vein**
5	Common carotid artery	14	Sternocleidomastoid (divided)
6	**Left brachiocephalic vein**	15	**External jugular vein**
7	**Inferior thyroid vein**	16	**Internal jugular vein**
8	Right brachiocephalic vein	17	Suprascapular vein
9	Internal thoracic vein		

18 Left venous angle with thoracic duct (divided)
19 Brachial plexus, subclavian artery
20 **Cephalic vein**
21 **Subclavian vein**
22 Thoracoepigastric vein
23 Left lung with pleura, internal thoracic artery

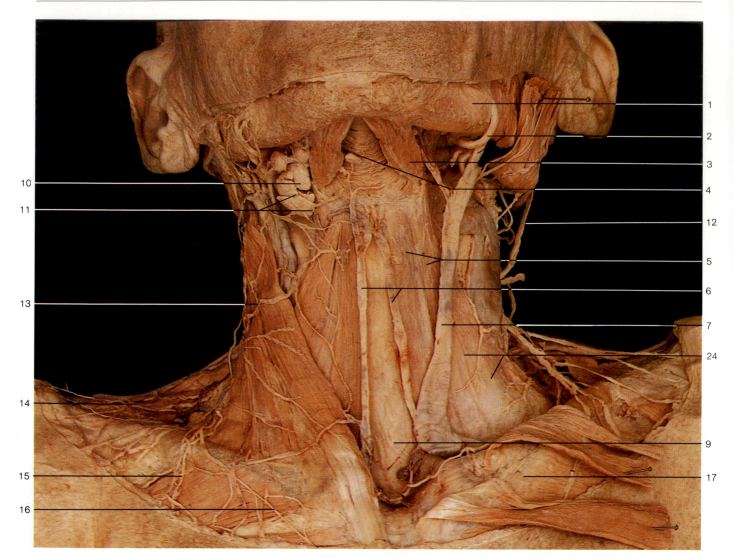

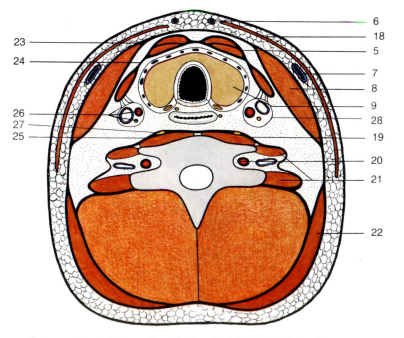

Neck (anterior aspect).
The superficial fascia has been removed.

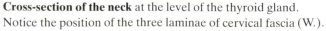

Cross-section of the neck at the level of the thyroid gland.
Notice the position of the three laminae of cervical fascia (W.).

1 Mandible
2 Facial artery and vein
3 Anterior belly of digastric
4 Mylohyoid
5 Infrahyoid muscles (sternohyoid, sternothyroid, omohyoid)
6 Anterior jugular veins
7 External jugular vein
8 Sternocleidomastoid
9 Thyroid gland
10 Submandibular gland
11 Cervical branch of facial nerve and communicating branch with transverse cervical nerve
12 Lesser occipital nerve ⎫
13 Transverse cervical nerves ⎪ Cutaneous
14 Posterior supraclavicular nerves ⎬ branches of cervical
15 Middle supraclavicular nerves ⎪ plexus
16 Anterior supraclavicular nerves ⎭
17 Clavicle
18 Platysma
19 Longus coli
20 Vertebral artery and vein
21 Scalene muscles
22 Trapezius
23 Superficial lamina of cervical fascia
24 Pretracheal lamina of cervical fascia
25 Prevertebral lamina of cervical fascia with sympathetic trunk
26 Carotid sheath with common carotid artery internal jugular vein and vagus nerve
27 Cervical part of sympathetic trunk
28 Carotid sheath

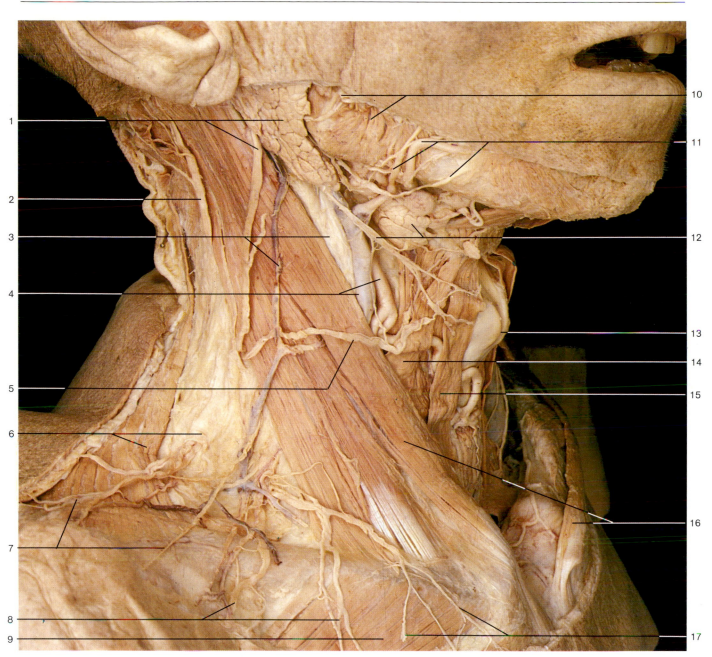

Posterior and carotid triangles (lateral aspect).
Superficial dissection.

1 Parotid gland, great auricular nerve
2 Lesser occipital nerve
3 Internal and external jugular veins
4 Retromandibular vein, superior thyroid artery
5 Transverse cervical nerve with communicating branch to cervical branch of facial nerve
6 Trapezius, superficial lamina of cervical fascia
7 Posterior supraclavicular nerves

8 Middle supraclavicular nerves
9 Pectoralis major
10 Buccal branch of facial nerve, masseter
11 Facial artery and vein, mandibular branch of facial nerve
12 Cervical branch of facial nerve
13 Thyroid cartilage
14 Omohyoid
15 Sternohyoid
16 Sternocleidomastoid
17 Anterior supraclavicular nerves

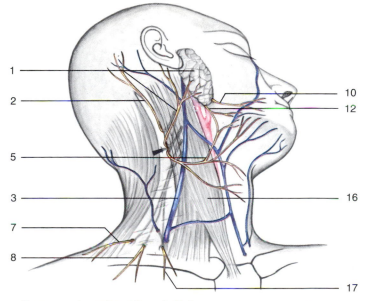

Cutaneous branches of cervical plexus. Erb's point is indicated by an arrowhead. (Schematic diagram.)

161

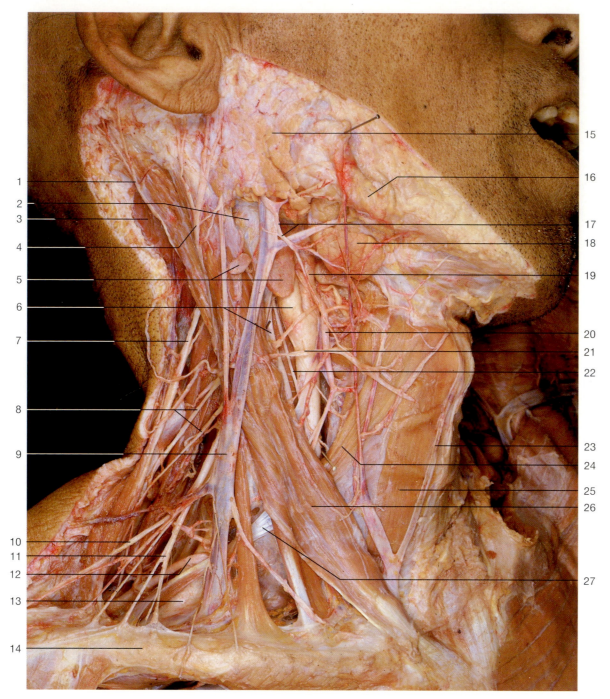

15	
16	
17	
18	
19	
20	
21	
22	
23	
24	
25	
26	
27	

Posterior and carotid triangles (lateral aspect). Superficial dissection. The superficial lamina of cervical fascia has been removed, to display the cutaneous branches of the cervical plexus and subcutaneous veins.

1	**Lesser occipital nerve**	11	**Middle supraclavicular nerves**
2	**Internal jugular vein**		
3	Splenius capitis	12	Suprascapular artery
4	**Great auricular nerve**	13	Pretracheal lamina of fascia of neck
5	Submandibular nodes	14	Clavicle
6	Internal carotid artery, vagus nerve	15	Parotid gland
7	**Accessory nerve**	16	Mandible
8	Muscular branches of cervical plexus	17	Cervical branch of facial nerve
9	External jugular vein	18	Submandibular gland
10	**Posterior supraclavicular nerves**	19	External carotid artery

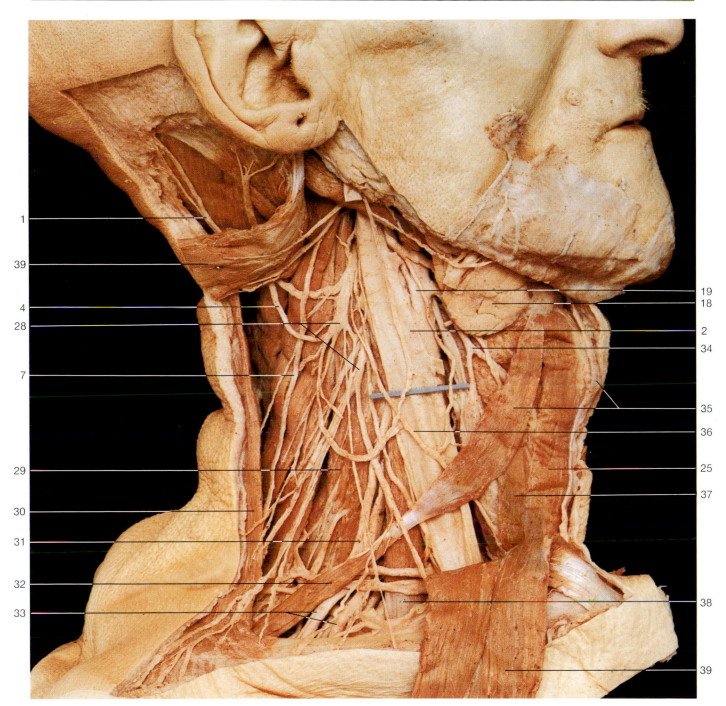

Posterior and carotid triangle (lateral aspect). The sternocleidomastoid has been severed and reflected to display the cervical and brachial plexus, the internal jugular vein and the carotid arteries. Note the position of the omohyoid muscle.

20 Superior thyroid artery
21 Transverse cervical nerve
22 Superior root of ansa cervicalis
23 Anterior jugular vein
24 Omohyoid muscle
25 Sternohyoid muscle
26 Sternocleidomastoid
27 Intermediate tendon of omohyoid muscle
28 Cervical plexus
29 Scalenus medius

30 Trapezius (lateral edge)
31 Brachial plexus
32 Omohyoid muscle (inferior belly)
33 Brachial plexus, subclavian artery
34 Superior thyroid artery
35 Omohyoid muscle (superior belly), anterior jugular vein
36 **Ansa cervicalis**
37 Sternothyroid muscle
38 Scalenus anterior
39 Sternocleidomastoid (reflected)

The Anterior Triangle of the Neck

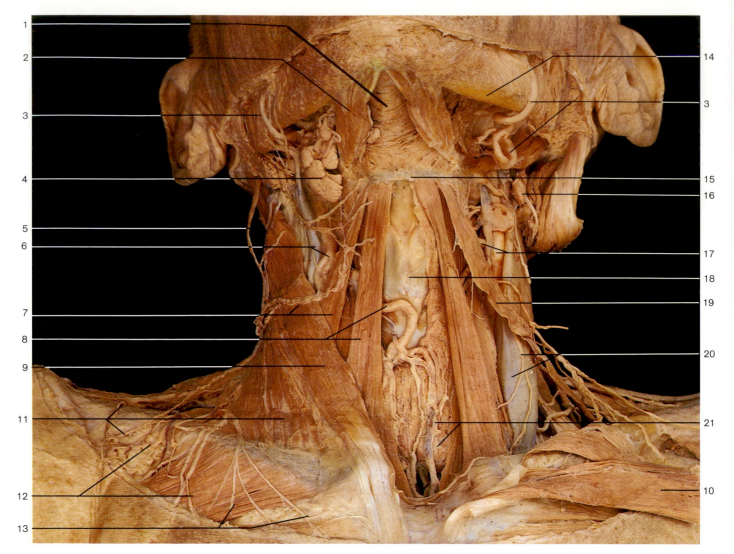

Anterior triangle (anterior aspect). The pretracheal lamina of cervical fascia and left sternocleidomastoid have been removed.

1 Mylohyoid
2 Anterior belly of digastric
3 Facial artery
4 Submandibular gland
5 Great auricular nerve
6 Internal jugular vein, common carotid artery
7 Transverse cervical nerve, omohyoid
8 Sternohyoid, superior thyroid artery
9 Sternocleidomastoid (sternal head)
10 Left sternocleidomastoid (reflected)
11 Sternocleidomastoid (clavicular head), posterior supraclavicular nerves
12 Middle supraclavicular nerves
13 Anterior supraclavicular nerves
14 Mandible
15 Hyoid bone
16 Superficial cervical lymph nodes
17 Left superior thyroid artery, external carotid artery
18 Thyroid cartilage
19 Omohyoid (superior belly)
20 Internal jugular vein, branches of ansa cervicalis
21 Thyroid gland, unpaired inferior thyroid vein

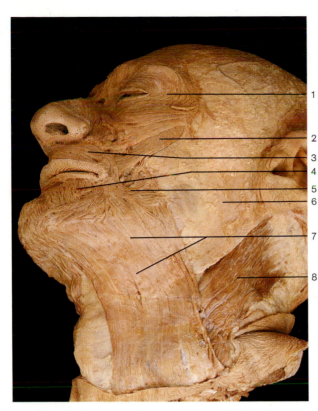

1 Orbicularis oculi
2 Zygomaticus major
3 Orbicularis oris
4 Depressor labii inferioris
5 Risorius
6 Parotid fascia
7 Platysma
8 Sternocleidomastoid

Platysma (oblique lateral aspect). Superficial lamina of cervical fascia partly removed.

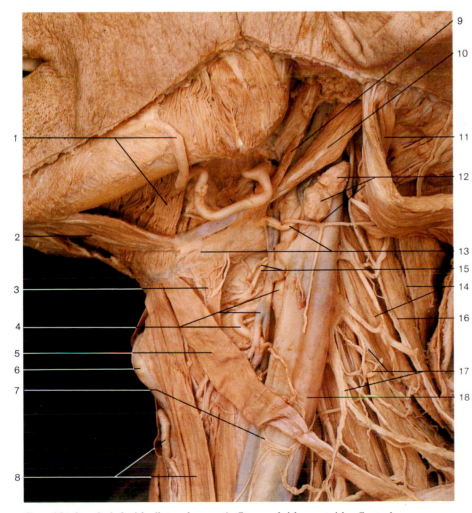

1 Mylohyoid muscle and facial artery
2 Anterior belly of digastric muscle
3 Thyrohyoid
4 External carotid artery, superior thyroid artery and vein
5 Omohyoid
6 Thyroid cartilage
7 Ansa cervicalis
8 Sternohyoid and superior thyroid artery
9 Stylohyoid
10 Posterior belly of digastric muscle
11 Sternocleidomastoid (reflected)
12 Superior cervical lymph nodes, sternocleidomastoid artery
13 Hyoid bone, hypoglossal nerve (n. XII)
14 Splenius capitis, levator scapulae
15 Superior laryngeal artery and nerve
16 Accessory nerve
17 Cervical plexus
18 Internal jugular vein

Carotid triangle left side (lateral aspect). Sternocleidomastoid reflected.

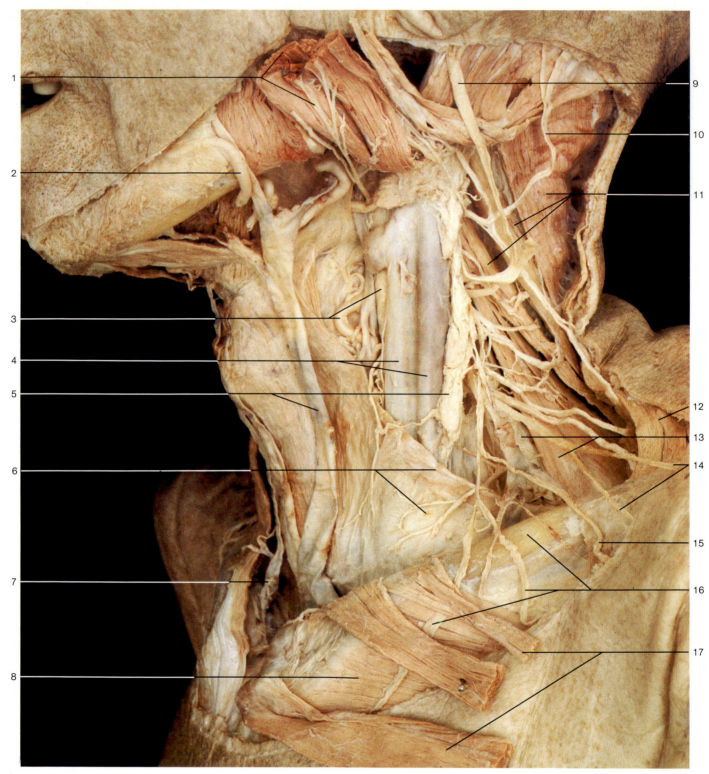

Neck, superficial dissection (lateral aspect). Sternocleidomastoid has been cut and reflected to display the pretracheal lamina of the cervical fascia.

1 Sternocleidomastoid (reflected) and branch of accessory nerve
2 Facial artery and vein
3 External carotid artery, superior thyroid artery
4 Internal jugular vein
5 Deep cervical lymph nodes and external jugular vein
6 Omohyoid and pretracheal lamina of cervical fascia
7 Anterior jugular vein
8 Pectoralis major
9 Great auricular nerve
10 Lesser occipital nerve
11 Splenius capitis, levator scapulae
12 Trapezius
13 Scalenus medius, branchial plexus
14 Posterior supraclavicular nerves
15 Middle supraclavicular nerve
16 Clavicle and anterior supraclavicular nerves
17 Sternocleidomastoid (reflected)

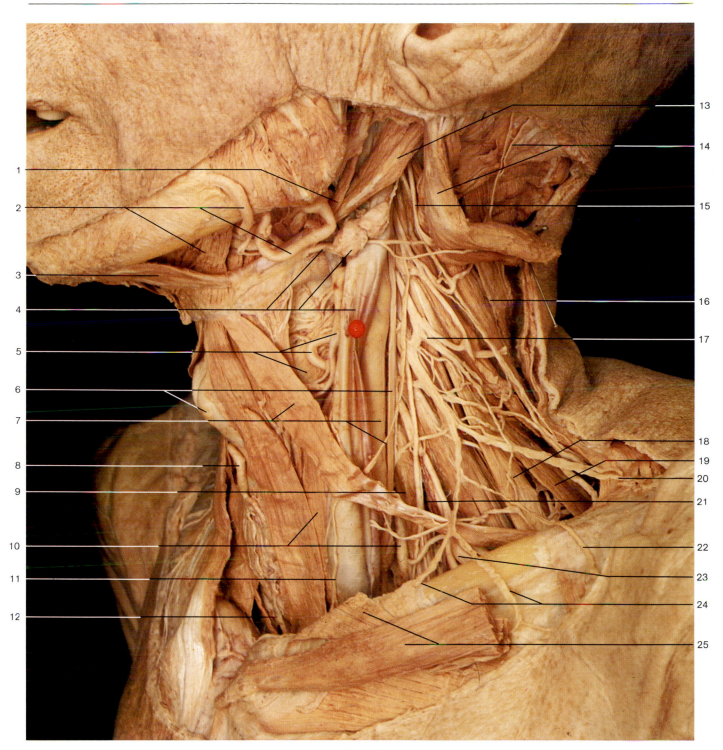

Neck, deep dissection (lateral aspect). The internal jugular vein has been reflected to expose the carotid artery and vagus nerve.

1 Stylohyoid
2 Facial artery, mylohyoid
3 Anterior belly of digastric muscle
4 Internal jugular vein, hypoglossal nerve, superficial cervical lymph nodes
5 Superior thyroid artery and vein, inferior pharyngeal constrictor
6 Thyroid cartilage, vagus nerve
7 Ansa cervicalis, omohyoid and common carotid artery
8 Right superior thyroid artery
9 Scalenus anterior
10 Sternothyroid, inferior thyroid artery
11 Muscular branches of ansa cervicalis to the infrahyoid muscles
12 Unpaired inferior thyroid vein

13 Posterior belly of digastric muscle
14 Sternocleidomastoid, lesser occipital nerve
15 Accessory nerve
16 Splenius capitis
17 Cervical plexus
18 Scalenus posterior
19 Levator scapulae
20 Posterior supraclavicular nerves
21 Phrenic nerve
22 Middle supraclavicular nerves
23 Brachial plexus
24 Anterior supraclavicular nerves
25 Sternocleidomastoid

The Ansa cervicalis

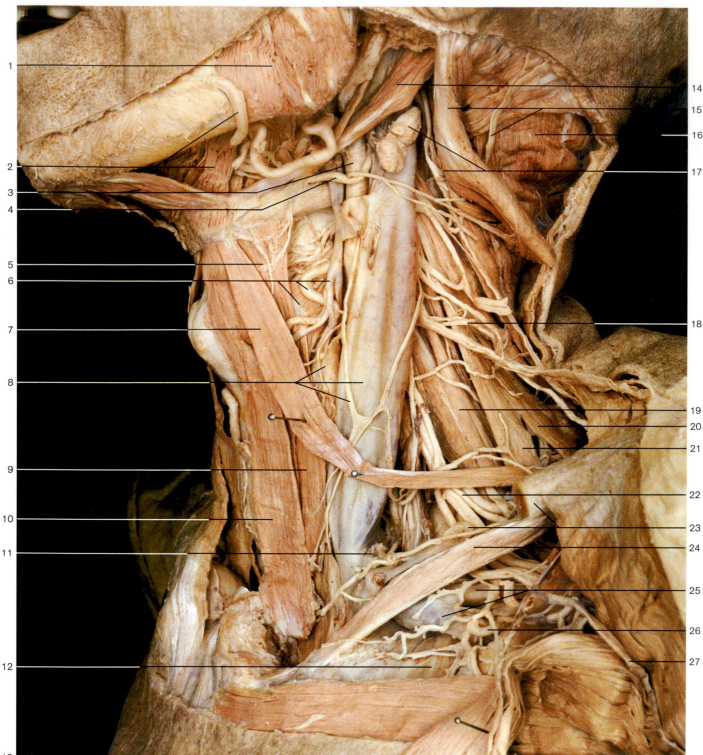

Neck, deeper dissection (lateral aspect). **Ansa cervicalis.** The cervical fascia and the clavicle partly removed. Ansa cervicalis and infrahyoid muscles displayed.

1 Masseter
2 Mylohyoid, facial artery
3 External carotid artery, anterior belly of digastric muscle
4 Hypoglossal nerve
5 Thyrohyoid
6 Superior thyroid artery and vein, inferior pharyngeal constrictor
7 Omohyoid (superior belly)
8 Ansa cervicalis, thyroid gland, internal jugular vein

9 Sternothyroid
10 Sternohyoid
11 Thoracic duct
12 Pectoralis minor
13 Pectoralis major
14 Posterior belly of digastric muscle
15 Sternocleidomastoid, lesser occipital nerve
16 Splenius capitis
17 Superficial cervical lymph nodes, accessory nerve

18 Cervical plexus
19 Scalenus medius
20 Levator scapulae
21 Scalenus posterior
22 Brachial plexus
23 Transverse cervical artery, clavicle
24 Subclavius
25 Subclavian artery and vein
26 Thoracoacromial artery
27 Cephalic vein

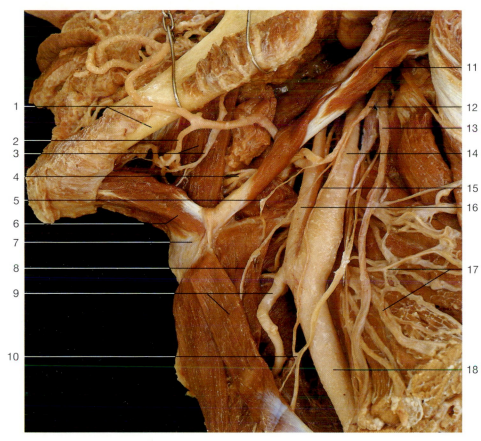

1	**Facial artery,** mandible
2	Submental artery
3	Mylohyoid muscle and nerve
4	Hypoglossal nerve, lingual branches
5	Geniohyoid branch of n. XII
6	Anterior belly of digastric muscle
7	Hyoid bone
8	Thyrohyoid branch of n. XII
9	Omohyoid muscle, superior thyroid artery
10	**Ansa cervicalis**
11	Posterior belly of digastric muscle
12	**Hypoglossal nerve** (n. XII)
13	**Vagus nerve** (n. X)
14	Internal carotid artery
15	Superior root of ansa cervicalis
16	**External carotid artery**
17	Cervical plexus
18	Common carotid artery

Neck, submandibular region (lateral aspect). **Hypoglossal nerve.** Mandible slightly elevated.

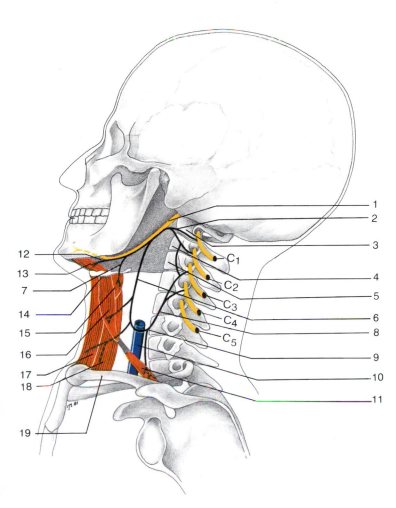

1	Hypoglossal nerve (n. XII)
2	Communication from the ventral ramus of the first cervical spinal nerve
3	Atlas
4	Axis
5	Third cervical vertebra
6	Superior root of ansa cervicalis
7	Thyroid branch of hypoglossal nerve
8	Inferior root of ansa cervicalis
9	Ansa cervicalis
10	Internal jugular vein
11	Inferior belly of omohyoid muscle
12	Geniohyoid branch of hypoglossal nerve
13	Geniohyoid muscle
14	Hyoid bone
15	Thyrohyoid
16	Superior belly of omohyoid muscle
17	Sternohyoid
18	Sternothyroid
19	Clavicle

Ansa cervicalis.
Innervation of infrahyoid muscles. Cervical plexus and its communication with the hypoglossal nerve. C_1–C_5 = ventral rami of cervical spinal nerves of the first five segments.

169

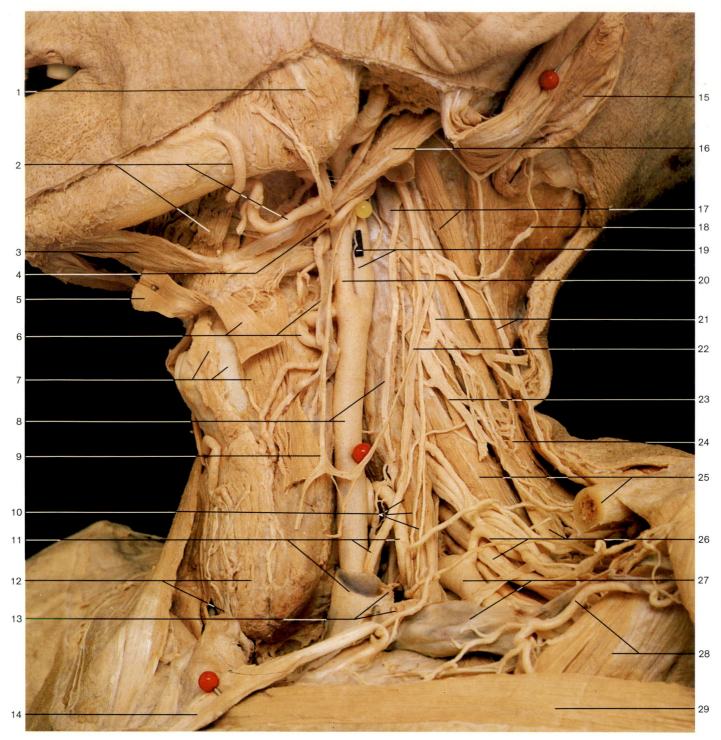

Neck, deep dissection (lateral aspect). Clavicle partly removed to show the slit between the scalene muscles. Internal jugular vein removed.

1 Masseter
2 Mylohyoid, facial artery
3 Anterior belly of digastric muscle
4 Hypoglossal nerve
5 Sternohyoid
6 Omohyoid, superior thyroid artery and vein
7 Sternothyroid, thyroid cartilage, pyramidal lobe
8 Common carotid artery, sympathetic trunk
9 Ansa cervicalis
10 Phrenic nerve and ascending cervical artery, scalenus anterior muscle

11 Inferior thyroid artery, vagus nerve, internal jugular vein
12 Thyroid gland, unpaired inferior thyroid vein
13 Thoracic duct, left subclavian trunk
14 Subclavius (reflected)
15 Sternocleidomastoid (reflected)
16 Posterior belly of digastric muscle
17 Superior cervical ganglion, splenius capitis muscle
18 Lesser occipital nerve
19 Internal carotid artery and branch of the glossopharyngeal nerve to the carotid body

20 External carotid artery
21 Cervical plexus, accessory nerve
22 Inferior root of ansa cervicalis
23 Supraclavicular nerve
24 Levator scapulae
25 Scalenus medius, clavicle
26 Transverse cervical artery, brachial plexus and scalenus posterior muscle
27 Subclavian artery and vein
28 Thoracoacromial artery, pectoralis minor
29 Pectoralis major

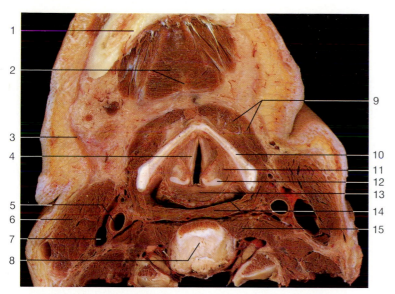

Horizontal section through the neck at the level of the fissure of glottis, viewed from below.

1 Mandible
2 Mylohyoid muscle, mylohyoid raphe
3 Platysma
4 **Vocal fold**
5 **Internal carotid artery**
6 Sternocleidomastoid
7 **Internal jugular vein**
8 Body of cervical vertebra
9 Infrahyoid muscles
10 **Thyroid cartilage**
11 Lateral cricoarytenoid muscle
12 Arytenoid cartilage
13 Transverse arytenoid muscle
14 Laryngopharynx, inferior constrictor of pharynx
15 Longus colli
16 Vertebral arch
17 Muscles of neck
18 **Fissure of glottis**
19 Pharynx

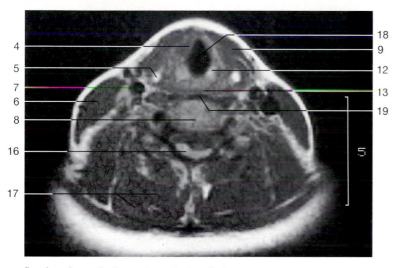

Section through the neck at the level of larynx. MR-Scan.
Bar = 5 cm.

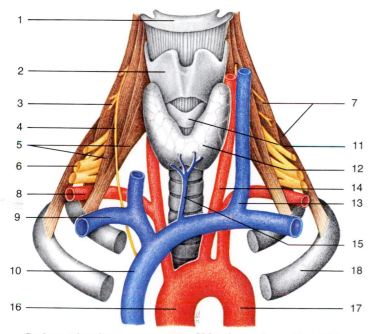

Scalene triangle, arrangements of blood vessels, and brachial plexus at the lower part of the neck (O.).

1 Hyoid bone
2 Thyroid cartilage
3 Cervical plexus (C_1–C_4)
4 Phrenic nerve
5 Scalenus anterior
6 Brachial plexus (C_5–T_1)
7 Middle and posterior scalenus muscles
8 Subclavian artery
9 Subclavian vein
10 Superior vena cava
11 Cricoid cartilage
12 Thyroid gland
13 Internal jugular vein
14 Common carotid artery
15 Unpaired inferior thyroid vein
16 Ascending aorta
17 Descending aorta
18 Second rib

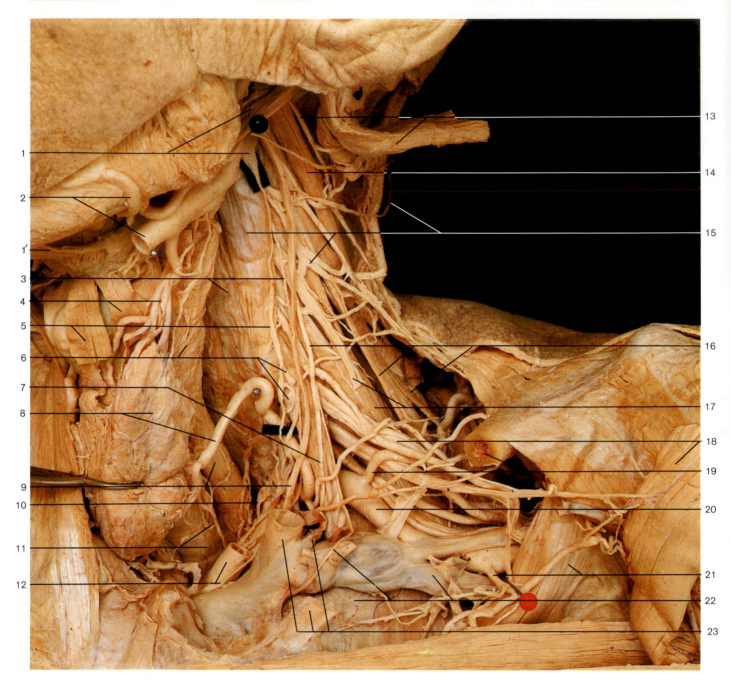

Neck, deepest dissection (anterolateral aspect). Thyroid gland reflected to expose the esophagus and the recurrent laryngeal nerve.

1   Superior cervical ganglion of sympathetic trunk, posterior belly of digastric muscle
1' Anterior belly of digastric muscle
2   Facial artery, common carotid artery (reflected anteriorly)
3   Ascending cervical artery, longus colli muscle
4   Omohyoid, superior thyroid artery
5   Sympathetic trunk, sternohyoid
6   Middle cervical ganglion, pharyngeal constrictor muscle
7   Scalenus anterior and phrenic nerve
8   Thyroid gland, inferior thyroid artery
9   Vagus, esophagus
10 Stellate ganglion
11 Recurrent laryngeal nerve, trachea

12 Common carotid artery, cervical cardiac branch of vagus nerve
13 Sternocleidomastoid, accessory nerve
14 Splenius capitis
15 Lesser occipital nerve, longus capitis, cervical plexus
16 Phrenic nerve, scalenus posterior, levator scapulae
17 Supraclavicular nerves, scalenus medius
18 Brachial plexus, pectoralis major (clavicular head)
19 Transverse cervical artery, clavicle
20 Subclavian artery
21 Thoracoacromial artery, pectoralis minor
22 First rib, accessory phrenic nerve, subclavian vein
23 Internal jugular vein, thoracic duct, subclavius muscle

Chapter IV
Trunk

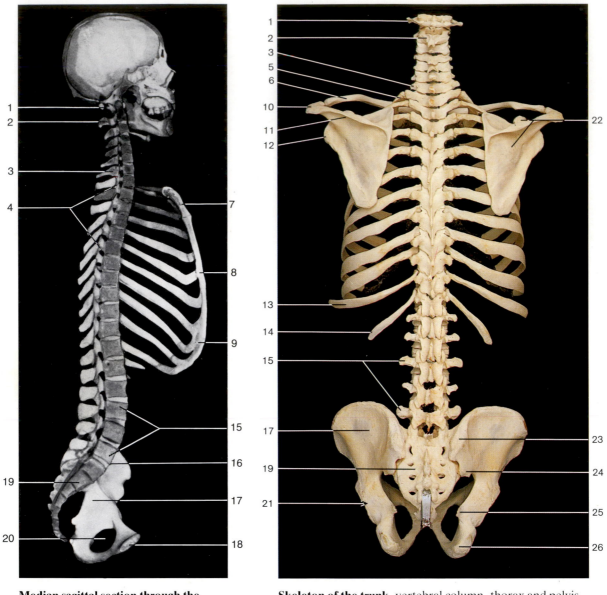

Median sagittal section through the vertebral column, head, and thorax of the adult.

Skeleton of the trunk, vertebral column, thorax and pelvis (posterior aspect).

The trunk is divided into segments best visible in the thoracic region, where each segment consists of a pair of ribs connected anteriorly by the sternum and posteriorly by a thoracic vertebra. In the lumbar part of the vertebral column only vestiges of ribs are present which form what appear to be the transverse processes. In cervical vertebrae, remnants of ribs are part of the transverse processes. Each segment also comprises muscles (e. g. intercostal muscles), nerves, and vessels. However, in the cervical and lumbar region the muscu-

1	Atlas	14	Twelfth rib
2	Axis	15	Lumbar vertebrae
3	Seventh cervical vertebra (vertebra prominens)	16	Sacral promontory
4	Vertebral canal	17	Hip bone
5	First rib	18	Symphysis pubis
6	Clavicle	19	Sacrum
7	Manubrium sterni	20	Obturator foramen
8	Body of sternum	21	Acetabulum
9	Costal arch	22	Scapula with coracoid process
10	Acromion	23	Posterior superior iliac spine
11	Spine of scapula	24	Posterior inferior iliac spine
12	Glenoid cavity, lateral angle of scapula	25	Ischial spine
13	Eleventh rib	26	Ischial tuberosity

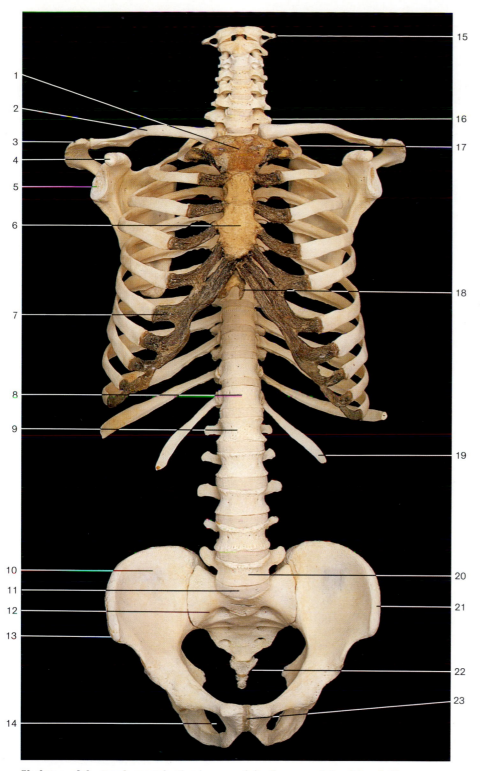

1 Manubrium sterni
2 Clavicle
3 Acromion
4 Coracoid process
5 Glenoid cavity
6 Body of sternum
7 Costal cartilage
8 Body of the twelfth thoracic vertebra
9 Body of the first lumbar vertebra
10 Hip bone
11 Sacral promontory
12 Sacrum
13 Anterior superior iliac spine
14 Obturator foramen
15 Atlas
16 Seventh cervical vertebra
17 First rib
18 Xiphoid process
19 Twelfth rib
20 Body of the fifth lumbar vertebra
21 Iliac crest
22 Coccyx
23 Symphysis pubis

Skeleton of the trunk, vertebral column, pelvis, thorax and shoulder girdle (anterior aspect).

lar segments fuse with each other forming large muscle plates, for example, the oblique muscles of the abdomen, while vessels and nerves still retain their segmental pattern.

Vertebrae

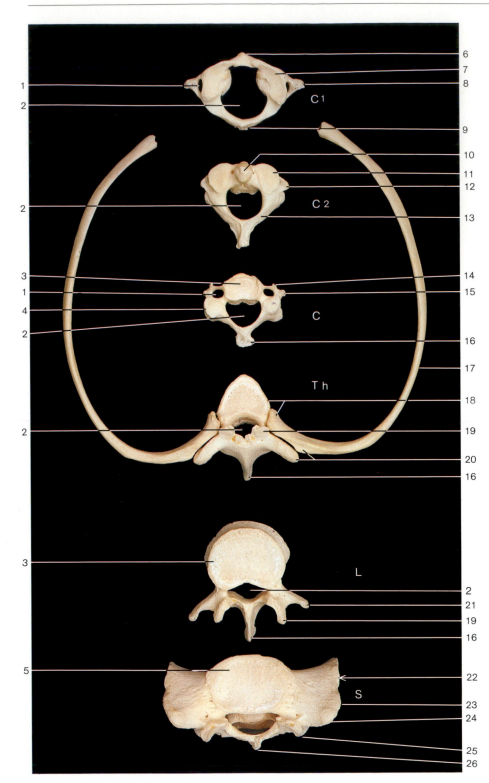

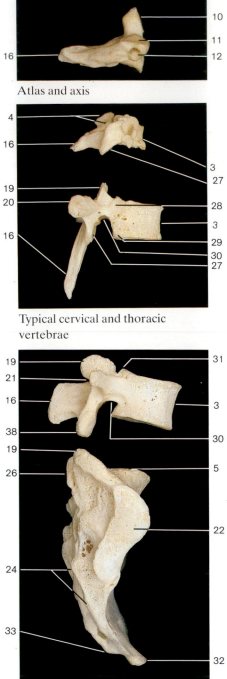

Atlas and axis

Typical cervical and thoracic vertebrae

Typical lumbar vertebra and sacrum

Representative vertebrae from each region of the vertebral column (superior aspect). From top to bottom: atlas (C_1), axis (C_2), cervical vertebra (C), thoracic vertebra (Th), lumbar vertebra (L), and sacrum (S).

Representative vertebrae from each region of the vertebral column (lateral aspect, ventral surface on the right).

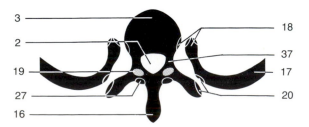

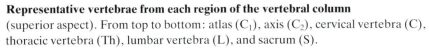

General organization of ribs and vertebrae. (Schematic diagram.)

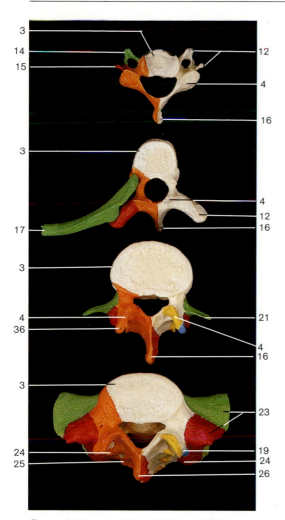

General characteristics of the vertebrae.
Typical cervical, thoracic, lumbar vertebrae
and sacrum.

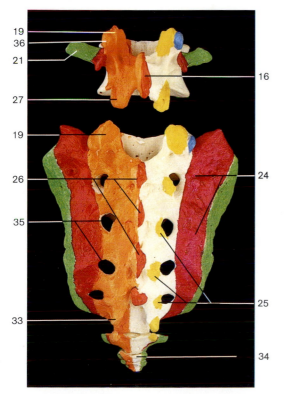

General characteristics of lumbar vertebrae
and sacrum (posterior aspect).

1 Vertebraterial foramen
2 Vertebral foramen
3 Body of vertebra
4 Superior articular facet
5 Base of sacrum
6 Anterior tubercle of atlas
7 Superior articular facet of atlas
8 Transverse process
9 Posterior tubercle of atlas
10 Dens of axis
11 Superior articular surface
12 Transverse process
13 Arch of vertebra
14 Anterior tubercle of transverse process
15 Posterior tubercle of transverse process
16 Spinous process
17 Shaft of rib
18 Body of vertebra and head of rib articulating with each other
   (costovertebral joint)
19 Superior articular process
20 Transverse process and tubercle of rib articulating with each other
   (costotransverse joint)
21 Transverse process
22 Auricular surface
23 Lateral part of sacrum
24 Lateral sacral crest
25 Intermediate sacral crest
26 Median sacral crest
27 Inferior articular facet
28 Superior demifacet for head of rib
29 Inferior demifacet for head of rib
30 Inferior vertebral notch
31 Superior vertebral notch
32 Apex of the sacrum
33 Sacral cornu
34 Coccyx
35 Dorsal sacral foramina
36 Mamillary process
37 Pedicle
38 Inferior articular process

Green = Ribs or homologous processes
Red   = Muscular processes (transverse and spinous processes)
Orange = Laminae and articular processes
Yellow = Articular facets

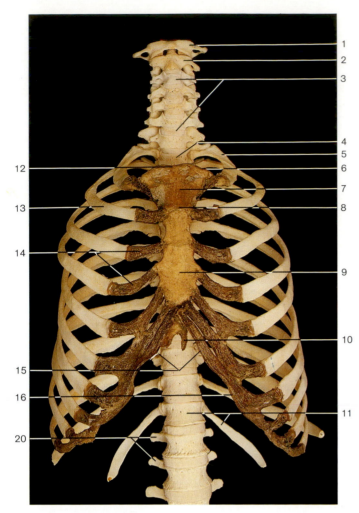

Skeleton of the thorax (anterior aspect).

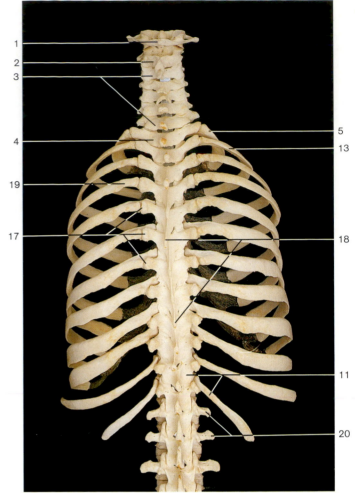

Skeleton of the thorax (posterior aspect).

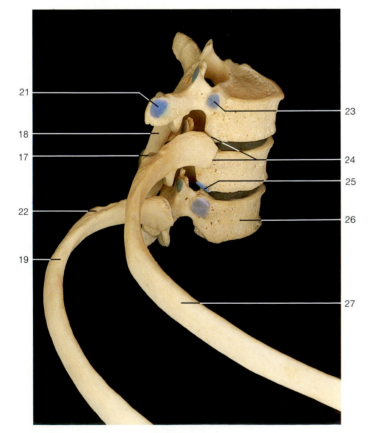

Costovertebral articulation (right lateral aspect).

1   Atlas
2   Axis
3   Cervical vertebrae
4   First thoracic vertebra
5   First rib
6   Facet for clavicle, clavicular notch
7   Manubrium sterni
8   Sternal angle
9   Body of sternum
10 Xiphoid process
11 Twelfth thoracic vertebra and rib
12 Jugular notch
13 Second rib
14 Costal cartilages
15 Infrasternal angle
16 Costal arch
17 Costotransverse joints between the transverse processes of thoracic vertebra and the tubercles of the ribs
18 Spinous processes
19 Costal angle
20 Transverse processes of lumbar vertebrae
21 Facet for articulation with rib
22 Tubercle of rib
23 Superior facet for articulation with head of rib
24 Articulation of head of rib with two vertebrae
25 Inferior facet for articulation with head of rib
26 Body of thoracic vertebra
27 Body or shaft of rib

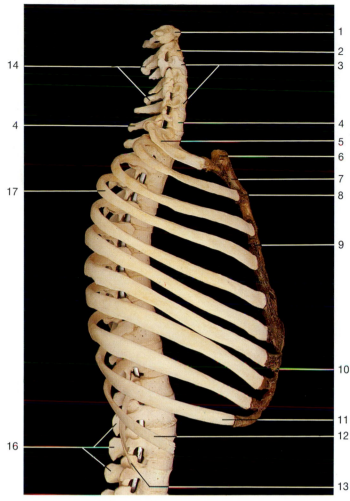

Skeleton of the thorax (right lateral aspect).

1   Atlas
2   Axis
3   Cervical vertebrae
4   Seventh cervical vertebra (vertebra prominens)
5   First rib
6   Facet for clavicle
7   Manubrium sterni
8   Sternal angle
9   Body of sternum
10 Costal arch
11 Tenth rib
12 Eleventh rib
13 Twelfth rib
14 Spinous processes of cervical vertebrae
15 Spinous processes of thoracic vertebrae
16 Spinous processes of lumbar vertebrae
17 Costal angle
18 Intervertebral foramina
19 Intervertebral discs
20 Cervical curvature
21 Thoracic curvature
22 Lumbar curvature
23 Sacrum

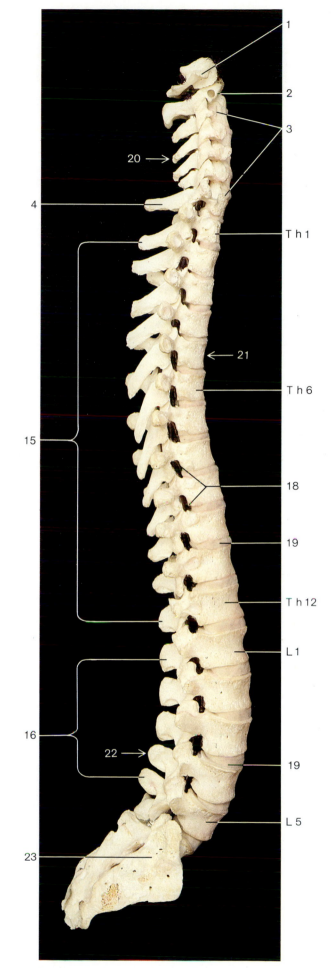

Vertebral column (right lateral aspect).

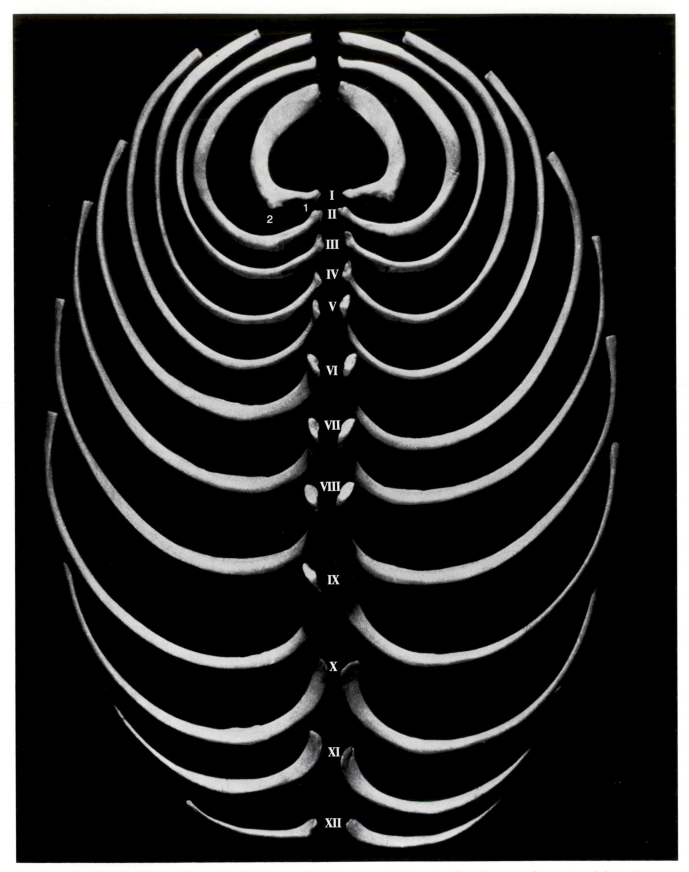

Disarticulated thorax skeleton. The twelve ribs arranged in a craniocaudal direction, first rib at top. Sternum and thoracic vertebrae omitted. I–XII = pairs of ribs; 1 = head of rib; 2 = neck of rib.

The head of a typical rib articulates with the bodies of adjacent vertebrae and the intervening intervertebral disc. The first seven ribs are directly connected through the costal cartilages (not depicted) to the sternum (true ribs) while the remaining five ribs (false ribs) are only indirectly connected to the sternum or end freely in the lateral wall of the trunk (floating ribs).

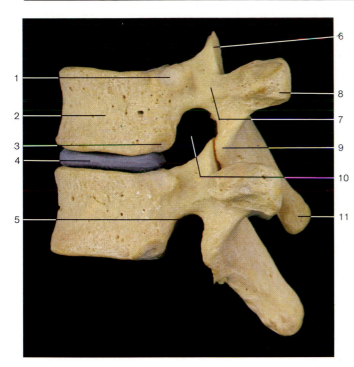

Two **thoracic vertebrae** (left lateral aspect).

1 Superior demifacet for head of rib
2 Body of vertebra
3 Inferior demifacet for head of rib
4 Intervertebral disc
5 Inferior vertebral notch
6 Superior articular facet and
   superior articular process
7 Pedicle
8 Transverse process and facet
   for tubercle of rib
9 Inferior articular process
10 Intervertebral foramen
11 Spinous process
12 Anterior longitudinal ligament
13 Intraarticular ligament
14 Radiate ligament
15 Superior costotransverse ligament
16 Neck of rib
17 Intertransverse ligament

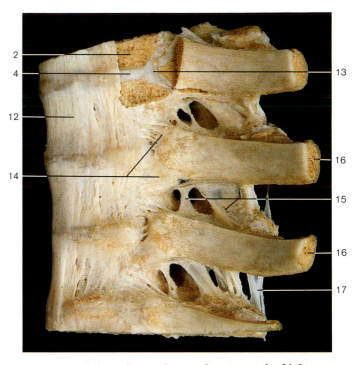

Ligaments of thoracic vertebrae and costovertebral joints
(left anterolateral aspect).
In the upper joint, most of the radiate ligament and the
anterior part of the head of the rib have been removed to
expose the two joint cavities and the interposed intraarticular ligament.

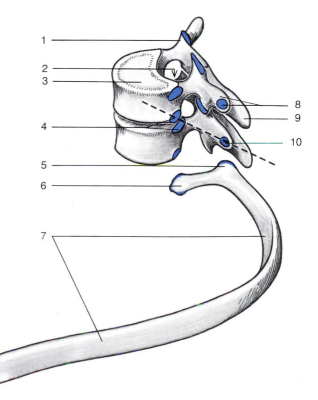

Costovertebral joints. (Schematic diagram) (W.).
Two thoracic vertebrae with an articulating rib (separated).
Axis of movement indicated by dotted line.
Blue = articular facets.

1 Superior articular process
2 Vertebral canal
3 Body of thoracic vertebra
4 Costovertebral joint (articular facets)
5 Tubercle of rib
6 Head of rib
7 Shaft of rib
8 Transverse process
   with articular facet
9 Spinous process
10 Costotransverse joint
   (articular facets)

181

Ligaments of the Vertebral Column

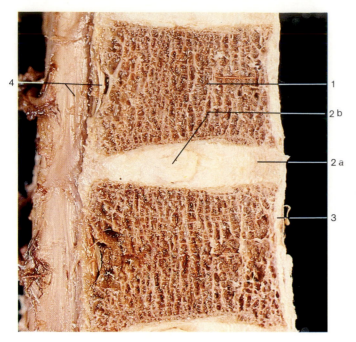

Median-sagittal section of the bodies of the vertebrae showing the **intervertebral discs,** each of which consists of an outer laminated portion and an inner core.

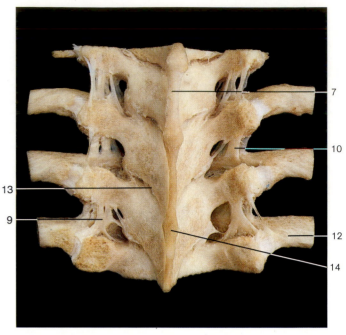

Ligaments of the vertebral column (dorsal aspect).

1 Body of vertebra
2 Intervertebral disc
  a Outer portion (anulus fibrosus)
  b Inner core (nucleus pulposus)
3 Anterior longitudinal ligament
4 Posterior longitudinal ligament and spinal dura mater
5 Transverse process of lumbar vertebra
6 Sacrum
7 Supraspinous ligament

8 Interspinous ligament
9 Intertransverse ligament
10 Superior costotransverse ligament
11 Transverse process of thoracic vertebra
12 Rib
13 Ligamentum flavum
14 Spinous process
15 Intervertebral foramen

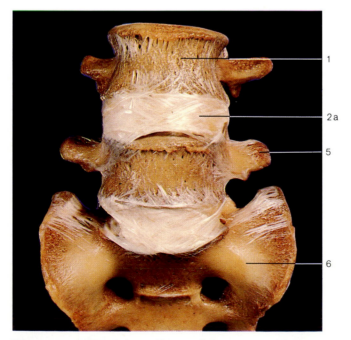

The two caudal lumbar vertebrae and the sacrum with their intervertebral discs (anterior aspect).

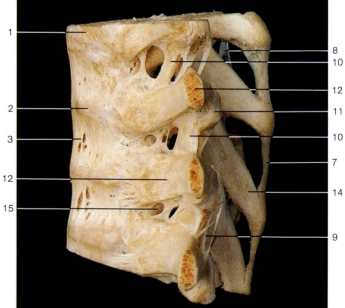

Ligaments of the vertebral column, thoracic part (left lateral aspect).

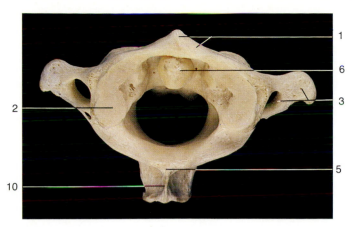

Atlas and axis (from above).

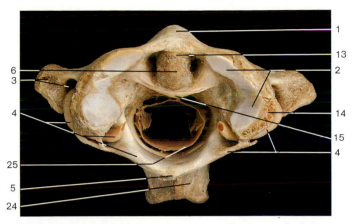

Median atlantoaxial joint and transverse ligament of atlas (from above). Dens of axis partly severed.

1	Anterior arch of atlas with anterior tubercle	14	Articular capsule of **atlantooccipital joint**
2	Superior articular facet of atlas	15	Transverse ligament of atlas
3	Vertebrarterial foramen and transverse process	16	Occipital bone
4	Posterior arch of atlas and vertebral artery	17	**Atlantooccipital joint**
5	Posterior tubercle of atlas	18	**Lateral atlantoaxial joint**
6	Dens of axis	19	Third cervical vertebra
7	Superior articular surface of axis	20	Superior longitudinal band of cruciform ligament
8	Body of axis	21	Alar ligaments
9	Pedicle and lamina of axis	22	Transverse ligament of atlas
10	Spinous process	23	Inferior longitudinal band of cruciform ligament
11	Inferior articular process	24	Spinous process of axis
12	Transverse process and vertebrarterial foramen	25	Dura mater
13	**Median atlantoaxial joint** (anterior part)		

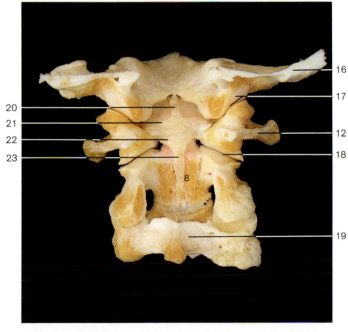

Atlantooccipital and atlantoaxial joints (posterior aspect). Posterior part of occipital bone, posterior arch of atlas and axis have been removed to show the cruciform ligament.

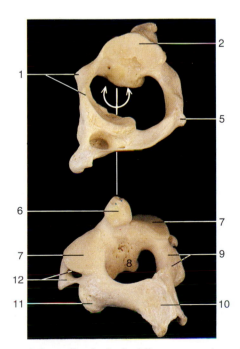

Atlas and axis. Left oblique posterolateral aspect, demonstrating the articulation of the dens of axis with atlas (cf. arrows).

183

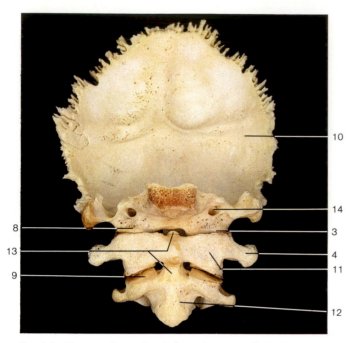

Occipital bone, atlas and axis (anterior aspect).

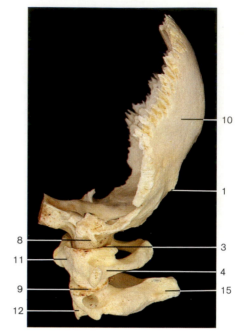

Occipital bone, atlas and axis (left lateral aspect).

1 External occipital protuberance
2 Foramen magnum
3 Atlantooccipital joint
4 Transverse process of atlas
5 Membrana tectoria
6 Posterior longitudinal ligament
7 Spinous process of third cervical vertebra
8 Occipital condyle

9 Lateral atlantoaxial joint
10 Occipital bone
11 Atlas
12 Axis
13 Dens of axis
14 Hypoglossal canal
15 Spinous processes of axis
16 Anterior longitudinal ligament

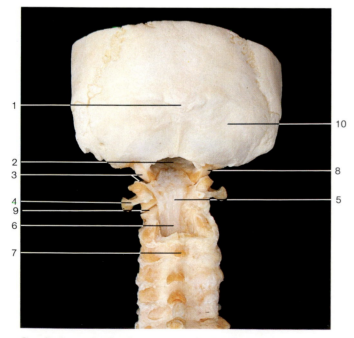

Cervical vertebral column and skull with ligaments
(posterior aspect). Posterior arch of atlas and axis removed
to show the membrana tectoria.

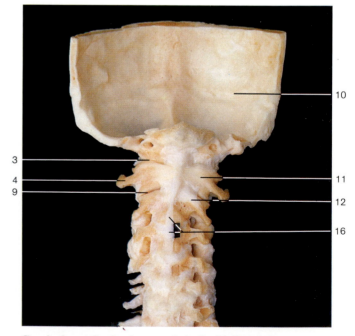

Cervical vertebral column and skull with ligaments
(anterior aspect). Anterior part of occipital bone removed.

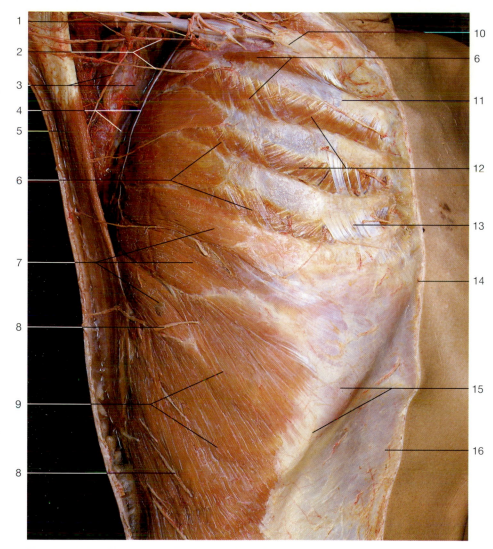

1	Axillary vein
2	Intercostobrachial nerves
3	Subscapular muscle, thoracodorsal nerve
4	Long thoracic nerve, lateral thoracic artery and vein
5	Latissimus dorsi muscle
6	External intercostal muscles
7	Serratus anterior muscle
8	Lateral cutaneous branches of intercostal nerves
9	External oblique muscle of abdomen
10	Clavicle (divided)
11	Second rib (costo-chondral junction)
12	Internal intercostal muscles
13	External intercostal membrane
14	Position of xiphoid process
15	Costal arch or margin
16	Anterior layer of rectus sheath

Muscles of the thorax, superficial layer (lateral aspect). Upper limb elevated. Pectoralis major and minor have been removed.

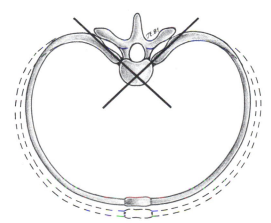

Effect of intercostal muscles on the costovertebral and costotransverse joints (Tr.). Axes of movement indicated by lines; direction of movements indicated by arrows.

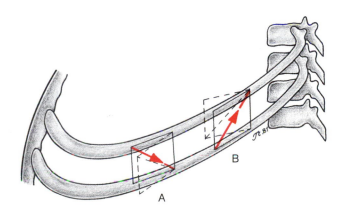

A   Action of internal intercostal muscles (expiration)
B   Action of external intercostal muscles (inspiration)

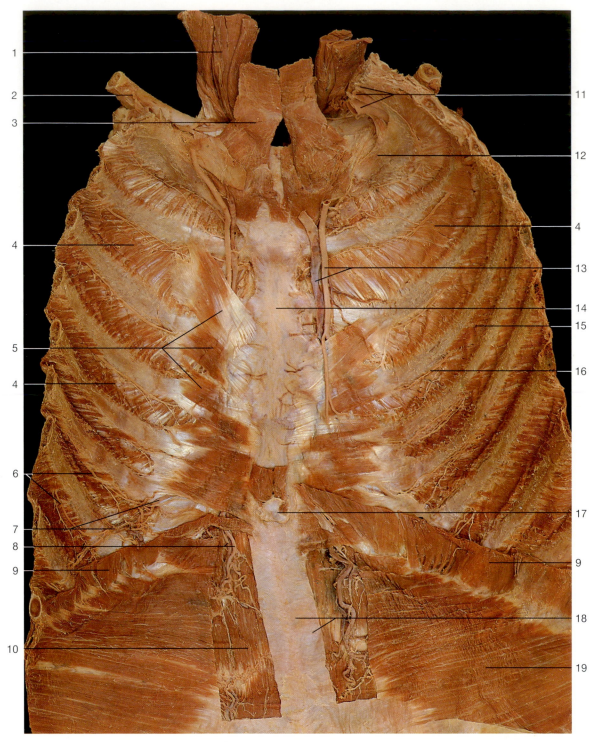

Anterior thoracic wall (posterior aspect). Diaphragm partly removed, posterior layer of rectus sheath fenestrated on both sides.

1 Sternocleidomastoid (divided)	11 Subclavian artery, brachial plexus
2 Clavicle	12 First rib
3 Sternothyroid muscle	13 Internal thoracic artery and vein
4 Internal intercostal muscle	14 Sternum
5 Transversus thoracis	15 Innermost intercostal muscle
6 Intercostal arteries and nerves	16 Intercostal artery and vein
7 Musculophrenic artery	17 Xiphoid process
8 Superior epigastric artery and vein	18 Linea alba, posterior layer of
9 Diaphragm (divided)	rectus sheath
10 Rectus abdominis muscle	19 Transversus abdominis

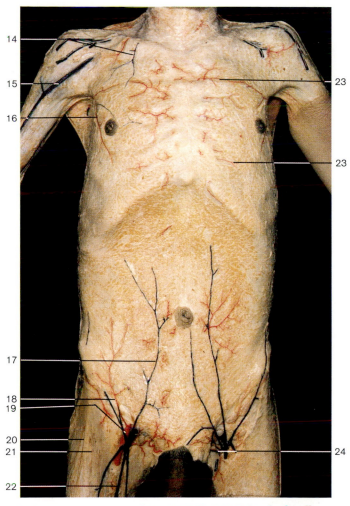

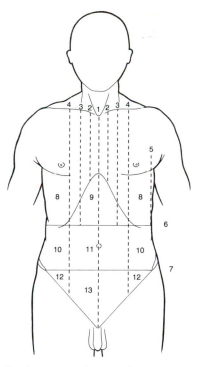

Regions and reference lines

for delineating surface projections. (Schematic diagram.)

Subcutaneous vessels of the thoracic and abdominal wall.

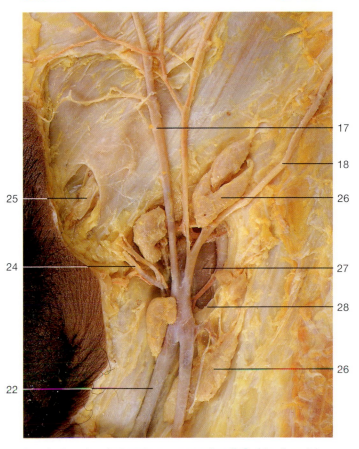

Inguinal region and saphenous opening (left side, female).

Reference lines and regions

1 Median line
2 Lateral sternal line
3 Parasternal line
4 Left lateral or midclavicular line
5 Midaxillary line
6 Transpyloric plane
7 Transtubercular plane
8 Hypochondriac region
9 Epigastric region
10 Lumbar region
11 Umbilical region
12 Iliac region
13 Hypogastric region

Subcutaneous vessels and nerves

14 Supraclavicular nerves
15 Cephalic vein
16 Thoracoepigastric vein
17 Superficial epigastric vein
18 Superficial circumflex iliac vein
19 Femoral artery and vein
20 Lateral femoral cutaneous nerve
21 Anterior femoral cutaneous nerves
22 Great saphenous vein
23 Anterior cutaneous branches of intercostal nerves
24 Superficial external pudendal vein
25 Round ligament and fat pad, superficial inguinal ring
26 Superficial inguinal nodes
27 Saphenous opening
28 Falciform margin

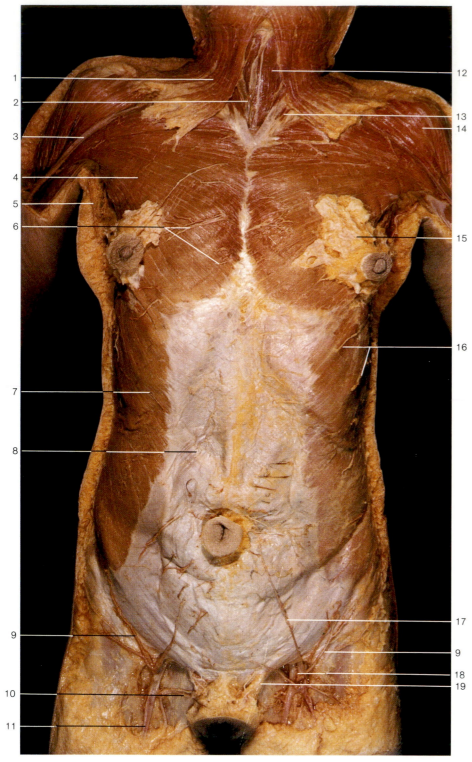

1 Platysma
2 Anterior jugular vein
3 Cephalic vein
4 Pectoralis major
5 Thoracoepigastric vein
6 Anterior cutaneous branches
  of intercostal nerves
7 External oblique muscle
8 Sheath of rectus abdominis;
  anterior layer
9 Superficial circumflex iliac artery
  and vein
10 Superficial external pudendal artery
   and vein
11 Great saphenous vein
12 Sternohyoid
13 Sternocleidomastoid
14 Deltoid
15 Mammary gland
16 Lateral cutaneous branches
   of intercostal nerves
17 Superficial epigastric vein
18 Femoral artery and vein
19 Round ligament

Superficial layer of the thoracic and abdominal wall (female).

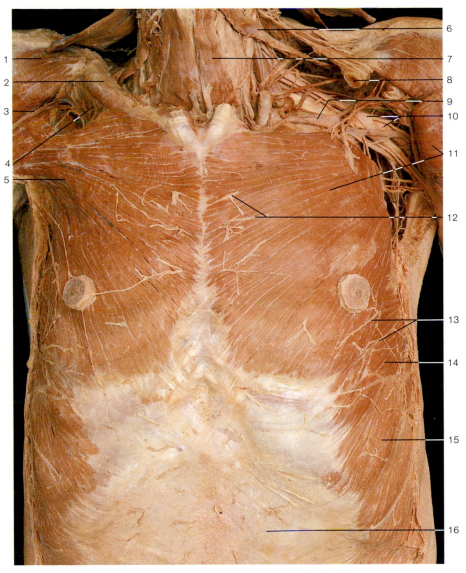

1 Deltoid
2 Right clavicle
3 Cephalic vein
4 Deltopectoral triangle
5 Right pectoralis major
6 Omohyoid
7 Sternohyoid
8 Left clavicle (divided)
9 Subclavian vein
10 Brachial plexus and subclavian artery
11 Left pectoralis major (reflected)
12 Anterior cutaneous branches of intercostal nerves and vessels
13 Lateral cutaneous branches of intercostal nerves
14 Serratus anterior
15 External oblique
16 Rectus sheath
17 Axillary artery
18 Intercostobrachial nerves
19 Thoracodorsal nerve
20 Long thoracic nerve
21 Latissimus dorsi
22 Serratus anterior muscle
23 Thoracoacromial artery
24 Clavicle
25 External intercostal muscle
26 Third rib
27 Internal intercostal muscle
28 Anterior intercostal artery and vein
29 Costal arch or margin

Thoracic wall I (anterior aspect). Left clavicle has been divided and pectoralis major and minor on the left side have been cut and reflected to show the brachial plexus.

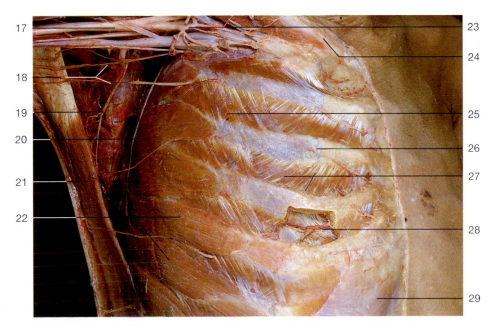

Thoracic wall (lateral aspect). Pectoralis major and minor removed. 4th rib fenestrated.

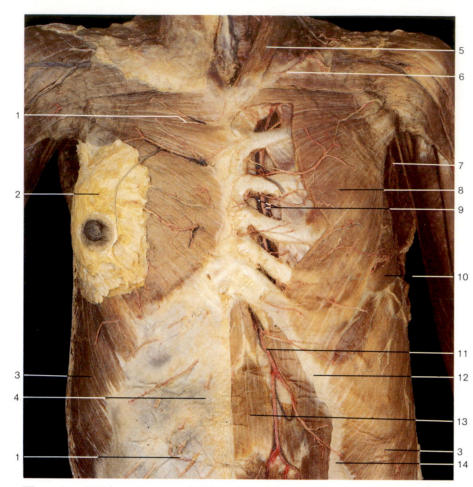

1 Anterior perforating branches of intercostal artery, vein and nerve
2 Mammary gland
3 External oblique
4 Rectus sheath
5 Sternocleidomastoid
6 Clavicle
7 Lateral thoracic artery and vein
8 Pectoralis major
9 Internal thoracic artery and vein
10 Serratus anterior
11 Superior epigastric artery and vein
12 Costal margin
13 Rectus abdominis
14 Cut edge of the anterior layer of the rectus sheath

Thoracic wall II (anterior aspect). Dissection of the **internal thoracic artery and vein.** Left pectoralis major partly removed. Anterior lamina of the rectus sheath on the left side removed.

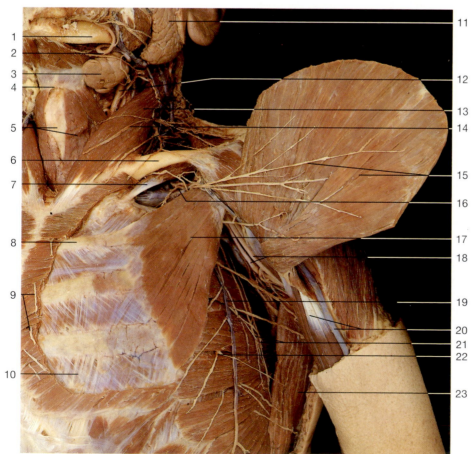

1 Mandible
2 Facial artery
3 Submandibular gland
4 Hyoid bone
5 Larynx, infrahyoid muscles
6 Clavicle
7 Subclavius muscle
8 Second rib
9 Anterior cutaneous branches of intercostal nerves
10 External intercostal membrane
11 Parotid gland
12 External carotid artery
13 Sternocleidomastoid, cutaneous branches of cervical plexus
14 Supraclavicular nerves
15 Pectoralis major, medial pectoral nerves
16 Thoracoacromial artery
17 **Pectoralis minor**
18 Median and ulnar nerve
19 Thoracoepigastric vein
20 Cephalic vein, long head of biceps muscle
21 Lateral thoracic artery, long thoracic nerve
22 Lateral cutaneous branches of intercostal nerve
23 Latissimus dorsi

Thoracic wall III (anterior aspect). Pectoralis major has been divided and reflected.

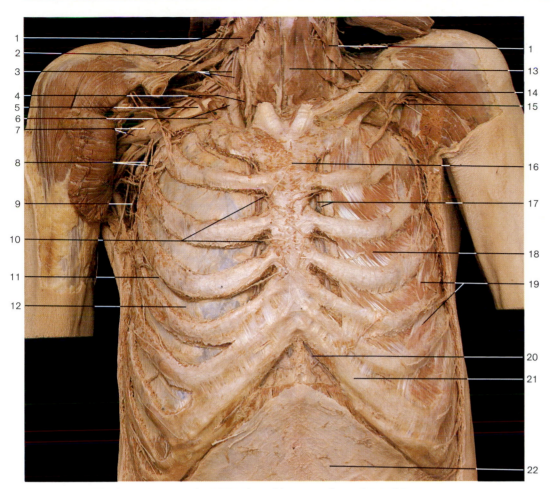

Thoracic wall IV (anterior aspect). Dissection of intercostal muscles and nerves. Internal and external intercostal muscles have been removed on the right side.

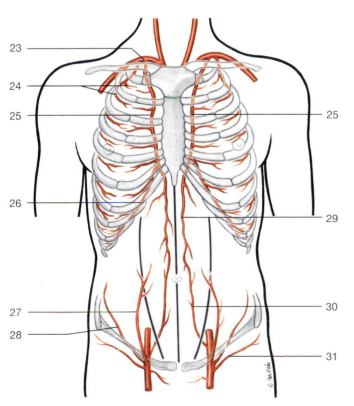

Main arteries of thoracic and abdominal wall (W.).

1　Omohyoid
2　Supraclavicular nerves
3　Phrenic nerve and ascending cervical artery
4　Thyrocervical trunk, transverse cervical artery
5　Brachial plexus and subclavian artery
6　Internal jugular and subclavian vein
7　Median nerve and brachial artery
8　Lateral thoracic artery and vein, long thoracic nerve
9　Thoracodorsal artery, vein and nerve
10　Anterior cutaneous branches of intercostal nerves and vessels
11　Intercostal nerve (T_4)
12　Endothoracic fascia, parietal pleura
13　Sternohyoid
14　Clavicle
15　Thoracoacromial artery and cephalic vein
16　Manubrium sterni
17　Internal thoracic artery and vein
18　Internal intercostal muscle
19　External intercostal muscle
20　Superior epigastric artery and vein
21　Costal margin
22　Rectus sheath
23　Subclavian artery
24　Highest intercostal artery
25　Internal thoracic artery
26　Musculophrenic artery
27　Superficial epigastric artery
28　Deep circumflex iliac artery
29　Superior epigastric artery
30　Inferior epigastric artery
31　Superficial circumflex iliac artery

Dissection of the Abdominal Wall

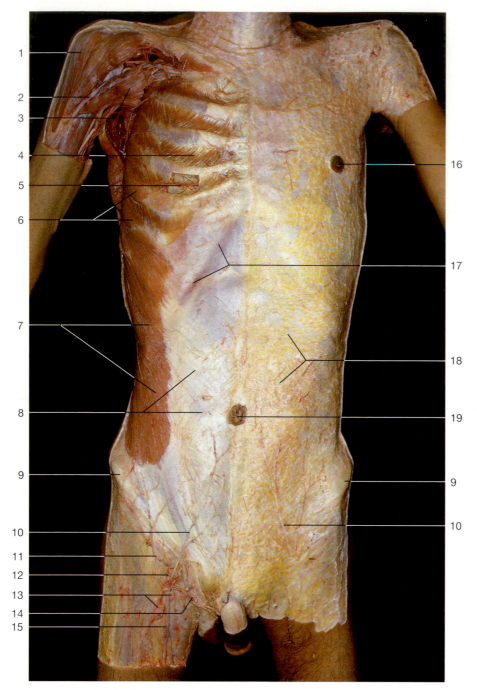

1   Deltoid muscle
2   Cephalic vein
3   Pectoralis major (divided)
4   Internal intercostal muscle
5   Intercostal artery and vein
    (intercostal space, fenestrated)
6   Serratus anterior muscle
7   External oblique muscle of
    abdomen
8   Anterior layer of rectus sheath
9   Iliac crest
10 Superficial epigastric vein
11 Superficial circumflex iliac vein
12 Saphenous opening
13 Superficial inguinal nodes
14 Superficial external pudendal veins
15 Great saphenous vein
16 Nipple
17 Costal margin
18 Subcutaneous fatty tissue
19 Umbilicus

Thoracic and abdominal wall I. Right pectoralis major and minor divided.
Muscles of thoracic and abdominal wall on right side are displayed.

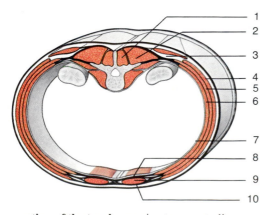

Cross-section of the trunk superior to arcuate line.
(Schematic drawing.)

1   Medial column of intrinsic muscles
    of the back
2   Lateral column of erector spinae
3   Thoracolumbar fascia with
    superficial and deep layer
4   External oblique
5   Internal oblique
6   Transversus abdominis
7   Fascia transversalis
8   Posterior layer of rectus sheath
9   Rectus abdominis
10 Anterior layer of rectus sheath

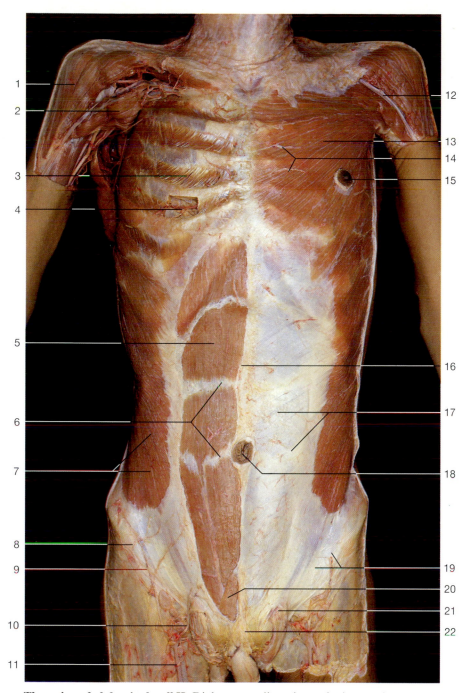

1	Deltoid muscle
2	Pectoralis major (divided)
3	Internal intercostal muscle
4	Intercostal artery and vein
5	**Rectus abdominis**
6	Tendinous intersections
7	**External oblique**
8	Anterior superior iliac spine
9	Superficial circumflex iliac vein
10	Superficial epigastric vein
11	Great saphenous vein
12	Cephalic vein
13	Pectoralis major
14	Anterior cutaneous branches of intercostal nerves
15	Nipple
16	Linea alba
17	Anterior layer of rectus sheath
18	Umbilicus
19	Inguinal ligament
20	Pyramidalis muscle
21	Superficial inguinal ring and spermatic cord
22	Suspensory ligament of penis
23	Longissimus and iliocostalis
24	Multifidus
25	Quadratus lumborum
26	Latissimus dorsi
27	Psoas major
28	Spinous process
29	Body of 1st lumbar vertebra
30	Diaphragm
31	Rib

Thoracic and abdominal wall II. Right pectoralis major and minor and anteroir layer of rectus sheath have been removed on the right side.

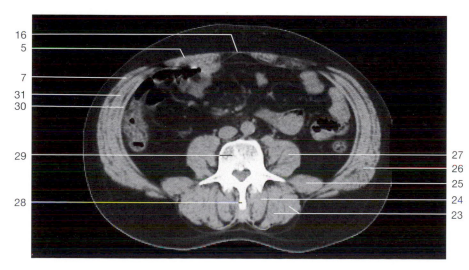

Horizontal section through the body at the level of 1st lumbar vertebra; seen from below. CT-Scan.

193

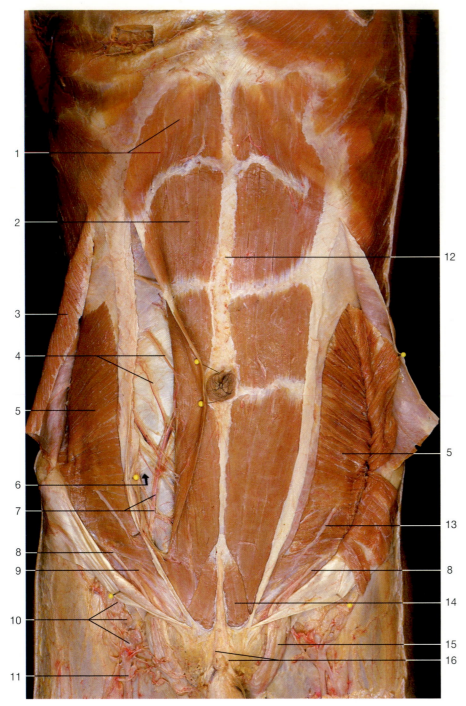

1 Costal margin
2 Rectus abdominis
3 External oblique (reflected)
4 Intercostal nerves with
   accompanying vessels
5 Internal oblique
6 Arcuate line (arrow)
7 Inferior epigastric artery and vein
8 Ilioinguinal nerve
9 Position of deep inguinal ring
10 Superficial inguinal nodes
11 Great saphenous vein
12 Linea alba
13 Iliohypogastric nerve
14 Pyramidalis muscle
15 Spermatic cord
16 Fundiform ligament of penis

Thoracic and abdominal wall III. External oblique muscle of abdomen has been divided and reflected on both sides. The right rectus has been reflected medially to display the posterior layer of rectus sheath.

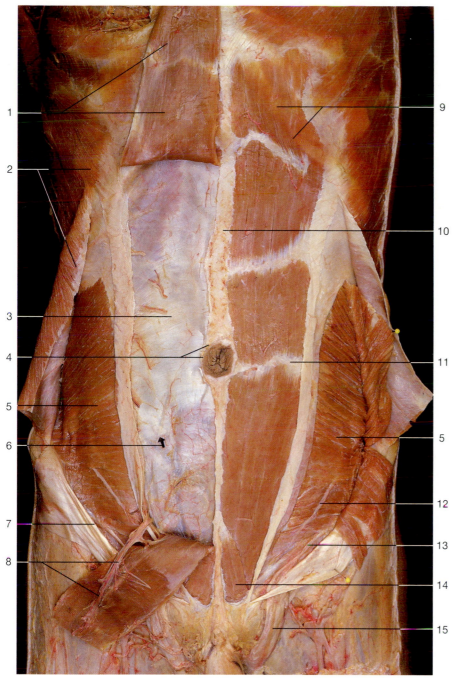

1 Rectus abdominis (reflected)
2 External oblique muscle of abdomen (divided)
3 Posterior layer of rectus sheath
4 Umbilical ring
5 Internal oblique muscle of abdomen
6 Arcuate line (arrow)
7 Inguinal ligament
8 Inferior epigastric artery and vein, rectus abdominis (divided and reflected)
9 Costal margin
10 Linea alba
11 Tendinous intersection
12 Iliohypogastric nerve
13 Ilioinguinal nerve
14 Pyramidalis muscle
15 Spermatic cord

Thoracic and abdominal wall IV. External oblique muscle of abdomen has been divided and reflected on both sides. The right rectus has been cut and reflected to display the posterior layer of rectus sheath.

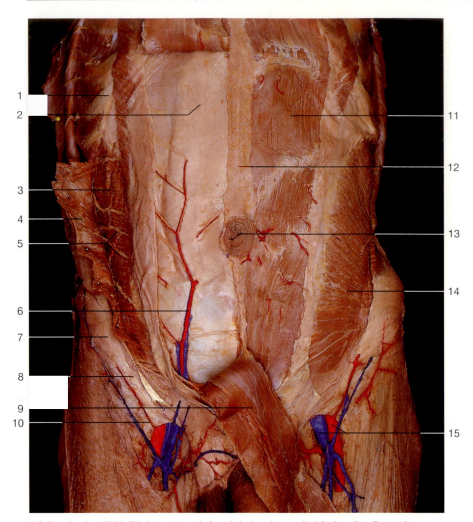

Abdominal wall V. Right rectus abdominis has been divided and reflected to display the inferior epigastric vessels. Right internal oblique has been reflected to show the segmental arrangement of abdominal wall nerves.

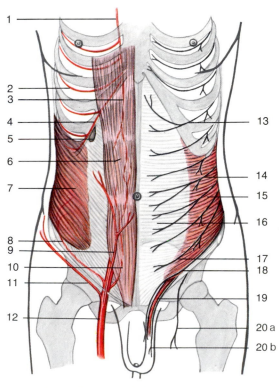

Arteries and nerves which supply the thoracic and abdominal wall. Note their segmental arrangement. (Schematic drawing.)

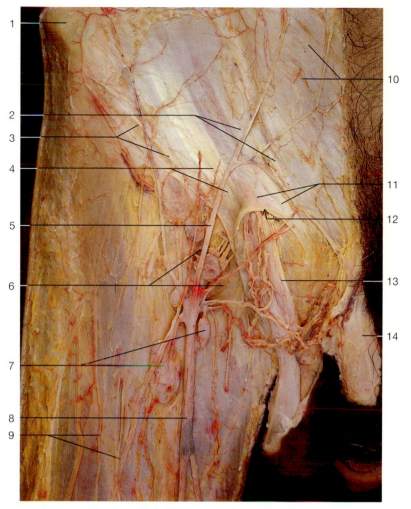

1 Anterior superior iliac spine
2 Medial crus of inguinal ring
3 Inguinal ligament
4 Lateral crus of inguinal ring
5 Superficial epigastric vein
6 Saphenous opening
7 Superficial inguinal nodes
8 Great saphenous vein
9 Anterior cutaneous nerves of femoral nerve
10 Anterior layer of rectus sheath
11 Intercrural fibers
12 Superficial inguinal ring
13 Spermatic cord, genital branch
   of genitofemoral nerve
14 Penis
15 Aponeurosis of external oblique (divided and
   reflected)
16 Internal oblique
17 Ilioinguinal nerve
18 Anterior cutaneous branches of iliohypogastric
   nerve
19 Superficial external pudendal veins

Inguinal canal in the male I. Dissection of superficial layer (anterior aspect, right side).

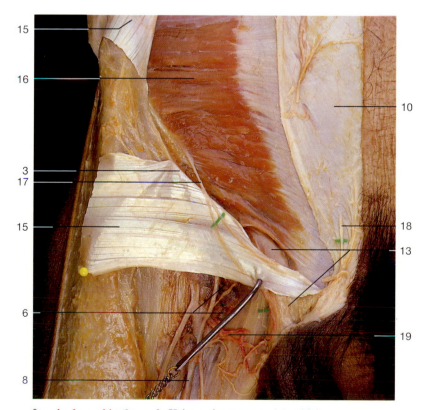

Inguinal canal in the male II (anterior aspect, right side).
The external oblique has been divided to display the inguinal canal.

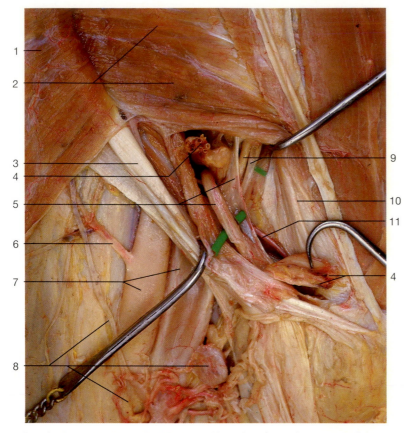

1 Internal oblique (reflected)
2 Transversus abdominis
3 Inguinal ligament
4 **Spermatic cord** with the exception of the ductus deferens (divided and reflected)
5 **Ductus deferens,** interfoveolar ligament
6 Superficial circumflex iliac artery
7 Femoral artery and vein
8 Superficial inguinal nodes, inguinal lymph vessel
9 **Inferior epigastric artery and vein**
10 Inguinal aponeurotic falx (cut)
11 Pubic branch of inferior epigastric artery
12 Superficial inguinal ring
13 Penis
14 External oblique
15 Anterior superior iliac spine
16 Intercrural fibers
17 Inguinal lymph nodes
18 Fascia lata and sartorius
19 Saphenous opening, great saphenous vein
20 Femoral artery and vein
21 Spermatic cord and cremaster muscle
22 Suspensory ligament of the penis
23 Internal spermatic fascia
24 Tunica vaginalis
25 Testis and epididymis

Inguinal canal in the male III. Deep dissection (anterior aspect, right side). Spermatic cord with exception of deferent duct (probe) has been divided and reflected.

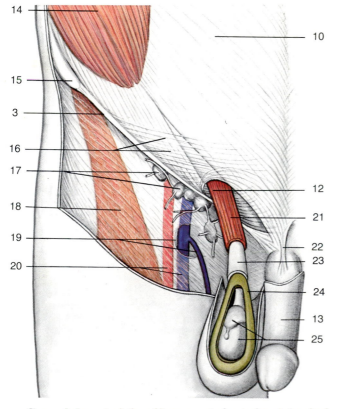

General characteristics of lower part of anterior abdominal wall and inguinal canal. (Schematic drawing.)

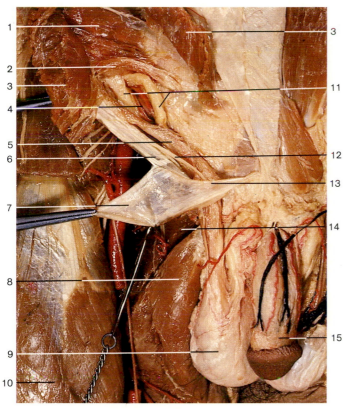

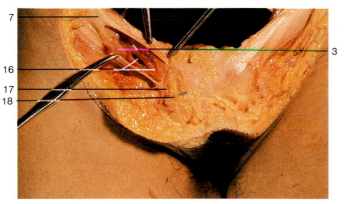

Inguinal canal in the male, right side, deep dissection (anterior aspect). Internal oblique divided and reflected.

1 Transversus abdominis
2 Deep inguinal ring
3 Internal oblique
4 Inferior epigastric vessels
5 Spermatic cord with ductus deferens
6 Inguinal ligament
7 Aponeurosis of external oblique
8 Adductor longus
9 Testis
10 Rectus femoris
11 Fatty tissue
12 Ilioinguinal nerve
13 Superficial inguinal ring
14 Pectineus
15 Penis
16 Round ligament
17 Genitofemoral nerve
18 Terminal fibers of the round ligament
19 External oblique
20 Skin of scrotum, dartos muscle, external spermatic fascia
21 Cremaster muscle, cremasteric fascia
22 Internal spermatic fascia (green)
23 Ductus deferens
24 Epididymis
25 Peritoneum (red)
26 Vestige of processus vaginalis (red dotted line)
27 Parietal and visceral layer of tunica vaginalis (red)

Inguinal canal in the female, right side (anterior aspect).

Inguinal herniae may either pass through the canal (indirect inguinal herniae) or directly penetrate the abdominal wall at the level of the superficial inguinal ring (direct herniae). Femoral herniae generally protrude through the femoral ring below the inguinal ligament. Proper assessment of the site of herniation requires the identification of both the inguinal ligament and the inferior epigastric artery.

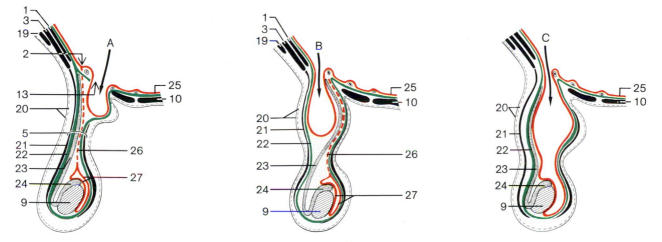

Different types of herniae. Note the different layers of different wall which surround each type of hernia.
A = direct inguinal hernia; B = indirect acquired inguinal hernia; C = congenital indirect inguinal hernia.

Dorsal Muscles of the Trunk

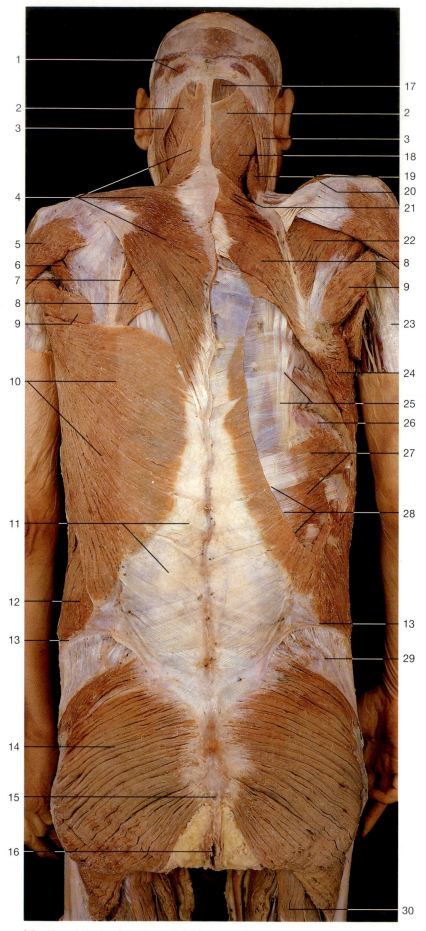

1 Occipital belly of occipitofrontalis muscle
2 Splenius capitis
3 Sternocleidomastoid
4 Trapezius
5 Deltoid muscle
6 Teres minor
7 Medial margin of scapula
8 Rhomboideus major
9 Teres major
10 Latissimus dorsi
11 Thoracolumbar fascia
12 External oblique
13 Iliac crest
14 Gluteus maximus
15 Position of last coccygeal vertebra
16 Anus
17 Semispinalis capitis
18 Splenius cervicis
19 Levator scapulae
20 Spine of scapula
21 Rhomboideus minor
22 Infraspinatus muscle
23 Triceps brachii
24 Serratus anterior
25 Iliocostalis
26 External intercostal muscle
27 Serratus posterior inferior
28 Latissimus dorsi (cut edge)
29 Fascia over gluteus medius
30 Long head of biceps femoris

Muscles of the back I. Superficial layer on the left, deeper layer on the right. Right latissimus dorsi and trapezius are removed.

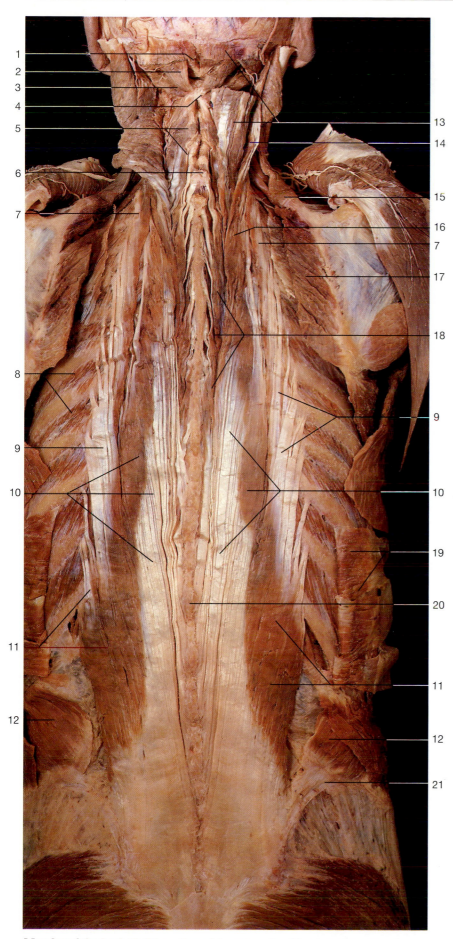

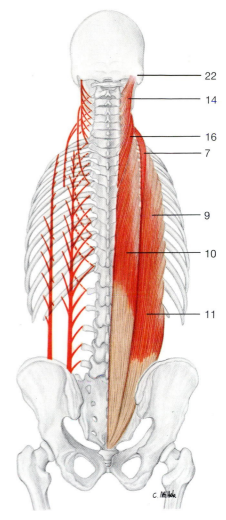

Origin and insertion of erector spinae muscles. (Schematic drawing) (W.).

Muscles of the back II. Dissection of deep muscles. Erector spinae muscle.

1   Rectus capitis posterior minor
2   Rectus capitis posterior major
3   Obliquus capitis inferior
4   Spinous process of axis
5   Semispinalis cervicis
6   Spinous process of seventh vertebra
7   **Iliocostalis cervicis**
8   External intercostal muscles
9   **Iliocostalis thoracis**
10 **Longissimus thoracis**
11 **Iliocostalis lumborum**
12 Internal oblique of abdomen
13 Semispinalis capitis (divided)
14 **Longissimus capitis**
15 Levator scapulae
16 **Longissimus cervicis**
17 Rhomboideus major
18 Spinalis thoracis
19 Inferior posterior serratus (reflected)
20 Spinous process of second lumbar vertebra
21 Iliac crest
22 Mastoid process

201

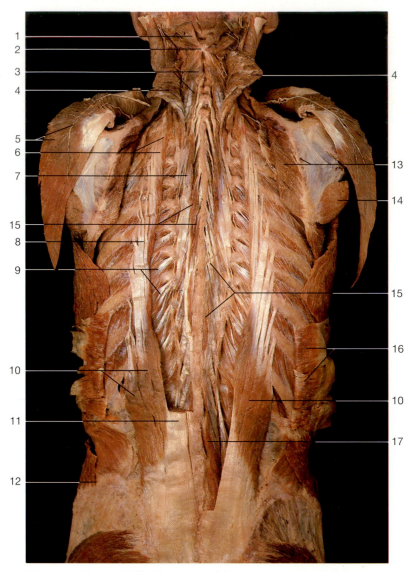

1	Rectus capitis posterior major
2	Spinous process of axis
3	Semispinalis cervicis
4	Semispinalis capitis (reflected)
5	Trapezius (reflected), accessory nerve
6	**Iliocostalis cervicis**
7	Semispinalis thoracis
8	**Iliocostalis thoracis**
9	Levatores costarum
10	**Iliocostalis lumborum**
11	Longissimus (divided)
12	Iliac crest
13	Rhomboideus major (divided), medial margin of scapula
14	Teres major
15	Spinalis thoracis
16	Serratus posterior inferior (reflected)
17	Multifidus
18	External intercostal muscle
19	Tendons of iliocostalis thoracis
20	Transverse process of thoracic vertebra
21	Rotatores (short)
22	Rotatores (long)
23	Supraspinous ligament above spinous processes
24	Intertransverse ligament

Muscles of the back III. Dissection of deep muscles, Longissimus removed on both sides. Semispinalis capitis has been divided and reflected.

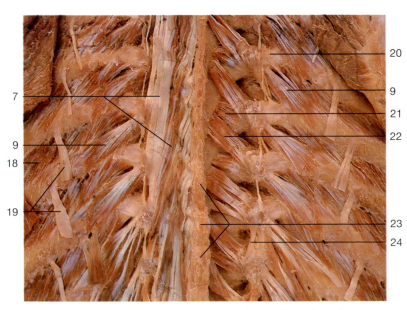

Muscles of the back IV. Short back muscles in the thoracic region. On the right, semispinalis has been removed.

On the back, the deepest muscles cover only 1 or 2 segments (e. g. rotatores muscles), whereas the muscles closer to the surface are longer and cover several segments (e. g. multifidus, semispinalis). The muscles closest to the surface (trapezius, latissimus) are girdle muscles of the upper limb.

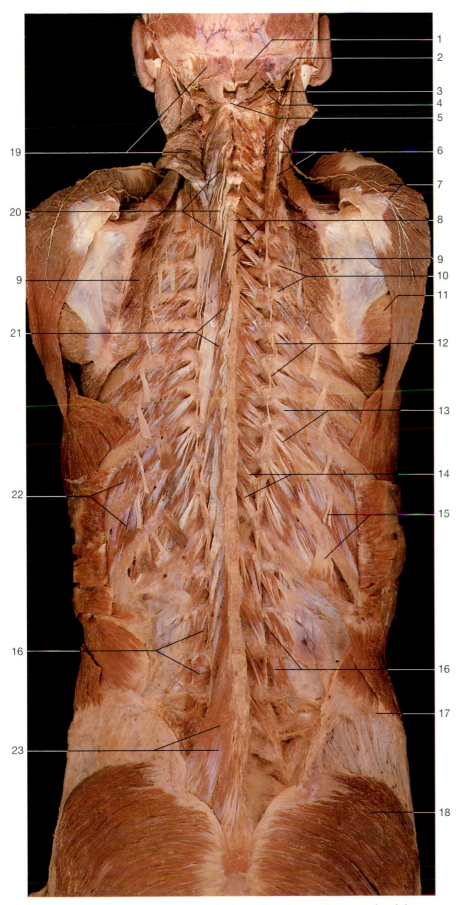

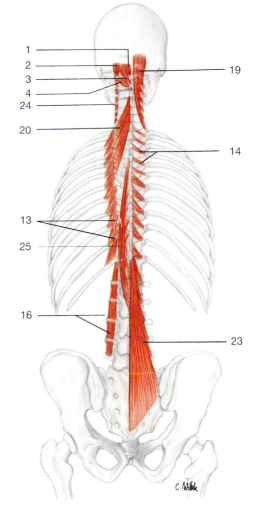

Medial column of intrinsic muscles of the back. Transversospinal and intertransversal system. (Schematic drawing) (W.).

1   Rectus capitis posterior minor
2   Obliquus capitis superior
3   Rectus capitis posterior major
4   Obliquus capitis inferior
5   Spinous process of axis
6   Longissimus capitis
7   Trapezius (reflected), accessory
    nerve (n. XI)
8   Spinous processes
9   Rhomboideus major
10 Transverse processes of thoracic
    vertebrae
11 Teres major
12 Intertransverse ligaments
13 Levatores costarum
14 Rotatores
15 Tendons of iliocostalis
16 Intertransversarii lumborum (lateral)
17 Iliac crest
18 Gluteus maximus
19 Semispinalis capitis
20 Semispinalis cervicis
21 Semispinalis thoracis
22 External intercostal muscles
23 Multifidus
24 Intertransversarii posterior cervicis
25 Spinalis thoracis

Muscles of the back V. Transversospinal muscles, deepest layer on the right, where all parts of semispinalis and multifidus have been removed.

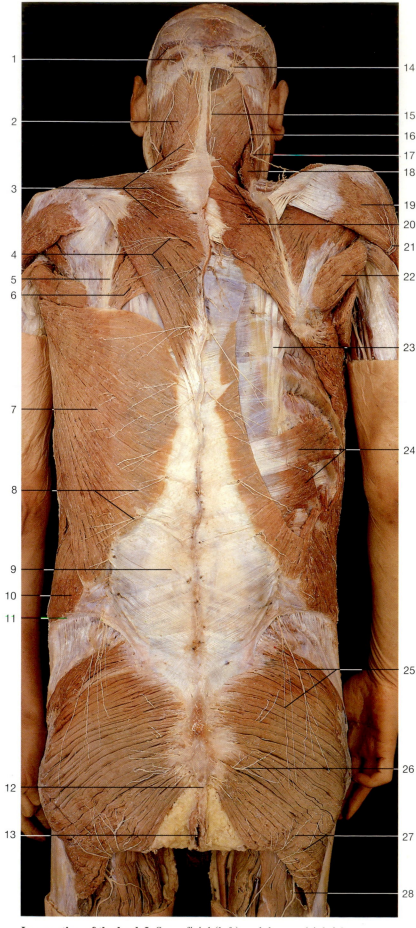

Innervation of the back I. Superficial (left) and deeper (right) layers (right). Right trapezius and latissimus dorsi removed.

1 Occipital belly of occipitofrontalis muscle
2 Splenius capitis
3 Trapezius
4 Medial cutaneous branches of dorsal rami of spinal nerves
5 Medial margin of scapula
6 Rhomboideus major
7 Latissimus dorsi
8 Lateral cutaneous branches of dorsal rami of spinal nerves
9 Thoracolumbar fascia
10 External oblique
11 Iliac crest
12 Last coccygeal vertebra
13 Anus
14 Greater occipital nerve
15 Third occipital nerve
16 Lesser occipital nerve
17 Cutaneous branches of cervical plexus
18 Levator scapulae
19 Deltoid muscle
20 Rhomboideus major and minor
21 Upper lateral cutaneous nerve of arm (branch of axillary nerve)
22 Teres major
23 Iliocostalis thoracis
24 Serratus posterior inferior muscle
25 Superior clunial nerves
26 Middle clunial nerves
27 Inferior clunial nerves
28 Posterior femoral cutaneous nerve

▷
To page 205:
1 Trapezius
2 Infraspinatus muscle
3 Left latissimus dorsi
4 Thoracolumbar fascia
5 Splenius cervicis
6 Serratus posterior superior
7 Medial branches of dorsal rami of thoracic spinal nerves
8 Lateral branches of dorsal rami of thoracic spinal nerves
9 Iliocostalis
10 Serratus posterior inferior
11 Latissimus dorsi

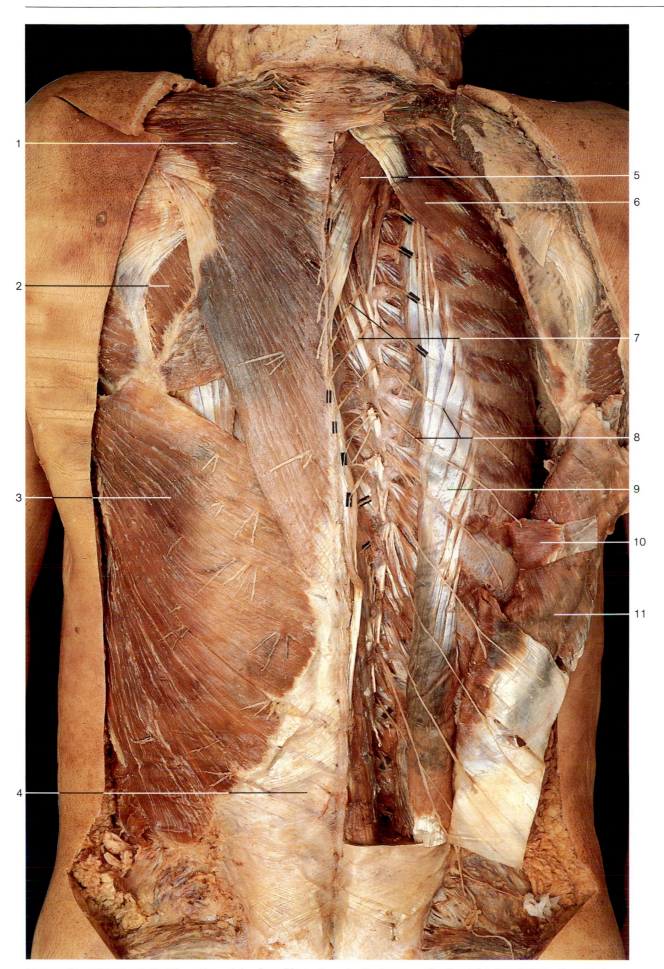

Innervation of the back II. Dissection of the dorsal branches of spinal nerves. On the right, longissimus thoracis has been removed and iliocostalis laterally reflected.

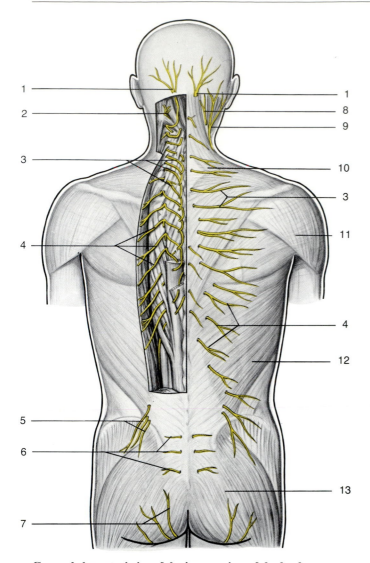

1 Greater occipital nerve (C_2)
2 Suboccipital nerve (C_1)
3 Medial branches of dorsal rami of spinal nerves
4 Lateral branches of dorsal rami of spinal nerves
5 Superior clunial nerves (L_1–L_3)
6 Middle clunial nerves (S_1–S_3)
7 Inferior clunial nerves, derived from branches of the sacral plexus (ventral rami)
8 Lesser occipital nerve
9 Great auricular nerve
10 Trapezius
11 Deltoid
12 Latissimus dorsi
13 Gluteus maximus
14 External intercostal muscle
15 Internal intercostal muscle
16 Innermost intercostal muscle
17 Dorsal ramus of spinal nerve
18 Spinal nerve and spinal ganglion
19 Sympathetic trunk with ganglion
20 Intercostal nerve
21 Lateral cutaneous branch ⎫ of intercostal nerve
22 Anterior cutaneous branch ⎭

General characteristics of the innervation of the back.
Distribution of dorsal branches of spinal nerves. Note the segmental arrangement of the innervation of the dorsal part of the trunk. (Schematic drawing.)

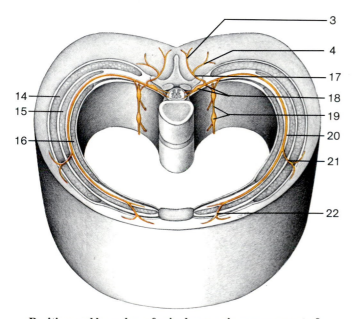

Position and branches of spinal nerves in one segment of thoracic wall (O.).

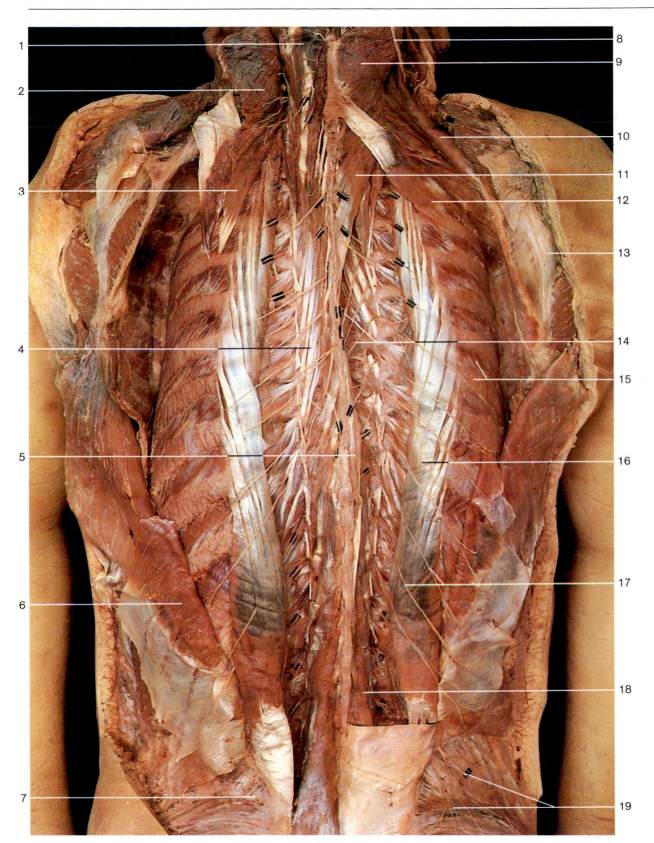

Innervation of the back III. Deeper layer (dorsal aspect).

1 Semispinalis capitis
2 Left splenius capitis (cut and reflected)
3 Left splenius cervicis (cut and reflected)
4 Semispinalis thoracis
5 Spinalis thoracis
6 Latissimus dorsi

7 Iliac crest
8 Lesser occipital nerve
9 Splenius capitis
10 Levator scapulae
11 Splenius cervicis
12 Serratus posterior superior
13 Scapula

14 Medial branches of dorsal rami of spinal nerves
15 Rib and external intercostal muscle
16 Iliocostalis thoracis
17 Lateral branches of dorsal rami of spinal nerves
18 Multifidus
19 Superior clunial nerves

207

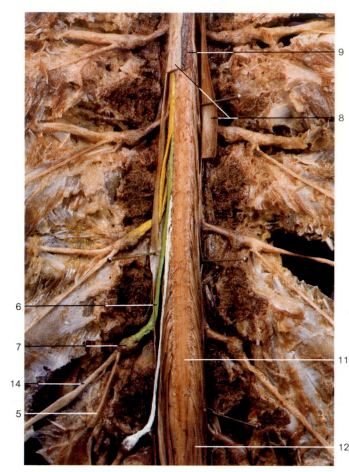

Lumbar portion of spinal cord. Note the relation between the nervous and muscular segments.

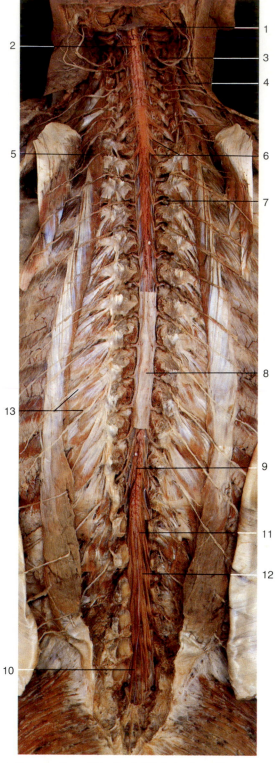

Innervation of the back IV. Spinal cord in the vertebral canal (opened). Longissimus dorsi removed and iliocostalis reflected.

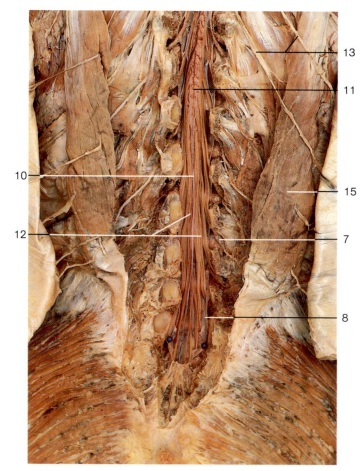

Terminal part of spinal cord. Dura removed.

1	Cerebellomedullary cistern and cerebellum	9	Spinal arachnoid mater
2	Medulla oblongata	10	Filum terminale
3	Greater occipital nerve (C_2)	11	Conus medullaris
4	Third cervical nerve (C_3)	12	Cauda equina
5	Dorsal primary ramus	13	Lateral branches of dorsal rami of spinal nerves
6	Dorsal roots	14	Ventral ramus of spinal nerve (intercostal nerve)
7	Spinal ganglion	15	Iliocostalis
8	Spinal dura mater		

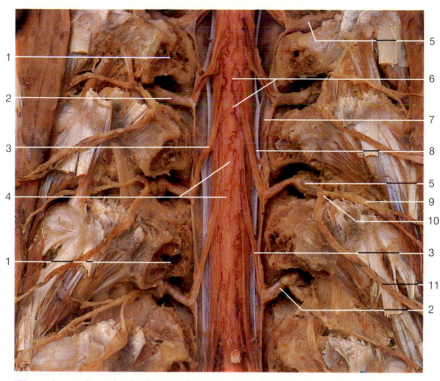

1 Arch of vertebra (divided)
2 Spinal nerve with meningeal coverings
3 Dorsal roots of thoracic spinal nerves
4 Spinal cord (thoracic portion)
5 Spinal ganglia with meningeal coverings
6 Pia mater with blood vessels
7 Dura mater (opened)
8 Denticulate ligament
9 Lateral branch of dorsal ramus
10 Dorsal ramus of spinal nerve
   (dividing into a medial and lateral
   branch)
11 Medial branch of dorsal ramus
   of spinal nerve
12 Spinal dura mater
13 Spinal nerves of sacral segments
14 Filum terminale

Thoracic portion of spinal cord (dorsal aspect). Vertebral canal and dura mater opened.

Terminal part of spinal cord with dura mater (dorsal aspect). Dorsal part of sacrum removed.

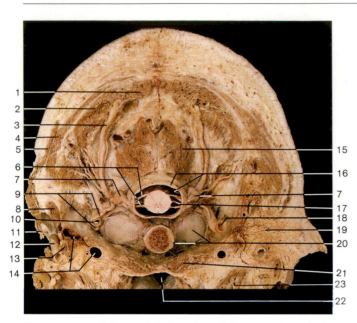

Cross-section of the neck. Dissection of the second cervical spinal nerve.

1. Trapezius
2. Semispinalis capitis
3. Dorsal ramus of spinal nerve
4. Sternocleidomastoid
5. Platysma
6. Dorsal and ventral roots of spinal nerves
7. Spinal ganglion
8. Posterior belly of digastric muscle
9. Ventral ramus of spinal nerve
10. Vertebral artery
11. Great auricular nerve
12. Superficial temporal artery
13. Styloid process
14. Internal jugular vein and internal carotid artery
15. Rectus capitis posterior major
16. Dura mater and subarachnoid space
17. Denticulate ligament
18. Vertebral artery
19. Parotid gland
20. Dens of axis (divided), inferior articular facet of atlas
21. Longus capitis
22. Pharyngeal cavity
23. Medial pterygoid
24. Periosteum of vertebral canal
25. Posterior spinal arteries
26. Anterior spinal artery

Meningeal coverings

27. Dura mater
28. Subdural space
29. Extradural or epidural space with venous plexus and fatty tissue
30. Arachnoid
31. Subarachnoid space
32. Pia mater
33. Nucleus pulposus
34. Crus of diaphragm
35. Intervertebral disc
36. Body of first lumbar vertebra
37. Spinal cord
38. Conus medullaris
39. Cauda equina
40. Filum terminale
41. Spinous process

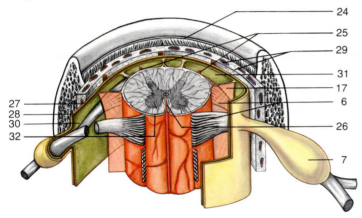

Meningeal coverings of the spinal cord (anterior aspect). (Schematic drawing.)

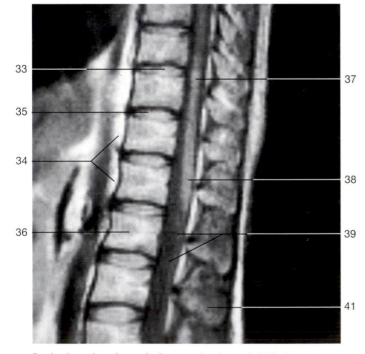

Sagittal section through the vertebral canal, MR-Scan. (Th$_9$–L$_2$.)

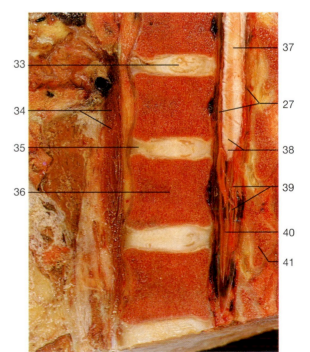

Sagittal section through vertebral canal (Th$_{12}$–L$_2$). Notice red bone marrow (unfixed).

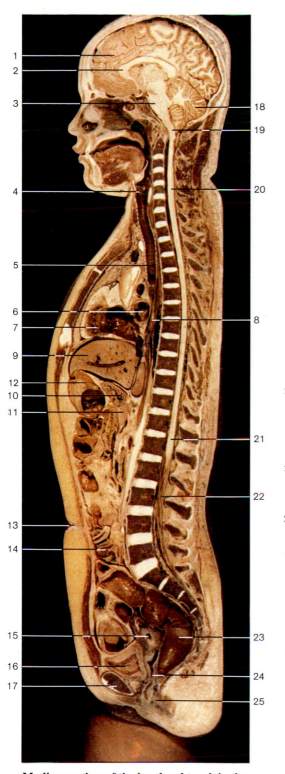

Median section of the head and trunk in the adult (female). The conus medullaris of the spinal cord is located a the level of L_1.

Median section of the head and trunk in the neonate. Note that in the neonate the conus medullaris of the spinal cord extends far more caudally than in the adult.

1	Cerebrum	11	Pancreas	21	Conus medullaris
2	Corpus callosum	12	Transverse colon	22	Cauda equina
3	Pons	13	Umbilicus	23	Rectum
4	Larynx	14	Small intestine	24	Vagina
5	Trachea	15	Uterus	25	Anus
6	Left atrium	16	Urinary bladder	26	Inferior vena cava
7	Right ventricle	17	Pubic symphysis	27	Aorta
8	Esophagus	18	Cerebellum	28	Umbilical cord
9	Liver	19	Medulla oblongata	29	Thymus
10	Stomach	20	Spinal cord		

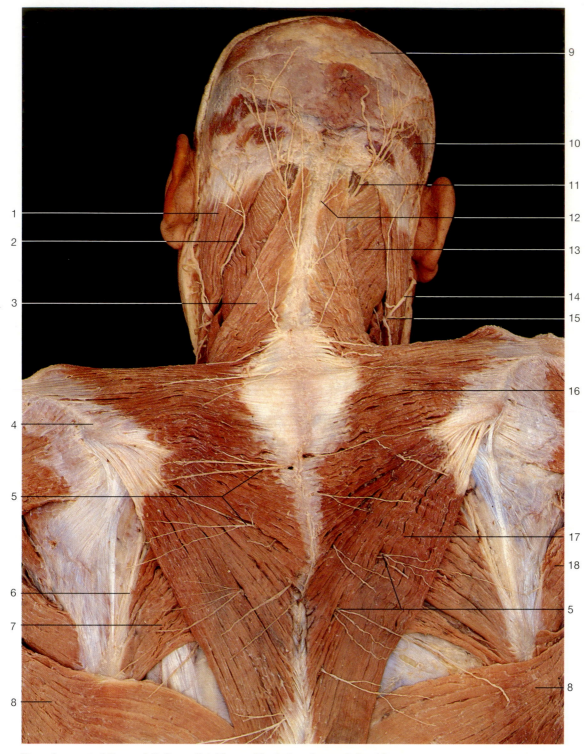

Dorsal aspect of the neck I. Superficial layer. Nuchal region and shoulder.

1 Sternocleidomastoid
2 Lesser occipital nerve
3 Descending fibers of trapezius
4 Spine of scapula
5 Medial cutaneous branches of dorsal rami of spinal nerves
6 Medial margin of scapula
7 Rhomboideus major
8 Latissimus dorsi
9 Galea aponeurotica

10 Occipital belly of occipitofrontalis muscle
11 Greater occipital nerve
12 Third occipital nerve
13 Splenius capitis
14 Great auricular nerve
15 Cutaneous nerves of cervical plexus
16 Transverse fibers of trapezius
17 Ascending fibers of trapezius
18 Teres major

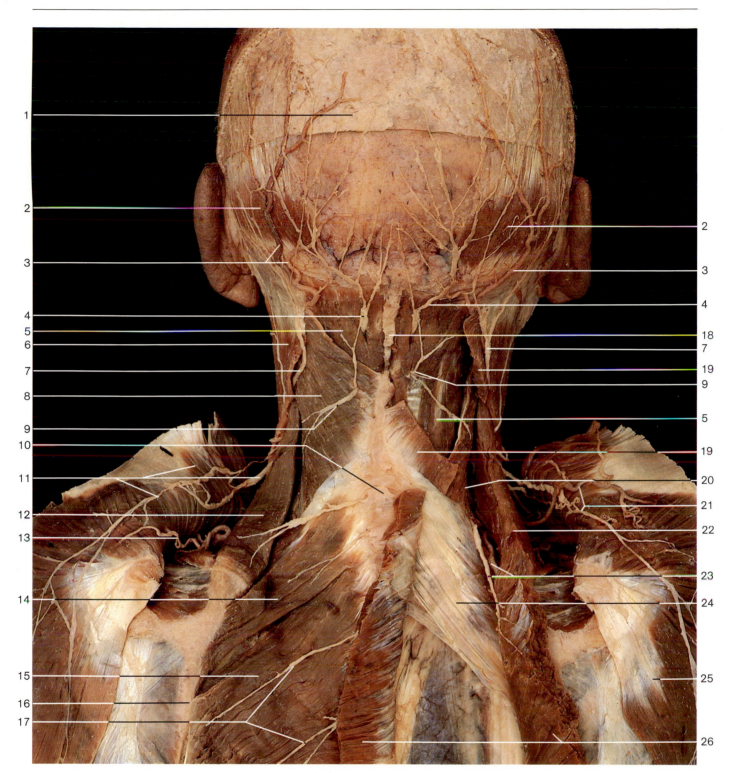

Dorsal aspect of neck II. Deeper layer. The left trapezius has been divided and reflected. On the right, trapezius, rhomboideus, and splenius have been divided. Right levator scapulae has been slightly reflected.

1 Galea aponeurotica
2 Occipital belly of occipitofrontalis
3 Occipital artery
4 Greater occipital nerve (C_2)
5 Semispinalis capitis
6 Sternocleidomastoid
7 Lesser occipital nerve
8 Left splenius capitis
9 Third occipital nerve (C_3)
10 Spinous process of vertebra prominens (C_7)
11 Left trapezius, accessory nerve
12 Levator scapulae
13 Superficial branch of transverse cervical artery
14 Rhomboideus minor
15 Rhomboideus major
16 Medial margin of scapula
17 Medial branches of dorsal rami of spinal nerves
18 Ligamentum nuchae
19 Splenius capitis (divided)
20 Splenius cervicis
21 Right accessory nerve, superficial branch of transverse cervical artery
22 Right levator scapulae
23 Dorsal scapular nerve, deep branch of transverse cervical artery
24 Serratus posterior superior
25 Right trapezius (divided and reflected)
26 Right rhomboideus major (divided and reflected)

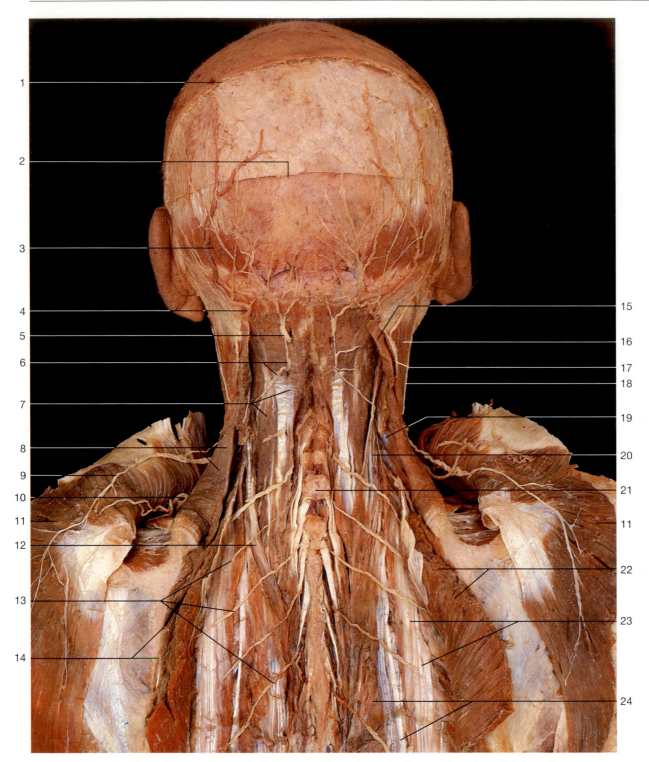

Dorsal aspect of neck III. Deepest layer. Nuchal region. Trapezius, splenius capitis and cervicis have been divided and partly removed or reflected.

1 Skin of scalp	9 Accessory nerve (n. XI)	17 Lesser occipital nerve
2 Galea aponeurotica	10 Superficial cervical artery	18 Great auricular nerve
3 Occipital belly of occipitofrontalis muscle	11 Trapezius (reflected)	19 Splenius cervicis
4 Occipital artery	12 Longissimus cervicis	20 Longissimus cervicis
5 Greater occipital nerve	13 Medial cutaneous branches of dorsal rami of spinal nerves	21 Spinous process of seventh cervical vertebra (vertebra prominens)
6 Third occipital nerve	14 Medial margin of scapula	22 Rhomboid muscles (divided)
7 Semispinalis capitis	15 Splenius capitis (divided)	23 Iliocostalis thoracis
8 Levator scapulae	16 Sternocleidomastoid	24 Longissimus thoracis

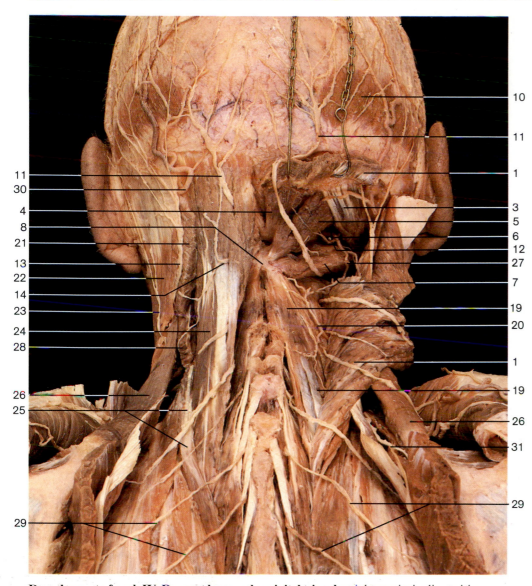

1 Semispinalis capitis (divided)
2 External occipital protuberance
3 Obliquus capitis superior
4 Rectus capitis posterior minor
5 Rectus capitis posterior major
6 Vertebral artery
7 Obliquus capitis inferior
8 Spinous process of axis
9 Third cervical vertebra
10 Occipital belly of occipitofrontalis
11 Greater occipital nerve
12 Suboccipital nerve (C₁)
13 Lesser occipital nerve
14 Third occipital nerve (C₃)
15 Mastoid process and splenius capitis
16 Atlas
17 Axis
18 Spinous process of third cervical vertebra
19 Right semispinalis cervicis
20 Deep cervical artery
21 Left splenius capitis (divided)
22 Left sternocleidomastoid
23 Great auricular nerve
24 Left semispinalis capitis
25 Left longissimus cervicis
26 Levator scapulae
27 Muscular branch of vertebral artery
28 Left semispinalis cervicis (divided)
29 Medial branches of dorsal rami of spinal nerves
30 Occipital artery
31 Dorsal scapular nerve

Dorsal aspect of neck IV. Deepest layer, suboccipital triangle; right semispinalis capitis divided and reflected.

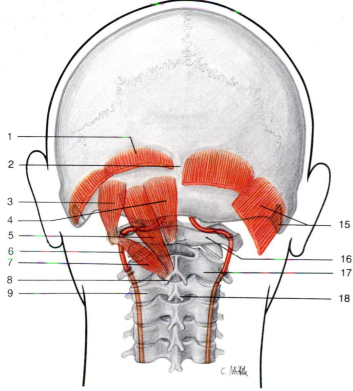

Suboccipital triangle and position of the vertebral artery. (Schematic drawing) (W.).

215

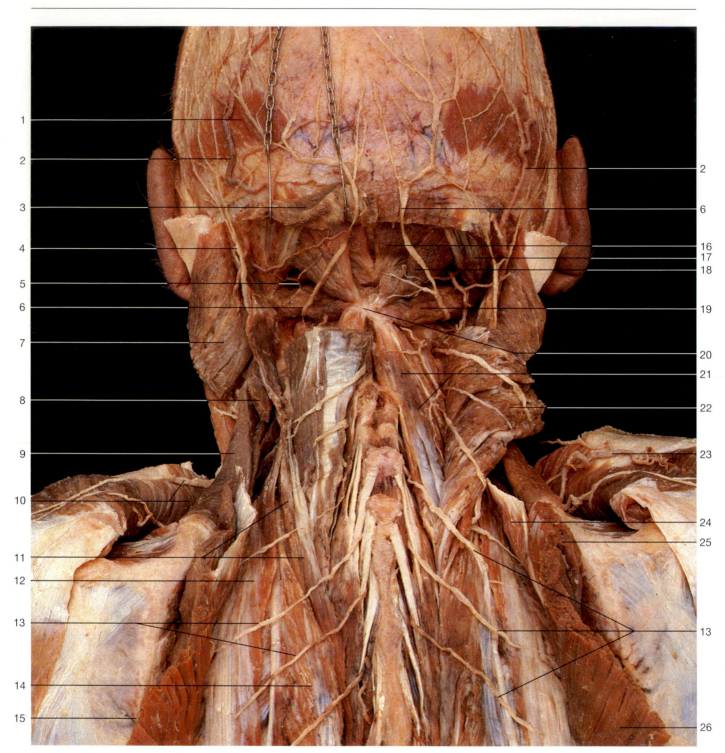

Dorsal aspect of neck V. Nuchal region. Deepest layer. Dissection of suboccipital triangle on both sides.

1 Occipital belly of occipitofrontalis muscle
2 Occipital artery
3 Insertion of semispinalis capitis (divided)
4 Lesser occipital nerve (from cervical plexus)
5 Suboccipital nerve (C₁)
6 Greater occipital nerve (C₂)
7 Splenius capitis (reflected)
8 Splenius cervicis
9 Levator scapulae
10 Accessory nerve (n. XI), trapezius

11 Longissimus cervicis
12 Iliocostalis cervicis
13 Medial cutaneus branches of dorsal rami of spinal nerves (C₇, C₈)
14 Longissimus thoracis
15 Medial margin of scapula
16 Rectus capitis posterior minor
17 Obliquus capitis superior
18 Rectus capitis posterior major
19 Obliquus capitis inferior
20 Spinous process of axis

21 Semispinalis cervicis
22 Semispinalis capitis (divided and reflected)
23 Transverse cervical artery, superficial branch
24 Serratus posterior superior (divided and reflected)
25 Rhomboideus minor (divided and reflected)
26 Rhomboideus major (divided and reflected)

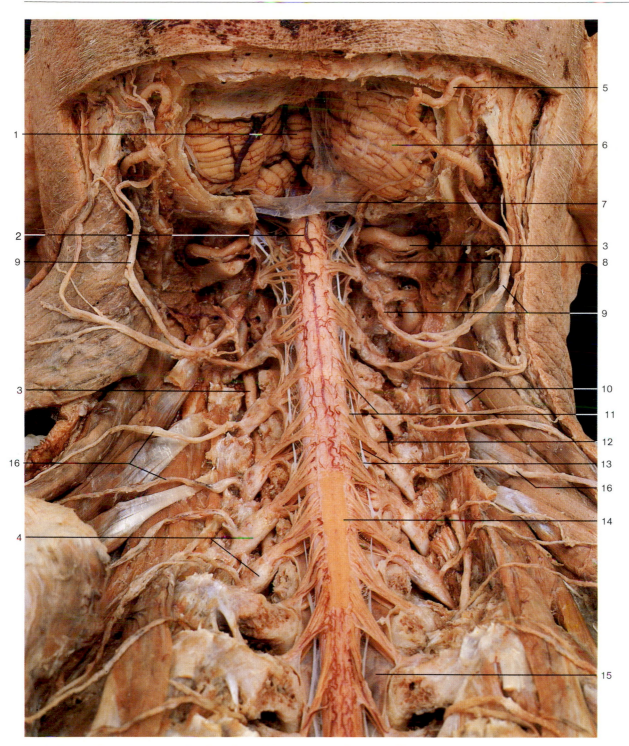

Neck, deepest layer. Spinal cord and medulla oblongata (dorsal aspect). Cranial cavity opened.

1 Vermis of the cerebellum
2 Medulla oblongata and posterior spinal artery
3 Vertebral artery
4 Spinal ganglion
5 Occipital artery
6 Cerebellum
7 Cerebellomedullary cistern
8 Atlas

9 Greater occipital nerve (C₂)
10 Levator scapulae, intertransverse ligament
11 Dorsal roots of spinal nerves
12 Vertebral arch
13 Denticulate ligament
14 Area where pia mater has been removed
15 Dura mater
16 Dorsal rami of spinal nerves

217

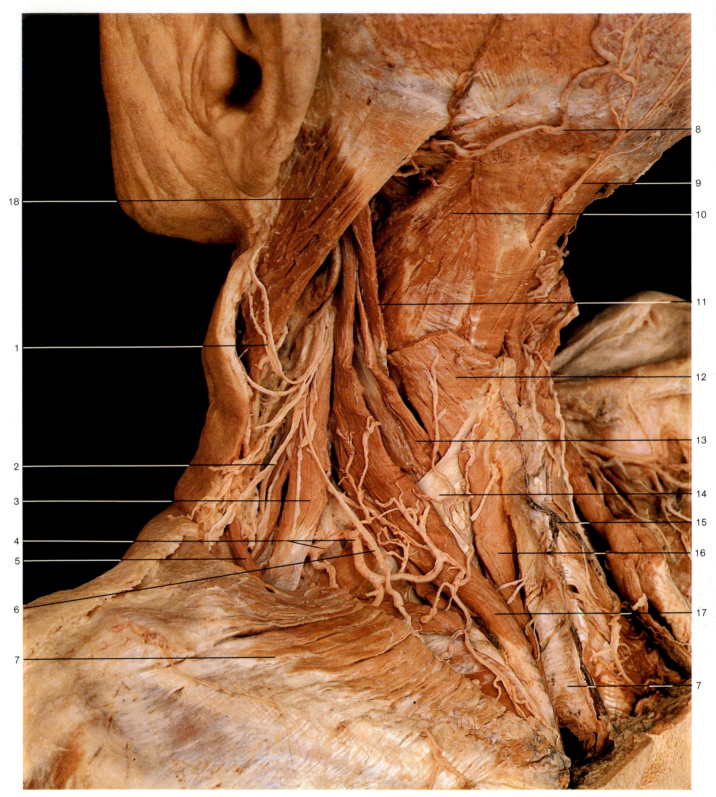

Deeper layer of the dorsal neck (oblique lateral aspect). Trapezius and semispinalis capitis have been divided and partly removed.

1	Great auricular nerve	10	Semispinalis capitis
2	Dorsal scapular nerve	11	Longissimus capitis
3	Scalenus posterior	12	Splenius capitis
4	Transverse cervical artery	13	Splenius cervicis
5	Omohyoid	14	Serratus posterior superior
6	Accessory nerve	15	Dorsal azygos vein (variant)
7	Trapezius	16	Rhomboideus minor
8	Occipital artery	17	Levator scapulae
9	Greater occipital nerve	18	Sternocleidomastoid

Chapter V
Thoracic Organs

Respiratory System,
Heart and Mediastinum

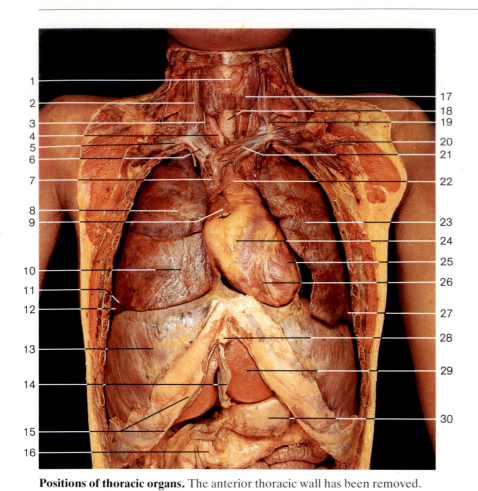

1 Larynx
2 Right internal jugular vein
3 Vagus nerve
4 Right common carotid artery
5 Right subclavian vein
6 Right brachiocephalic vein
7 Superior vena cava
8 Upper lobe of right lung
9 Right auricle
10 Middle lobe of right lung
11 Oblique fissure of right lung
12 Lower lobe of right lung
13 Diaphragm
14 Falciform ligament
15 Costal margin
16 Transverse colon
17 Thyroid gland
18 Trachea
19 Left internal jugular vein
20 Left cephalic vein
21 Left brachiocephalic vein
22 Pericardium (cut edge)
23 Upper lobe of left lung
24 Right ventricle
25 Left ventricle
26 Anterior interventricular sulcus
27 Lower lobe of left lung
28 Xiphoid process
29 Liver
30 Stomach
31 Pectoralis major

Positions of thoracic organs. The anterior thoracic wall has been removed.

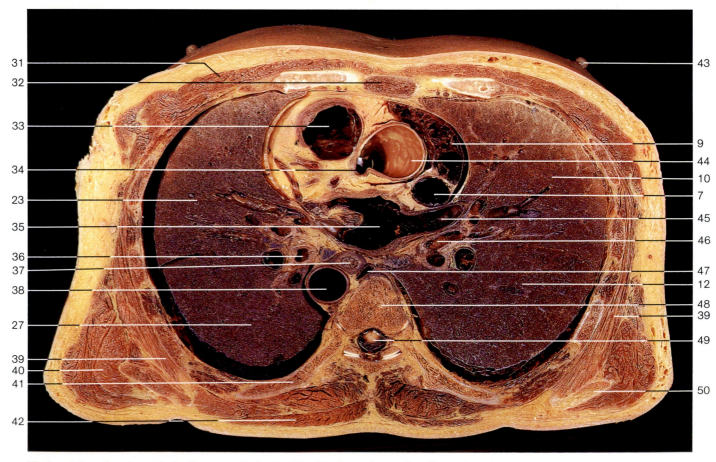

Horizontal section through the thorax at the level of the 7th thoracic vertebra (from above).

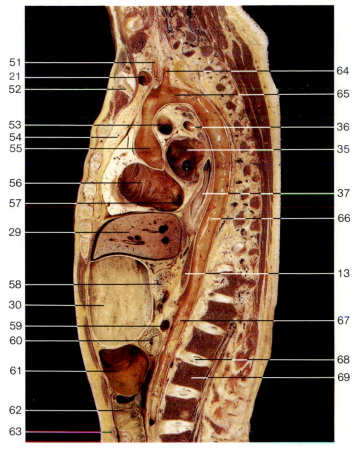

Sagittal section through the left thorax, 2 cm lateral to the median plane.

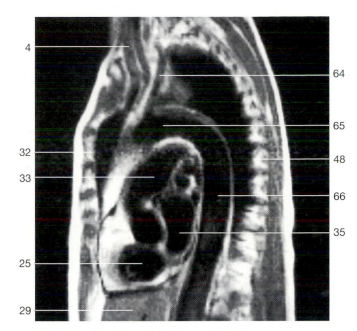

Sagittal section through the torax. MR-Scan.

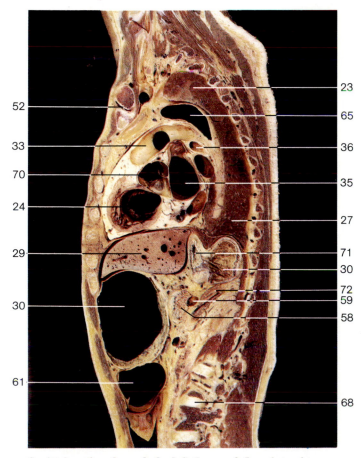

Sagittal section through the left thorax, 3.5 cm lateral to the median plane.

32 Sternum
33 Pulmonary trunk
34 Left coronary artery
35 Left atrium
36 Left main bronchus
37 Esophagus
38 Descending aorta
39 Serratus anterior
40 Teres major
41 Rib
42 Trapezius
43 Nipple
44 Ascending aorta
45 Right pulmonary veins
46 Right main bronchus
47 Azygos vein
48 Body of vertebra
49 Spinal cord
50 Scapula
51 Left common carotid artery
52 Sternoclavicular articulation with disc
53 Right pulmonary artery
54 Remnants of thymus
55 Aortic bulb
56 Right atrium
57 Entrance of inferior vena cava in right atrium
58 Pancreas
59 Portal vein
60 Duodenum
61 Transverse colon (dilated)
62 Small intestine
63 Umbilicus
64 Left subclavian artery
65 Aortic arch
66 Thoracic aorta
67 Abdominal aorta
68 Intervertebral disc
69 Body of lumbar vertebra
70 Aortic valve
71 Cardia of stomach
72 Suprarenal gland

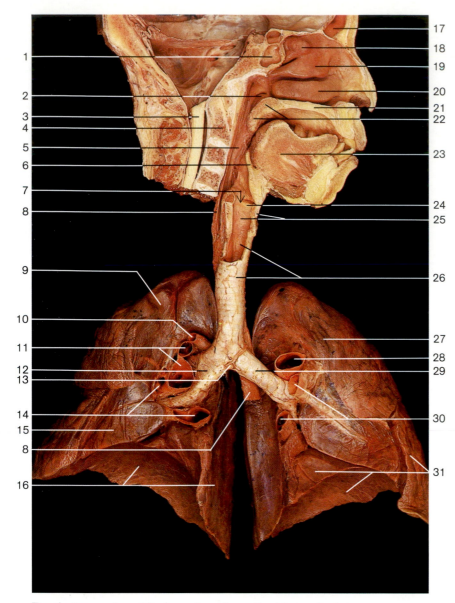

Respiratory system. The lungs have been fixed in expiration.

1	Sphenoid sinus
2	Pharyngeal opening of auditory tube
3	Spinal cord
4	Dens of axis
5	Oropharynx, oropharyngeal isthmus
6	Epiglottis
7	Entrance of larynx
8	Esophagus
9	Upper lobe of right lung
10	Azygos vein
11	Branches of pulmonary artery
12	Right main bronchus
13	Bifurcation of trachea
14	Tributaries of right pulmonary veins
15	Middle lobe of right lung
16	Lower lobe of right lung
17	Frontal sinus
18	Superior nasal concha
19	Middle nasal concha
20	Inferior nasal concha
21	Hard palate
22	Soft palate with uvula
23	Tongue
24	Vocal fold
25	Larynx
26	Trachea
27	Upper lobe of left lung
28	Left pulmonary artery
29	Left main bronchus
30	Left pulmonary veins
31	Lower lobe of left lung

▷

To page 223:

1	Nasal cavity
2	Pharynx
3	Larynx (thyroid cartilage)
4	Trachea
5	Upper lobe of right lung
6	Bifurcation of trachea
7	Right main bronchus
8	Horizontal fissure of right lung
9	Middle lobe of right lung
10	Oblique fissures of lungs
11	Lower lobe of right lung
12	Clavicle
13	Upper lobe of left lung
14	Left main bronchus
15	Bronchi supplying bronchopulmonary segments
16	Lower lobe of left lung
17	Costal margin
18	Hyoid bone
19	Right superior lobe bronchus
20	Right middle lobe bronchus
21	Right inferior lobe bronchus
22	Left superior lobe bronchus
23	Left inferior lobe bronchus
24	Segmental bronchi

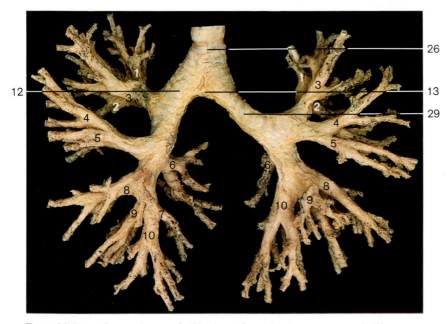

Bronchial tree (ventral aspect). The lung tissue has been removed. The bronchopulmonary segments are numbered 1–10.

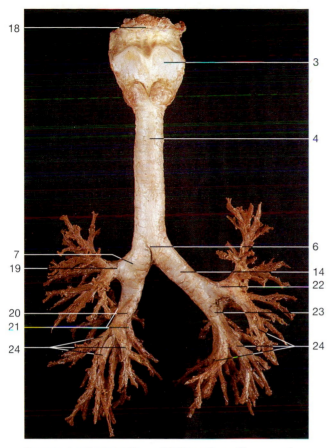

Larynx, trachea and bronchial tree (anterior aspect).

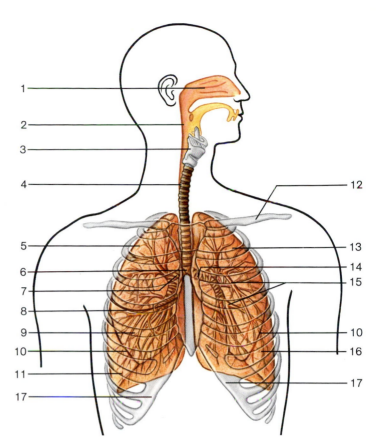

Organization and positions of respiratory organs. (Schematic drawing) (W.).

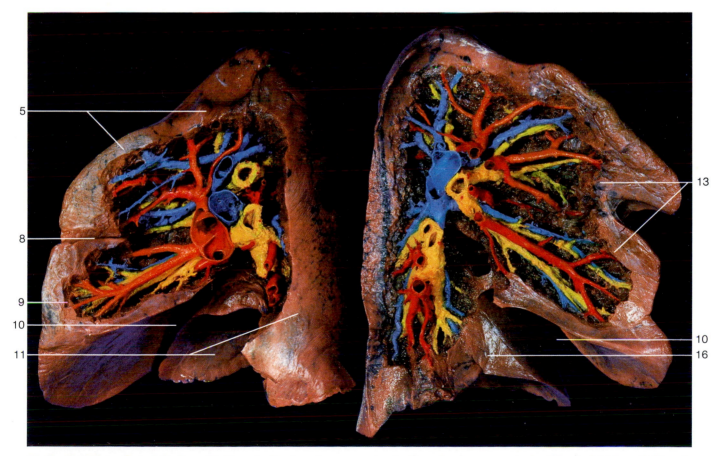

Mediastinal dissection of the bronchial tree (yellow), pulmonary veins (red), and pulmonary arteries (blue), right lung (left) and left lung (right) (medial aspect).

Projections of the Lungs and Pleura

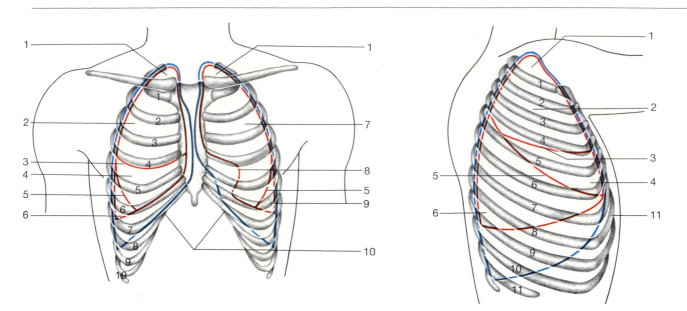

Surface projections of lungs and pleura on the thoracic wall. Left: anterior aspect; right: right-lateral aspect.
Red = margins of the lung; blue = margins of pleura. The numbers indicate ribs.

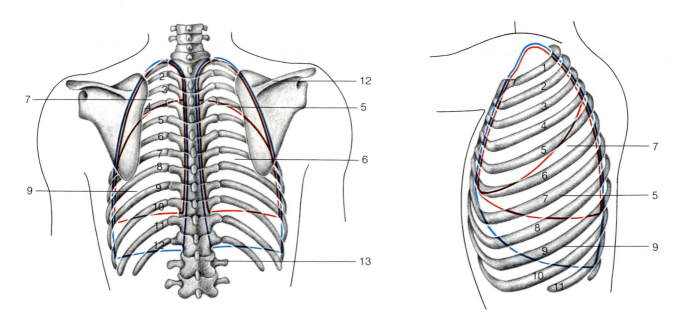

Surface projections of lungs and pleura on thoracic wall. Left: posterior aspect; right: left-lateral aspect.
Red = margins of lung; blue = margins of pleura. The number indicate ribs.

1 Apex of lung
2 Upper lobe of right lung
3 Horizontal fissure of right lung
4 Middle lobe of right lung
5 Oblique fissures of lungs

6 Lower lobe of right lung
7 Upper lobe of left lung
8 Cardiac notch of left lung
9 Lower lobe of left lung
10 Infrasternal angle

11 Costal margin
12 Spine of scapula
13 1st lumbar vertebra

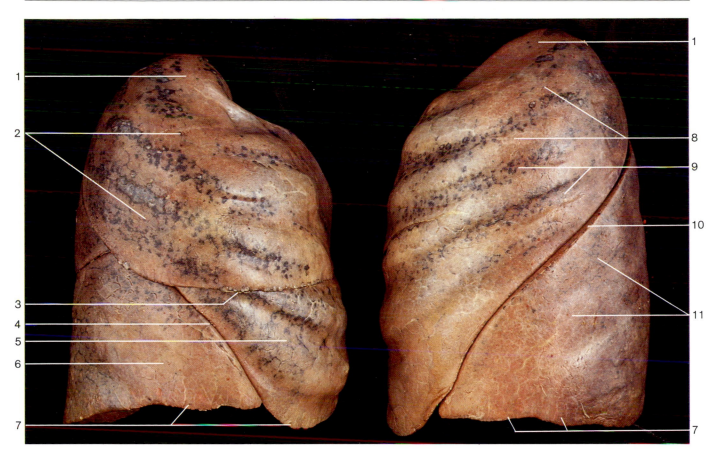

Right lung (lateral aspect).　　　　**Left lung** (lateral aspect).

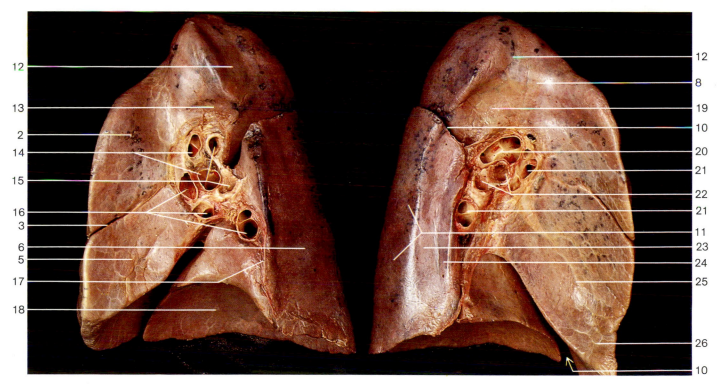

Right lung (medial aspect).　　　　**Left lung** (medial aspect).

1	Apex of lung	8	Upper lobe of left lung
2	Upper lobe of right lung	9	Impressions of ribs
3	Horizontal fissure of right lung	10	Oblique fissure of left lung
4	Oblique fissure of right lung	11	Lower lobe of left lung
5	Middle lobe of right lung	12	Groove for subclavian artery
6	Lower lobe of right lung	13	Groove for azygos vein
7	Inferior border	14	Branches of right pulmonary artery

15	Bronchi	22	Left main bronchus
16	Right pulmonary veins	23	Groove for thoracic aorta
17	Pulmonary ligament	24	Groove for esophagus
18	Diaphragmatic surface	25	Cardiac impression
19	Groove for aortic arch	26	Lingula
20	Left pulmonary artery		
21	Branches of left pulmonary veins		

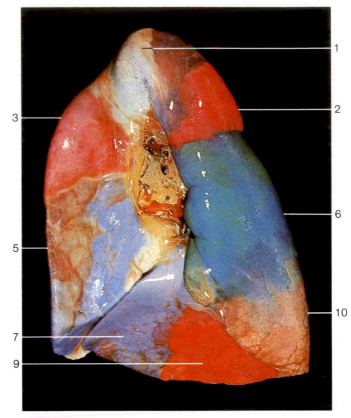

Right lung (medial aspect).

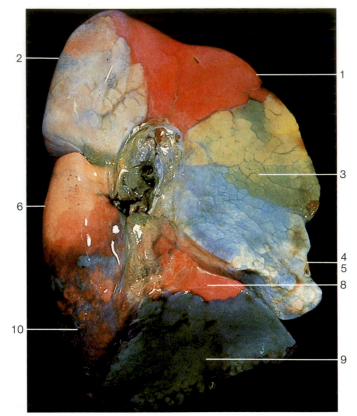

Left lung (medial aspect).

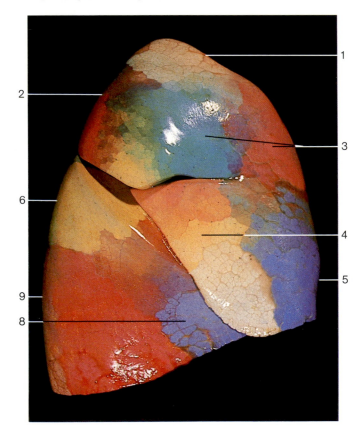

Right lung (lateral aspect).

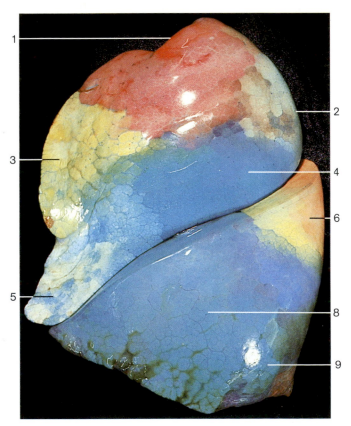

Left lung (lateral aspect).

The bronchopulmonary segments of the lungs are differentiated by the various colors. Notice, that the 7th segment of the left lung is absent. Compare with the schematic drawing on the facing page.

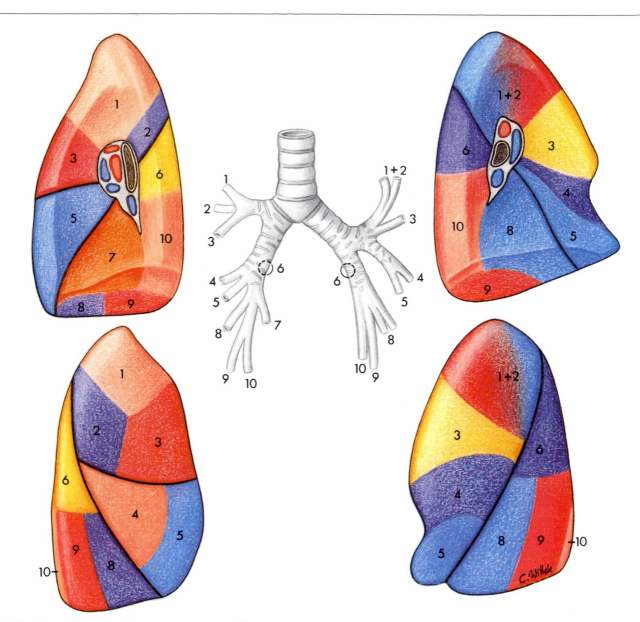

Distribution of bronchopulmonary segments of the lungs and their relation to the bronchial tree (after J. F. HUBER).

Right lung

1	Apical segment	Upper lobe bronchus
2	Posterior segment	
3	Anterior segment	
4	Lateral segment	Middle lobe bronchus
5	Medial segment	
6	Superior (apical) segment	Lower lobe bronchus
7	Medial basal segment	
8	Anterior basal segment	
9	Lateral basal segment	
10	Posterior basal segment	

Left lung

1+2	Apico-posterior segment	Superior division	Upper lobe bronchus
3	Anterior segment		
4	Superior lingular segment	Inferior division	
5	Inferior lingular segment		
6	Superior (apical) segment	Lower lobe bronchus	
7	Absent		
8	Anteromedial basal segment		
9	Lateral basal segment		
10	Posterior basal segment		

The Heart

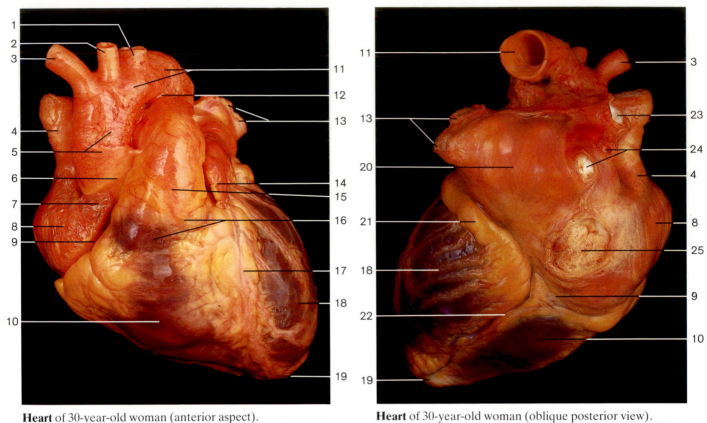

Heart of 30-year-old woman (anterior aspect).

Heart of 30-year-old woman (oblique posterior view).

1	Left subclavian artery	9	Coronary sulcus	18	Left ventricle
2	Left common carotid artery	10	Right ventricle	19	Apex of the heart
3	Brachiocephalic trunk	11	Aortic arch	20	Left atrium
4	Superior vena cava	12	Ligamentum arteriosum	21	Coronary sinus
5	Ascending aorta	13	Left pulmonary veins	22	Posterior interventricular sulcus
6	Bulb of the aorta	14	Left auricle	23	Right pulmonary artery
7	Right auricle	15	Pulmonary trunk	24	Right pulmonary veins
8	Right atrium	16	Sinus of pulmonary trunk	25	Inferior vena cava
		17	Anterior interventricular sulcus		

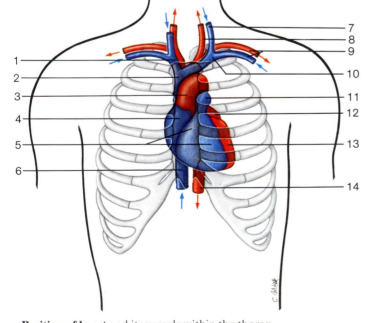

Position of heart and its vessels within the thorax.
(Schematic drawing) (W.).

1 Right brachiocephalic vein
2 Superior vena cava
3 Ascending aorta
4 Right atrium
5 Right ventricle
6 Inferior vena cava
7 Left internal jugular vein
8 Left common carotid artery
9 Left subclavian artery and vein
10 Left brachiocephalic vein
11 Pulmonary trunk
12 Left atrium
13 Left ventricle
14 Descending aorta

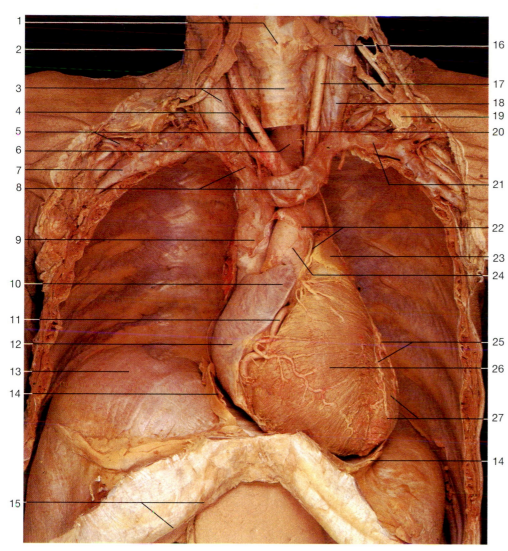

1	Larynx
2	Sternocleidomastoid (divided)
3	Trachea (divided), right internal jugular vein
4	Vagus nerve
5	Right common carotid artery, cephalic vein
6	Esophagus
7	Right subclavian vein
8	Right and left brachiocephalic veins
9	Superior vena cava
10	Right auricle
11	Right coronary artery
12	Right atrium
13	Diaphragm
14	Pericardium (cut edges)
15	Costal margin
16	Omohyoid muscle
17	Left common carotid artery
18	Left internal jugular vein
19	Clavicle (divided)
20	Recurrent laryngeal nerve
21	Left subclavian vein
22	Pericardial reflection
23	Pulmonary trunk
24	Ascending aorta
25	Anterior interventricular sulcus, interventricular branch of left coronary artery
26	Right ventricle
27	Left ventricle
28	Aortic valve
29	Tricuspid or right atrioventricular valve
30	Inferior vena cava
31	Pulmonary veins
32	Pulmonary valve
33	Left atrioventricular (bicuspid or mitral) valve

Heart and related vessels in situ (anterior aspect). Anterior thoracic wall, pericardium and epicardium have been removed, trachea divided.

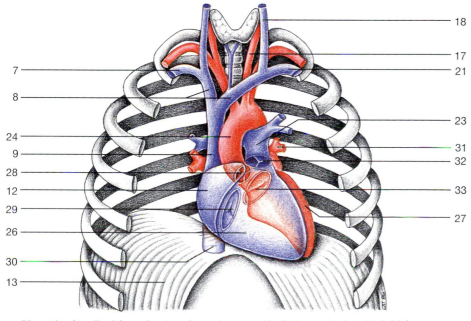

Heart in situ. Position of valves (anterior aspect). (Schematic drawing) (O.).

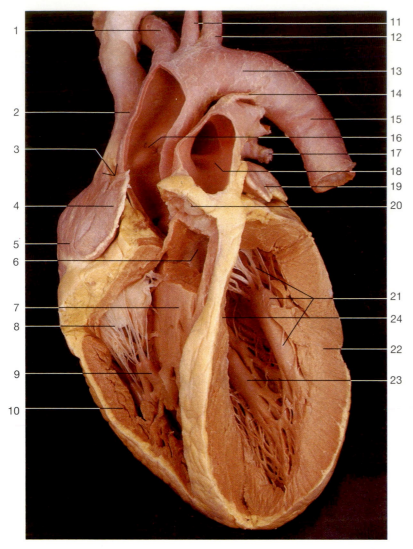

1 Brachiocephalic trunk
2 Superior vena cava
3 Sulcus terminalis
4 Right auricle
5 Right atrium
6 Aortic valve
7 Conus arteriosus (infundibulum)
8 Right atrioventricular (tricuspid) valve
9 Anterior papillary muscle
10 Myocardium of right ventricle
11 Left common carotid artery
12 Left subclavian artery
13 Aortic arch
14 Ligamentum arteriosum (remnant of ductus arteriosus)
15 Thoracic aorta (descending aorta)
16 Ascending aorta
17 Left pulmonary vein
18 Pulmonary trunk
19 Left auricle
20 Pulmonary valve
21 Anterior papillary muscle
22 Myocardium of left ventricle
23 Posterior papillary muscle
24 Interventricular septum
25 Right and left brachiocephalic veins
26 Chordae tendineae
27 Papillary muscles of right ventricle
28 Left atrium
29 Infundibulum
30 Left ventricle
31 Left atrioventricular (bicuspid or mitral) valve
32 Apex of heart

Anterior aspect of the heart. The anterior walls of the ventricles and of the aorta and pulmonary trunk have been fenestrated to show the aortic valve.

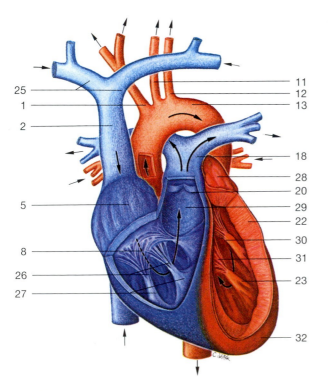

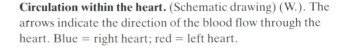

Circulation within the heart. (Schematic drawing) (W.). The arrows indicate the direction of the blood flow through the heart. Blue = right heart; red = left heart.

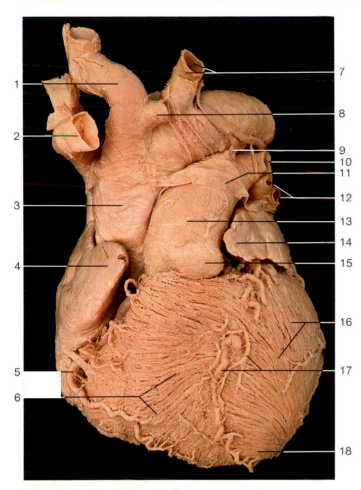

1 Brachiocephalic trunk (variant)
2 Brachiocephalic vein
3 Ascending aorta
4 Right auricle
5 Right coronary artery
6 Myocardium of right ventricle
7 Left subclavian artery
8 Left common carotid artery (variant)
9 Ligamentum arteriosum
10 Left pulmonary artery
11 Border of pericardium
12 Left pulmonary veins
13 Pulmonary trunk
14 Left auricle
15 Sinus of pulmonary trunk
16 Myocardium of left ventricle
17 Anterior interventricular artery and vein, anterior interventricular sulcus
18 Apex of the heart
19 Muscular vortex (right ventricle)
20 Posterior interventricular sulcus
21 Anterior interventricular sulcus
22 Muscular vortex (left ventricle)
23 Aorta
24 Left atrium
25 Coronary sinus
26 Superior vena cava
27 Right pulmonary vein
28 Right atrium
29 Inferior vena cava
30 Coronary sulcus

Myocardium (anterior aspect).

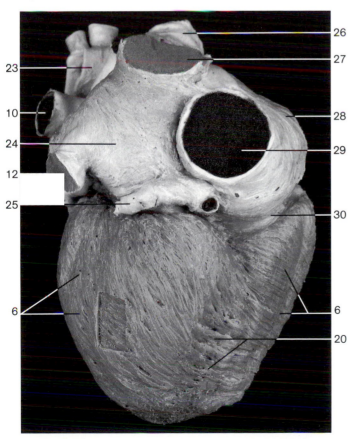

Myocardium (posterior aspect). The left ventricle has been opened to show the muscle fiber bundles of the deeper layer with their more circular course.

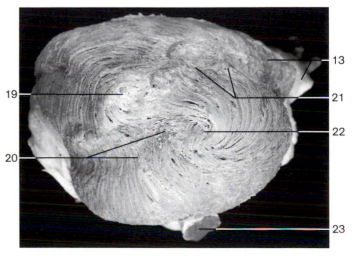

Vortex of cardiac muscle fibers (from below).

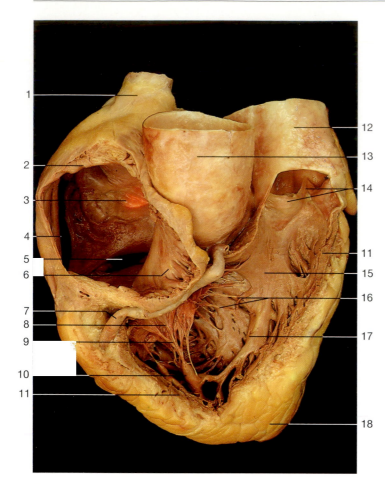

1	Superior vena cava
2	Crista terminalis
3	Fossa ovalis
4	Opening of inferior vena cava
5	Opening of coronary sinus
6	Right auricle
7	Right coronary artery, coronary sulcus
8	**Anterior cusp** of **tricuspid valve**
9	Chordae tendineae
10	**Anterior papillary muscle**
11	Myocardium
12	Pulmonary trunk
13	Ascending aorta
14	**Pulmonary valve**
15	Conus arteriosus (infundibulum)
16	Septal papillary muscles
17	Septomarginal or moderator band
18	Apex of heart
19	Left auricle
20	**Aortic valve**
21	**Left ventricle**
22	Pulmonary veins
23	Position of fossa ovalis
24	**Left atrium**
25	**Left atrioventricular** (bicuspid or **mitral**) **valve**
26	Coronary sinus
27	Left coronary artery
28	Posterior papillary muscle
29	Left subclavian artery
30	Descending aorta
31	Left pulmonary artery

Right heart (anterior aspect). Anterior wall of right atrium and ventricle removed.

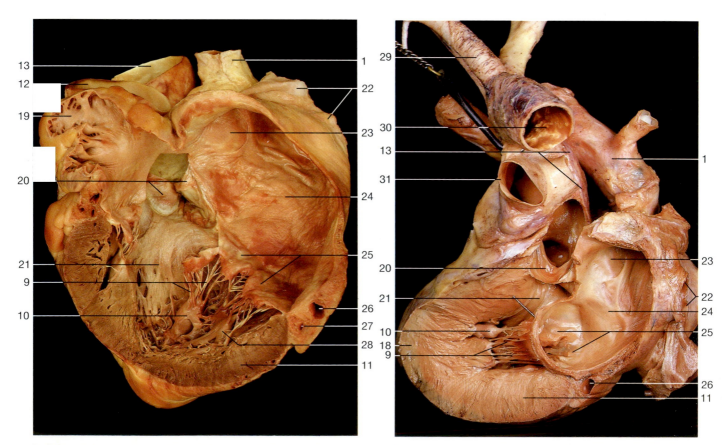

Left heart. Left atrium and ventricle opened. Aortic valve fenestrated.

Left heart. Systole. Aortic valve fenestrated. Atrium and ventricle opened.

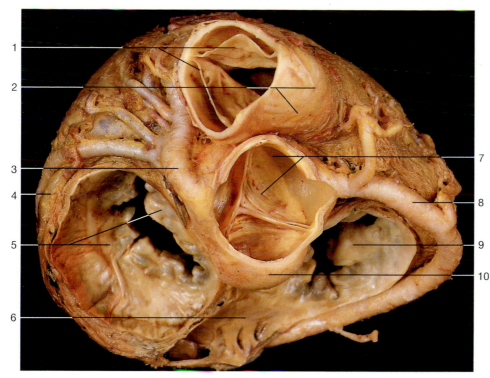

1 Pulmonary valve
2 Sinus of pulmonary trunk
3 Left coronary artery
4 Great cardiac vein
5 Left atrioventricular (mitral) valve
6 Coronary sinus
7 Aortic valve
8 Right coronary artery
9 Right atrioventricular (tricuspid) valve
10 Bulb of aorta
11 Anterior semilunar cusp of pulmonary valve
12 Left semilunar cusp of pulmonary valve
13 Right semilunar cusp of pulmonary valve
14 Left semilunar cusp of aortic valve
15 Right semilunar cusp of aortic valve
16 Posterior semilunar cusp of aortic valve
17 Right atrium
18 Anterior cusp of tricuspid valve
19 Chordae tendineae
20 Trabeculae carneae
21 Interventricular septum
22 Septal cusp of tricuspid valve
23 Anterior papillary muscle
24 Myocardium of right ventricle

Valves of heart (superior aspect). Left and right atrium removed. Dissection of coronary arteries. Above: anterior wall of the heart.

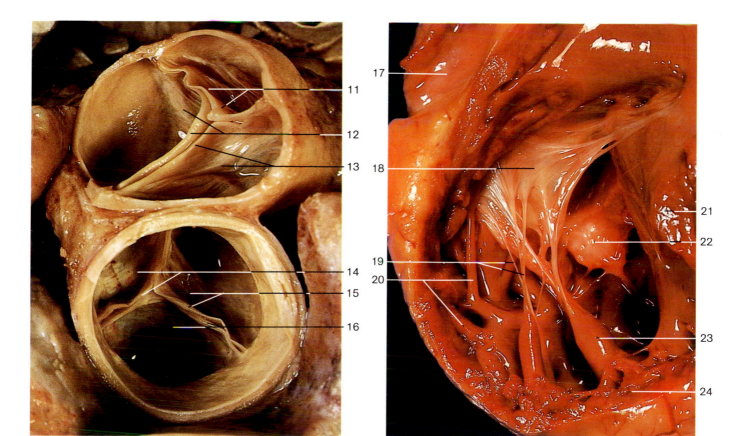

Pulmonary and aortic valves (from above; anterior wall of the heart at the top). Both valves are closed.

Right atrioventricular (tricuspid) valve (anterior aspect after removal of the anterior wall of the right ventricle).

233

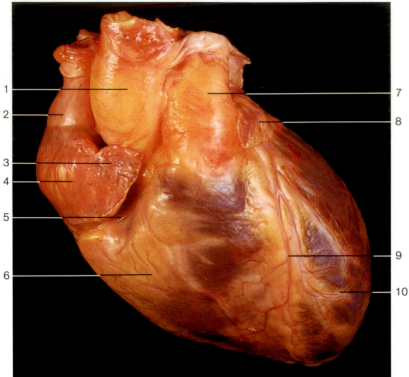

1 Ascending aorta
2 Superior vena cava
3 Right auricle
4 Right atrium
5 Coronary sulcus
6 Right ventricle
7 Pulmonary trunk
8 Left auricle
9 Anterior interventricular sulcus
10 Left ventricle
11 Right pulmonary artery
12 Sulcus terminalis with sinuatrial node
13 Position of valves
14 Myocardium of right atrium
15 Inferior vena cava
16 Pulmonary valve
17 Tricuspid valve
18 Myocardium of right ventricle

Heart, fixed in **diastole** (anterior aspect). The ventricles are dilated, atria contracted.

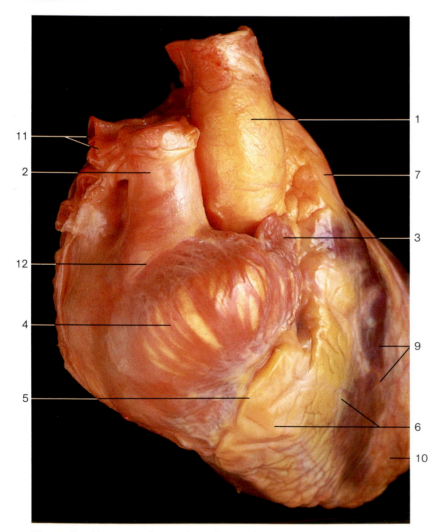

Heart, fixed in **systole** (anterolateral aspect). The ventricles are contracted, atria dilated.

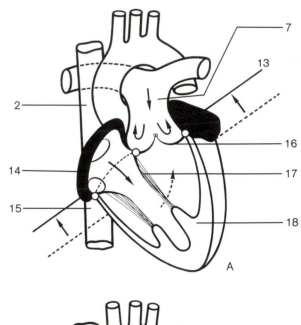

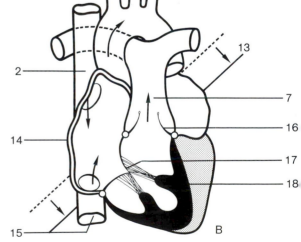

Morphological changes during heart movements. (Schematic drawing after GAUER) (W.). Note the changes in position of the valves (arrows). Contracted portions of heart are indicated in black.

A Diastole, muscle of ventricles dilated
B Systole, muscles of ventricles contracted

234

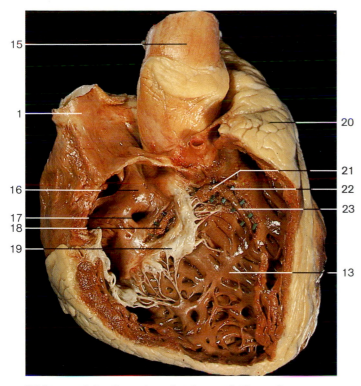

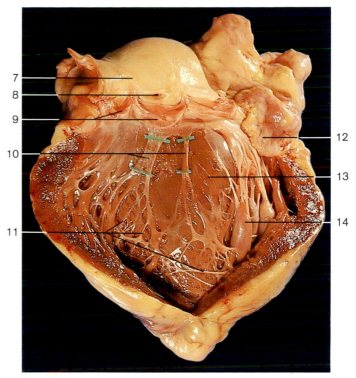

Right ventricle, dissection of **atrioventricular node, atrioventricular bundle (bundle of His)** and right limb or bundle branch (probes).

Left ventricle, dissection of the left limb or bundle branch of conducting system (probes).

1	Superior vena cava	5	Muscle fiber bundles of right atrium
2	Sulcus terminalis	6	Coronary sulcus (with right coronary artery)
3	Bulb of aorta	7	Aortic sinus
4	Sinuatrial node (arrows)	8	Entrance to left coronary artery

9 Aortic valve
10 Branches of left bundle branch
11 Purkinje fibers
12 Left auricle
13 Interventricular septum
14 Papillary muscles
15 Ascending aorta
16 Right atrium
17 Opening of coronary sinus
18 Atrioventricular node
19 Septal cusp of tricuspid valve
20 Pulmonary trunk
21 Atrioventricular bundle (bundle of His)
22 Bifurcation of atrioventricular bundle
23 Right bundle branch
24 Inferior vena cava
25 Left atrium
26 Left bundle branch
27 Papillary muscles with Purkinje fibers

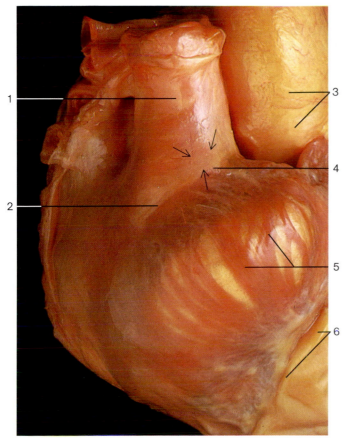

Right atrium, anterior wall, showing the location of the **sinuatrial node** (arrows).

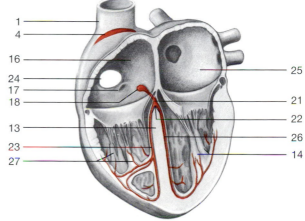

Conducting system of the heart.
(Schematic drawing) (W.).

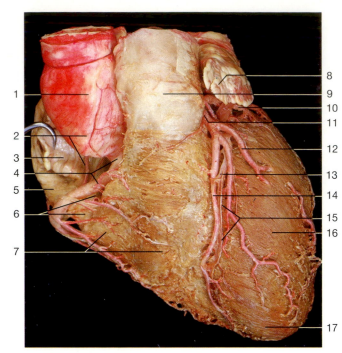

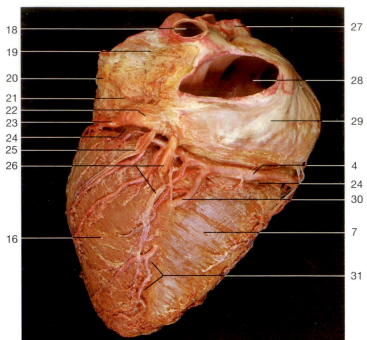

Coronary arteries (anterior aspect). The epicardium and subepicardial fatty tissue have been removed. The arteries have been injected with red resin from the aorta.

Right coronary artery and veins of the heart (dorsal aspect). The epicardium and subepicardial fatty tissue have been removed.

1   Ascending aorta
2   Aortic bulb and (in the above specimen) sinuatrial branch of right coronary artery
3   Right auricle لاتوى
4   **Right coronary artery**
5   Right atrium دمع
6   Coronary sulcus
7   Right ventricle نطن
8   Left auricle
9   Pulmonary trunk

10   Circumflex branch of left coronary artery
11   **Left coronary artery**
12   Diagonal branch of left artery
13   Anterior interventricular vein
14   Anterior interventricular artery
15   Anterior interventricular sulcus
16   Left ventricle
17   Apex of heart
18   Right pulmonary vein
19   Left atrium
20   Left pulmonary veins
21   Oblique vein of left atrium (Marshall's vein)
22   **Coronary sinus**
23   **Great cardiac vein**
24   Coronary sulcus (posterior portion)
25   Posterior vein of left ventricle
26   **Middle cardiac vein**
27   Left pulmonary artery
28   Inferior vena cava
29   Right atrium
30   Posterior interventricular branch of right coronary artery
31   Posterior interventricular sulcus
32   Superior vena cava
33   Right marginal branch

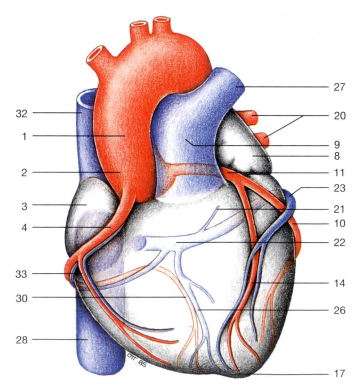

Vessels of the heart. Coronary arteries, veins of the heart (anterior aspect) (O.).

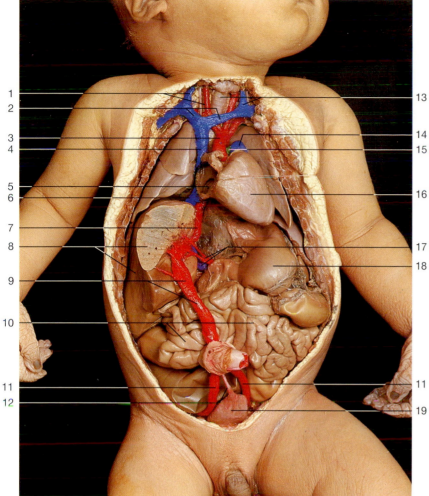

1 Internal jugular vein, right common carotid artery
2 Right and left brachiocephalic vein
3 Aortic arch
4 Superior vena cava
5 **Foramen ovale**
6 Inferior vena cava
7 **Ductus venosus**
8 Liver
9 **Umbilical vein**
10 Small intestine
11 **Umbilical artery**
12 Urachus
13 Trachea, left internal jugular vein
14 Left pulmonary artery
15 **Ductus arteriosus**
16 Right ventricle
17 Hepatic arteries (red), portal vein (blue)
18 Stomach
19 Urinary bladder
20 Portal vein
21 Pulmonary veins
22 Descending aorta
23 Placenta

Thoracic and abdominal organs in the newborn. The main vessels are colored to demonstrate the fetal circulatory system (anterior aspect). The right atrium has been opened to show the foramen ovale. The left lobe of the liver has been removed.

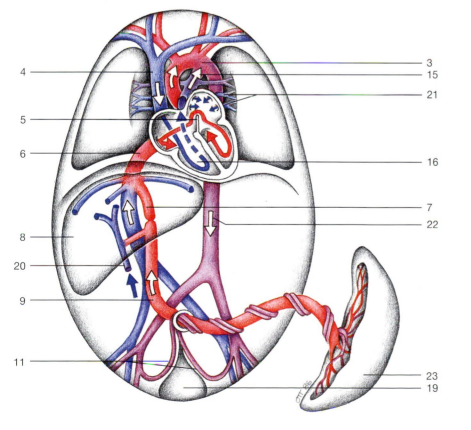

Fetal circulatory system. (Schematic drawing) (O.). The oxygen gradient is indicated by color.

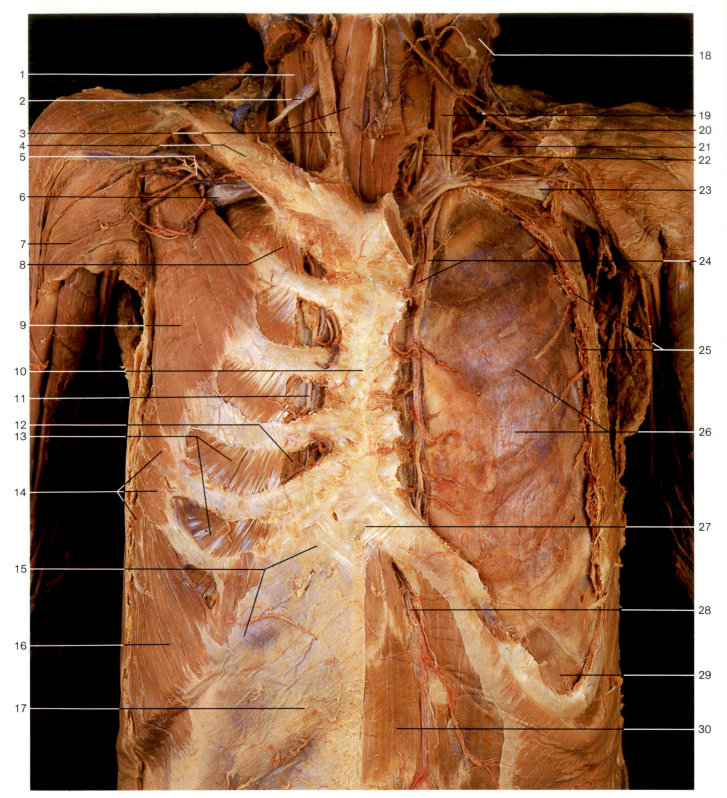

Thoracic wall and organs (ventral aspect). The left clavicle and ribs have been partially removed, and the right intercostal spaces have been opened to show the internal thoracic vein and artery.

1	Right internal jugular vein	11	Right internal thoracic artery and vein	21	Brachial plexus
2	Omohyoid muscle	12	Fascicles of transversus thoracis	22	Vagus nerve
3	Sternohyoid muscle and external jugular vein	13	Internal intercostal muscles	23	Left subclavian vein
4	Clavicle	14	Serratus anterior	24	Left internal thoracic artery and vein
5	Thoracoacromial artery	15	Costal arch	25	Ribs and thoracic wall (cut)
6	Right subclavian vein	16	External oblique muscle	26	Costal pleura
7	Pectoralis major	17	Anterior sheath of rectus abdominis	27	Xiphoid process
8	External intercostal muscle	18	Sternocleidomastoid	28	Superior epigastric artery
9	Pectoralis minor	19	Left internal jugular vein	29	Diaphragm
10	Body of sternum	20	Transverse cervical artery	30	Rectus abdominis

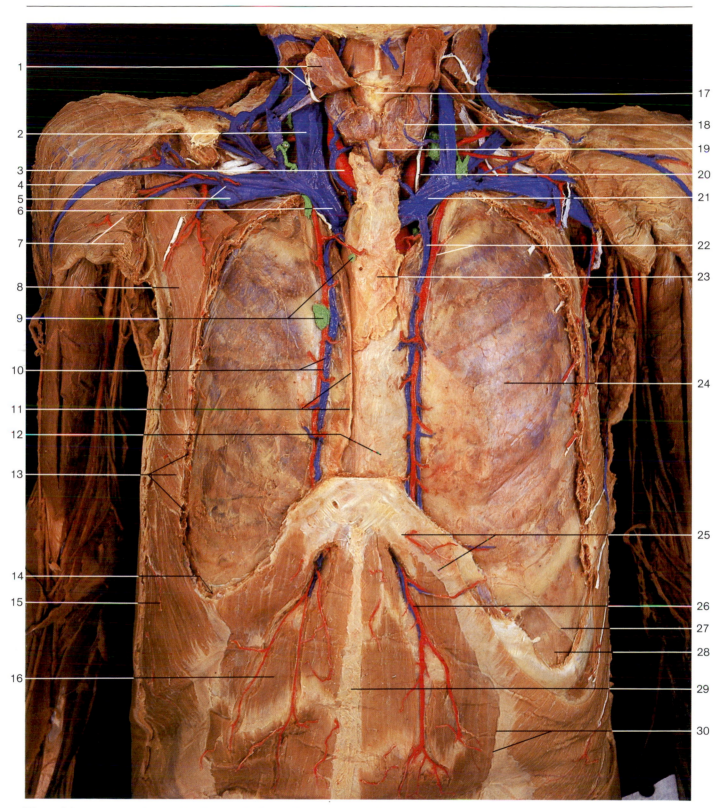

Thoracic organs, anterior mediastinum and pleura. Ribs, clavicle and sternum have been partly removed.
Red = arteries; blue = veins; green = lymph vessels and nodes.

1 Sternothyroid muscle and its nerve,
   a branch of the ansa cervicalis
2 Right internal jugular vein
3 Right common carotid artery
4 Cephalic vein
5 Right subclavian vein
6 Right brachiocephalic vein
7 Pectoralis major (divided)
8 Pectoralis minor (divided)
9 Anterior mediastinal lymph nodes
10 Internal thoracic artery and vein

11 Anterior margin of costal pleura
12 Pericardium
13 5th and 6th ribs (divided)
   and serratus anterior
14 Costodiaphragmatic recess
15 External oblique muscle
16 Rectus abdominis
17 Larynx
18 Thyroid gland
19 Trachea
20 Left vagus nerve

21 Left brachiocephalic vein
22 Left internal thoracic artery and vein
23 Thymus
24 Costal pleura
25 Costal margin
26 Superior epigastric artery
27 Margin of costal pleura
28 Diaphragm
29 Linea alba
30 Cut edge of anterior sheath of rectus
   abdominis

239

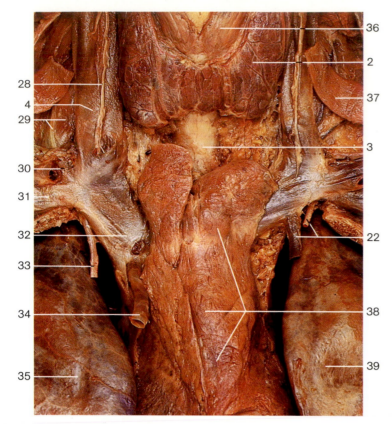

The **thymus** above the heart, showing its position and size.

1 Larynx
2 Thyroid gland
3 Trachea
4 Internal jugular vein
5 Brachial plexus
6 Right brachiocephalic vein, common carotid artery
7 Right phrenic nerve
8 Ascending aorta
9 Pectoralis minor (divided)
10 Pulmonary trunk (covered by pericardium)
11 Costal pleura
12 Pericardium and heart
13 Serratus anterior
14 Xiphoid process
15 Costal margin
16 External oblique muscle
17 Sternothyroid muscle (divided and reflected)
18 Vagus nerve
19 Left common carotid artery
20 Left sympathetic trunk
21 Recurrent laryngeal nerve
22 Left internal thoracic artery and vein (divided)
23 Margin of costal pleura
24 Intercostal nerves and vessels
25 Superior epigastric artery
26 Rectus abdominis
27 Diaphragm
28 Ansa cervicalis
29 Phrenic nerve and scalenus anterior
30 External jugular vein (divided)
31 Right subclavian vein
32 Right brachiocephalic vein
33 Internal thoracic artery (divided)
34 Internal thoracic vein (divided)
35 Right lung
36 Cricothyroid muscle
37 Omohyoid muscle
38 **Thymus**
39 Left lung

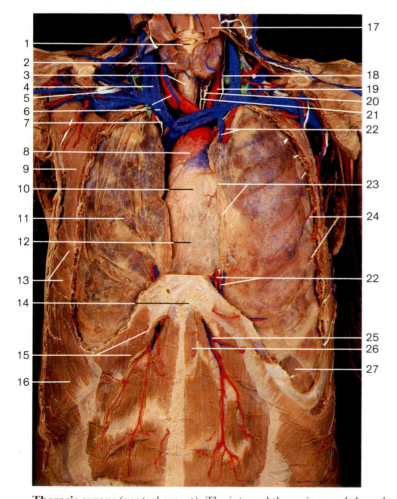

Thoracic organs (ventral aspect). The internal thoracic vessels have been removed, and the anterior margins of the pleura and lungs have been slightly reflected to display the **anterior** and **middle mediastinum,** including the **heart** and **great vessels.**

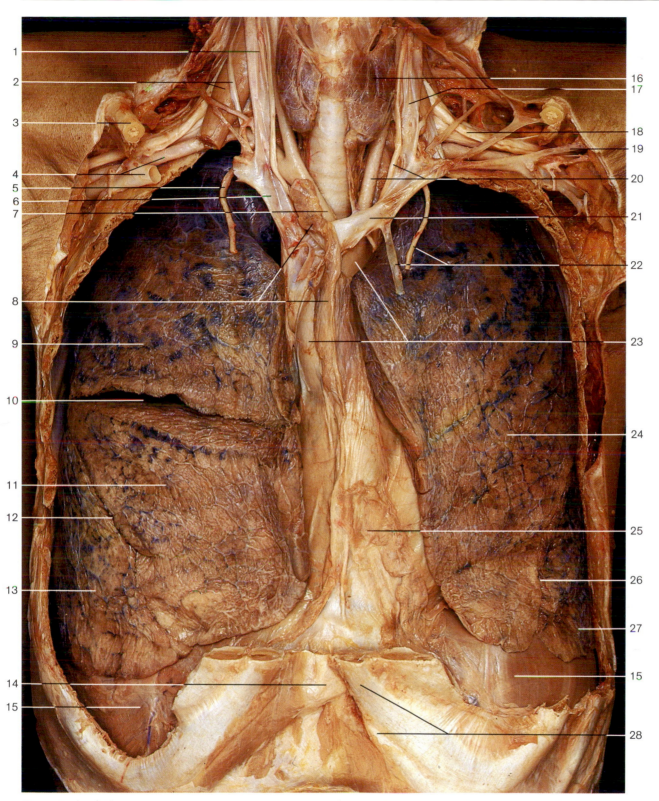

Thoracic organs (ventral aspect). The pleura has been opened and the lungs exposed. Remnants of the thymus and pericardium are seen.

1	Right internal jugular vein	11	Middle lobe of right lung	20	Left common carotid artery,
2	Phrenic nerve and scalenus anterior	12	Oblique fissure of right lung		vagus nerve
3	Clavicle (divided)	13	Lower lobe of right lung	21	Left brachiocephalic vein
4	Right subclavian artery and vein	14	Xiphoid process	22	Internal thoracic artery and vein (divided)
5	Internal thoracic artery	15	Diaphragm	23	Ascending aorta and aortic arch
6	Right brachiocephalic vein	16	Thyroid gland	24	Upper lobe of left lung
7	Brachiocephalic trunk	17	Left internal jugular vein	25	Pericardium
8	Thymus (atrophic)	18	Brachial plexus	26	Oblique fissure of left lung
9	Upper lobe of right lung	19	Left cephalic vein	27	Lower lobe of left lung
10	Horizontal fissure of right lung (incomplete)			28	Costal margin

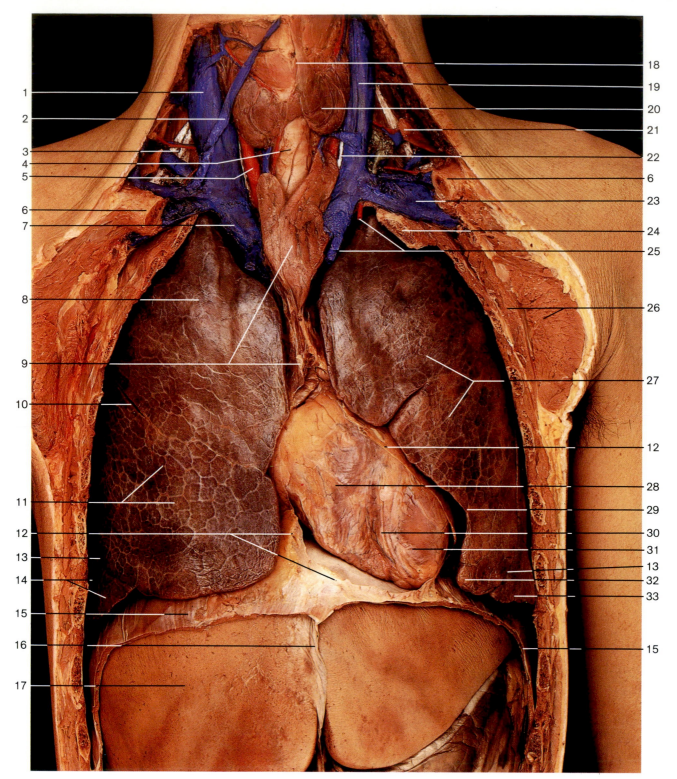

Thoracic organs (ventral aspect). The thoracic wall, costal pleura, pericardium and diaphragm have been partly removed.

1 Internal jugular vein	12 Pericardium (cut edges)	23 Left subclavian vein
2 External jugular vein	13 Oblique fissure of right lung	24 1st rib (divided)
3 Brachial plexus	14 Lower lobe of right lung	25 Internal thoracic artery and vein
4 Trachea	15 Diaphragm	26 Pectoralis major and pectoralis minor (cut edges)
5 Right common carotid artery	16 Falciform ligament	27 Upper lobe of left lung
6 Clavicle (divided)	17 Liver	28 Right ventricle
7 Right brachiocephalic vein	18 Larynx	29 Cardiac notch of left lung
8 Upper lobe of right lung	19 Left internal jugular vein	30 Interventricular sulcus of heart
9 **Thymus** (atrophic)	20 Thyroid gland	31 Left ventricle
10 Horizontal fissure of right lung	21 Omohyoid muscle (divided)	32 Lingula
11 Middle lobe of right lung	22 Vagus nerve	33 Lower lobe of left lung

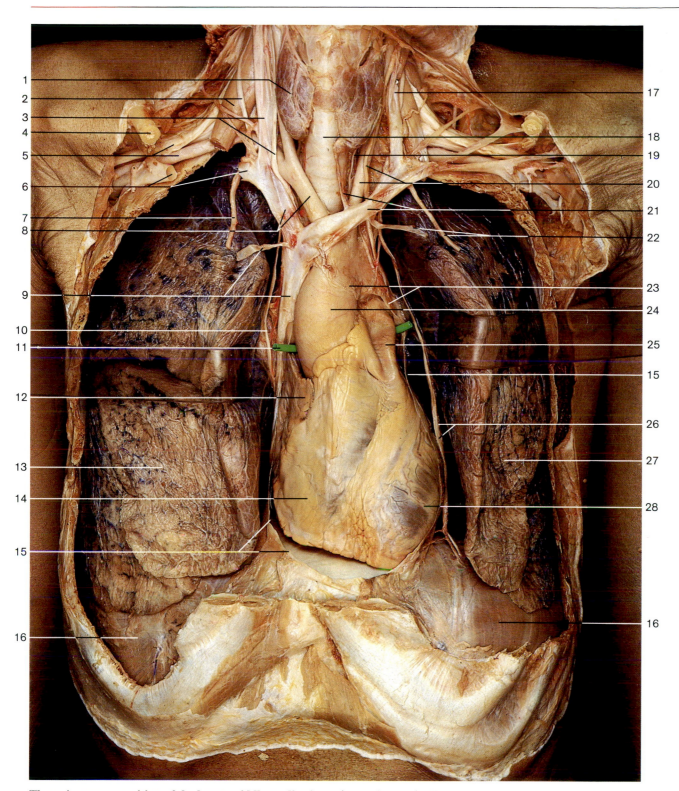

Thoracic organs, position of the heart, middle mediastinum (ventral aspect). The anterior wall of the thorax, the costal pleura and the pericardium have been removed and the lungs slightly reflected.

1 Thyroid gland	11 Transverse pericardial sinus (probe)	21 Left brachiocephalic vein, inferior thyroid vein
2 Phrenic nerve and scalenus anterior	12 Right auricle	
3 Vagus nerve, internal jugular vein	13 Middle lobe of right lung	22 Left internal thoracic artery and vein (divided)
4 Clavicle (divided)	14 Right ventricle	
5 Brachial plexus, subclavian artery	15 Cut edge of pericardium	23 Upper margin of pericardial sac
6 Subclavian vein	16 Diaphragm	24 Ascending aorta
7 Internal thoracic artery	17 Internal jugular vein	25 Pulmonary trunk
8 Brachiocephalic trunk and right brachiocephalic vein	18 Trachea	26 Left phrenic nerve, left peri-cardiacophrenic artery and vein
	19 Recurrent laryngeal nerve	
9 Superior vena cava, thymic vein	20 Left common carotid artery, vagus nerve	27 Upper lobe of left lung
10 Right phrenic nerve		28 Left ventricle

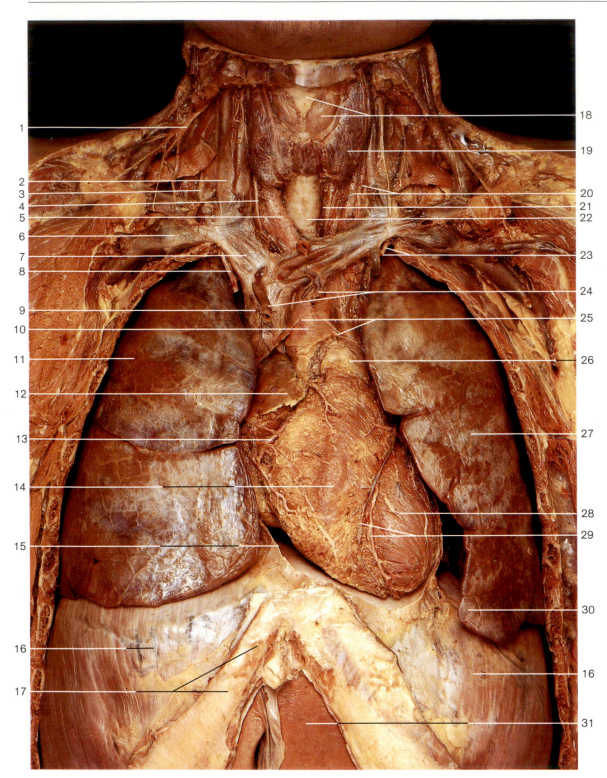

Thoracic organs, position of heart, dissection of coronary vessels in situ (ventral aspect). The anterior wall of thorax, costal pleura and pericardium have been removed.

1 Intermediate supraclavicular nerve	12 Right atrium	21 Recurrent laryngeal nerve
2 Internal jugular vein	13 Right coronary artery and	22 Trachea
3 Right phrenic nerve	small cardiac vein	23 Left internal thoracic artery and vein (divided)
4 Right vagus nerve	14 Right ventricle	24 Thymic veins
5 Right common carotid artery	15 Cut edge of pericardium	25 Margin of pericardial sac
6 Right subclavian vein	16 Diaphragm	26 Pulmonary trunk
7 Right brachiocephalic vein	17 Costal arch	27 Left lung
8 Right internal thoracic artery	18 Larynx, cricothyroid muscle	28 Left ventricle
9 Superior vena cava	19 Thyroid gland	29 Anterior interventricular artery and vein
10 Ascending aorta	20 Left common carotid artery,	30 Lingula
11 Right lung	left vagus nerve	31 Liver

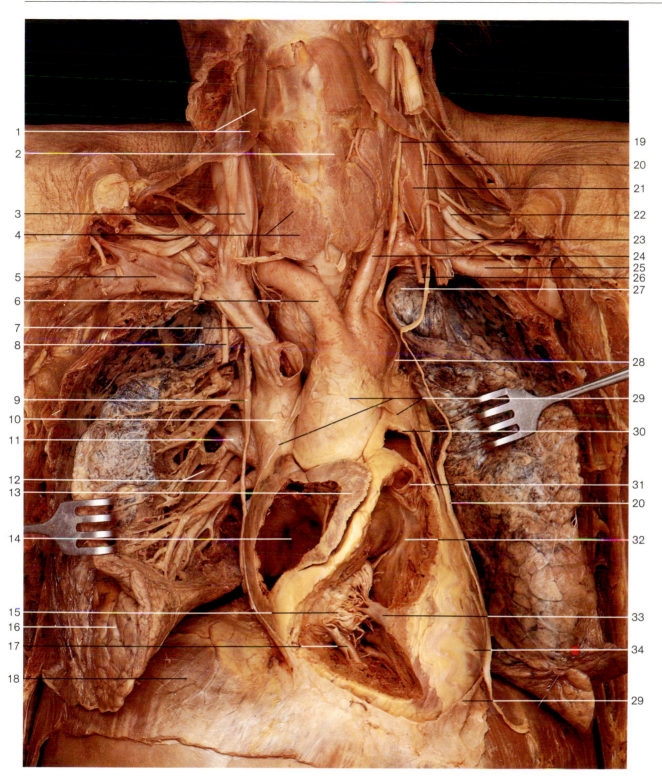

Thoracic organs, heart with valves in situ (ventral aspect). Anterior wall of thorax, pleura and anterior portion of pericardium have been removed. The right atrium and ventricle have been opened to show the right atrioventricular and pulmonary valves.

1 Omohyoid muscle	12 Branch of pulmonary artery	24 Left common carotid artery
2 Pyramidal lobe of thyroid gland	13 Right auricle	25 Left subclavian artery
3 Internal jugular vein	14 Right atrium	26 Left internal thoracic artery
4 Thyroid gland	15 Right atrioventricular (tricuspid) valve	27 Apex of left lung
5 Right subclavian vein	16 Right lung	28 Left recurrent laryngeal nerve
6 Brachiocephalic trunk	17 Posterior papillary muscle	29 Cut edge of pericardium
7 Right brachiocephalic vein	18 Diaphragm	30 Pulmonary trunk (fenestrated)
8 Right internal thoracic artery	19 Left vagus nerve	31 Pulmonary valve
9 Right phrenic nerve	20 Left phrenic nerve	32 Conus arteriosus
10 Superior vena cava	21 Scalenus anterior	33 Anterior papillary muscle
11 Pulmonary vein	22 Brachial plexus	34 Left ventricle
	23 Thyrocervical trunk	

245

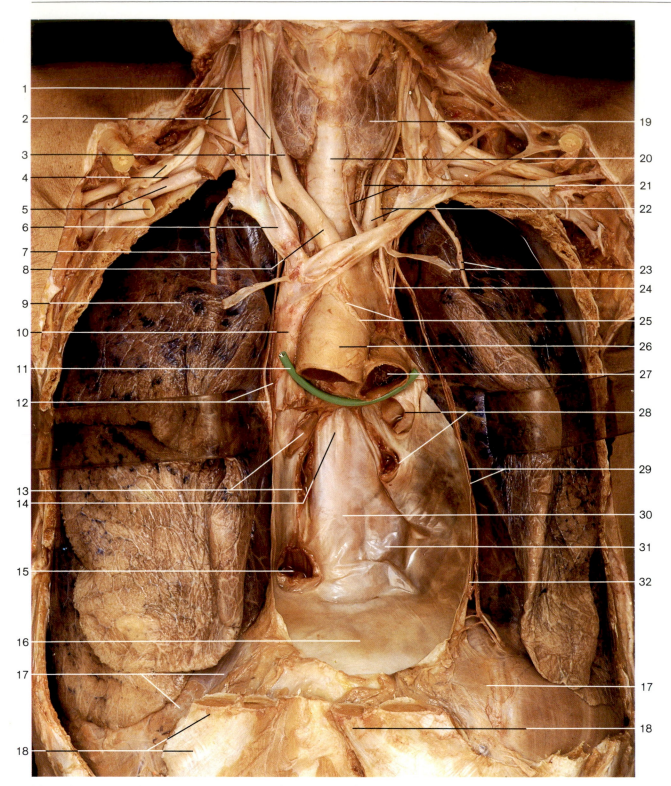

Thoracic organs, pericardium and **mediastinum** (ventral aspect). Anterior wall of thorax and heart have been removed and the lungs slightly reflected. Note probe within transverse pericardial sinus.

1 Right internal jugular vein, right vagus nerve	12 Right phrenic nerve, right pericardiacophrenic artery and vein	22 Left common carotid artery, left vagus nerve
2 Right phrenic nerve, scalenus anterior	13 Right pulmonary veins	23 Left internal thoracic artery and vein (divided)
3 Right common carotid artery	14 Oblique sinus of pericardium	24 Vagus nerve at aortic arch
4 Brachial plexus	15 Inferior vena cava	25 Cut edge of pericardium
5 Right subclavian artery and vein	16 Diaphragmatic part of pericardium	26 Ascending aorta
6 Right brachiocephalic vein	17 Diaphragm	27 Pulmonary trunk (divided)
7 Right internal thoracic artery (divided)	18 Costal margin	28 Left pulmonary veins
8 Brachiocephalic trunk	19 Thyroid gland	29 Left phrenic nerve, left pericardiacophrenic artery and vein
9 Upper lobe of right lung	20 Trachea	30 Contour of esophagus beneath pericardium
10 Superior vena cava	21 Recurrent laryngeal nerve, inferior thyroid vein	31 Contour of aorta beneath pericardium
11 Transverse pericardial sinus (probe)		32 Pericardium (cut edge)

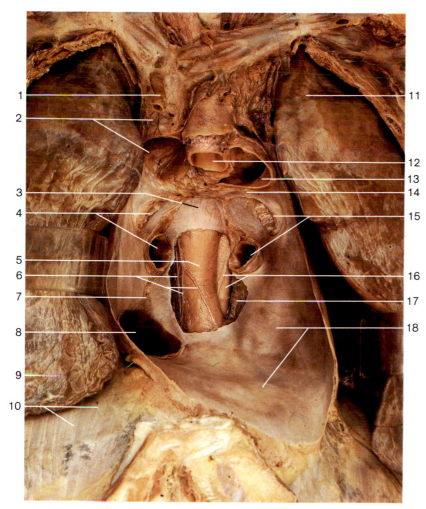

1 Internal thoracic vein
2 Superior vena cava
3 Oblique sinus of pericardium
4 Right pulmonary veins
5 Esophagus
6 Branches of right vagus nerve
7 Mesocardium
8 Inferior vena cava
9 Middle lobe of right lung
10 Diaphragm
11 Upper lobe of left lung
12 Ascending aorta
13 **Pulmonary trunk**
14 Transverse pericardial sinus (green probe)
15 Left pulmonary veins
16 Descending aorta, left vagus nerve
17 Left lung (adjacent to pericardium)
18 **Pericardium**
19 Left subclavian artery
20 Vagus nerve
21 Recurrent laryngeal nerve
22 Descending aorta
23 Pulmonary artery
24 **Left atrium**
25 **Left ventricle**
26 Coronary sinus
27 Left common carotid artery
28 Brachiocephalic trunk
29 Azygos vein
30 **Right atrium**
31 **Right ventricle**
32 Aortic arch

Pericardial sac (ventral aspect). The heart has been removed, and the posterior wall of the pericardium has been opened to show the adjacent esophagus and aorta.

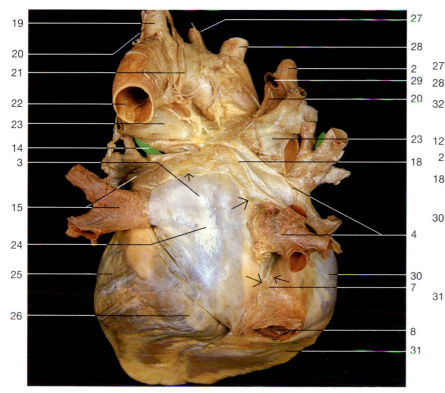

Heart with epicardium (posterior aspect). Arrows: oblique sinus.

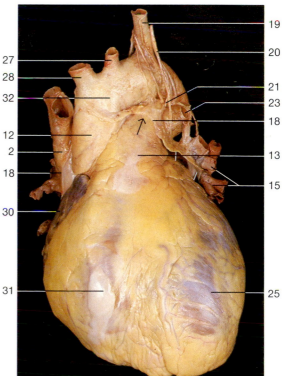

Heart with epicardium (anterior aspect). Arrow: pericardial reflection.

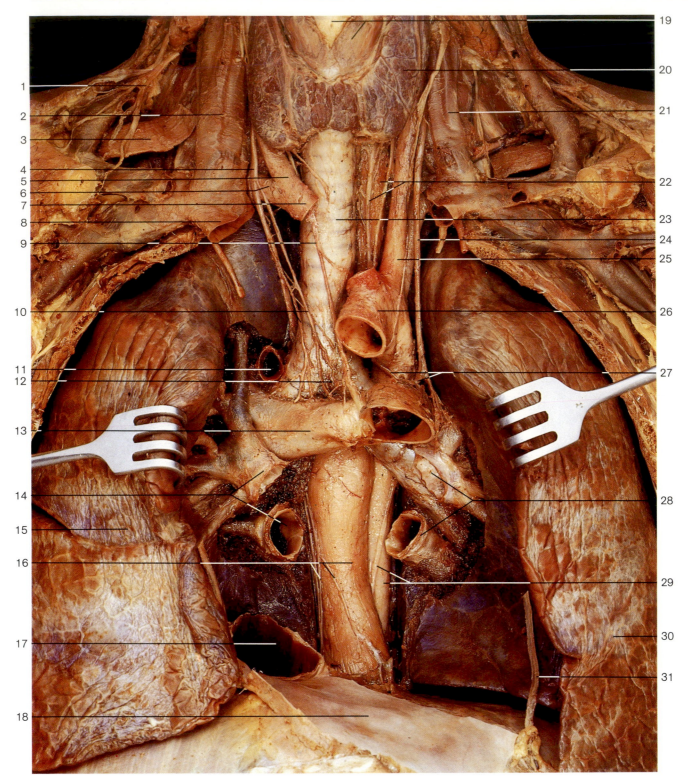

Mediastinal organs after removal of heart and pericardium (ventral aspect). Both lungs have been slightly reflected.

1 Supraclavicular nerves
2 Internal jugular vein
3 Omohyoid muscle
4 Right vagus nerve
5 Right common carotid artery
6 Right subclavian artery
7 Brachiocephalic trunk
8 Right brachiocephalic vein
9 Superior cervical cardiac branch
   of vagus nerve
10 Inferior cervical cardiac branches
   of vagus nerve

11 Azygos vein (divided)
12 Bifurcation of trachea
13 Right pulmonary artery
14 Right pulmonary veins
15 Right lung
16 Esophagus, branches
   of vagus nerve
17 Inferior vena cava
18 Pericardium
19 Larynx, cricothyroid muscle
20 Thyroid gland
21 Internal jugular vein

22 Esophagus, left recurrent
   laryngeal nerve
23 Trachea
24 Left vagus nerve
25 Left common carotid artery
26 Aortic arch
27 Left recurrent laryngeal nerve
   branching off from vagus nerve
28 Left pulmonary veins
29 Thoracic aorta, vagus nerve
30 Left lung
31 Left phrenic nerve (divided)

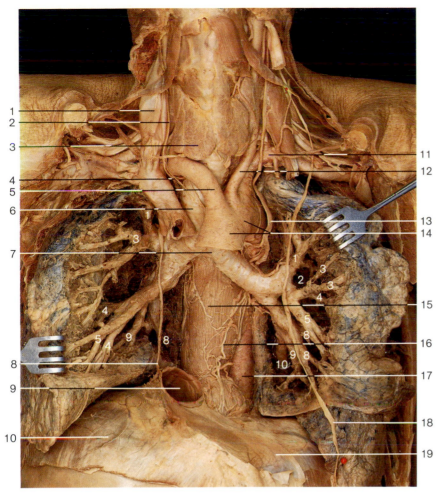

Bronchial tree in situ (ventral aspect). Heart and pericardium have been
removed; the bronchi of the bronchopulmonary segments are dissected.
1–10 = numbers of segments.

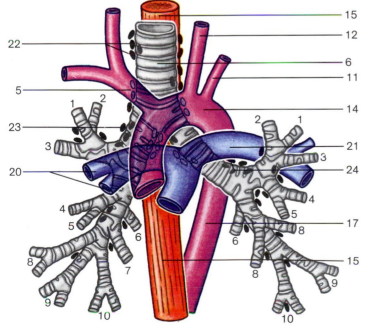

**Relation of aorta, pulmonary trunk and esophagus to trachea
and bronchial tree.** (Schematic drawing) (W.).
1–10 = numbers of segments.

249

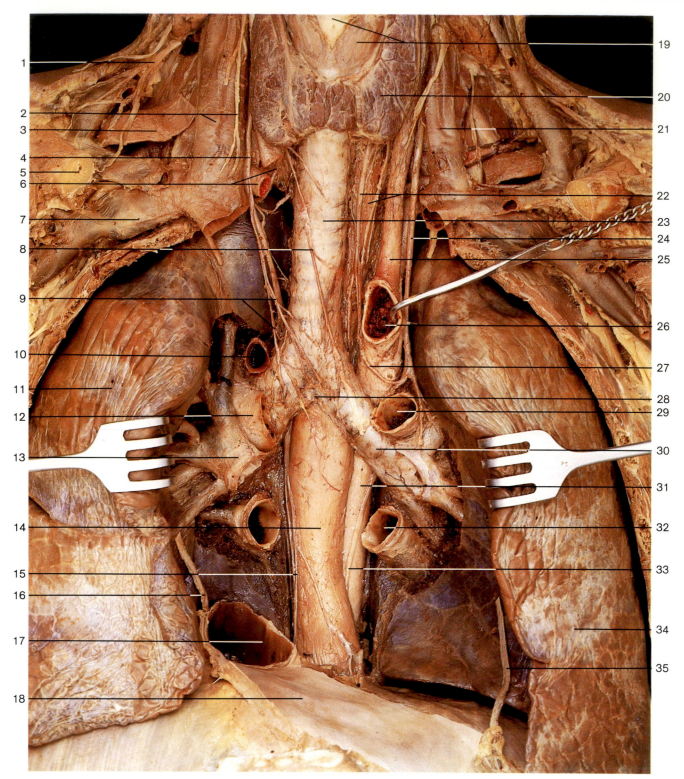

Organs of posterior mediastinum (ventral aspect). The heart with the pericardium has been removed, and the lungs and aortic arch have been slightly reflected to show the vagus nerves and their branches.

1 Supraclavicular nerves
2 Right internal jugular vein with ansa cervicalis
3 Omohyoid muscle
4 **Right vagus nerve**
5 Clavicle
6 Right subclavian artery and recurrent laryngeal nerve
7 Right subclavian vein
8 Superior cervical cardiac branch of vagus nerve
9 Inferior cervical cardiac branch of vagus nerve
10 Azygos vein (divided)
11 Right lung

12 Right pulmonary artery
13 Right pulmonary veins
14 Esophagus
15 Esophageal plexus
16 Right phrenic nerve (divided)
17 Inferior vena cava
18 Pericardium covering the diaphragm
19 Larynx, cricothyroid muscle
20 Thyroid gland
21 Left internal jugular vein
22 Esophagus, left inferior laryngeal nerve
23 Trachea

24 **Left vagus nerve**
25 Left common carotid artery
26 Aortic arch
27 Left recurrent laryngeal nerve
28 Bifurcation of trachea
29 Left pulmonary artery
30 Left main bronchus
31 Descending aorta
32 Left pulmonary veins
33 Branch of left vagus nerve
34 Left lung
35 Left phrenic nerve (divided)

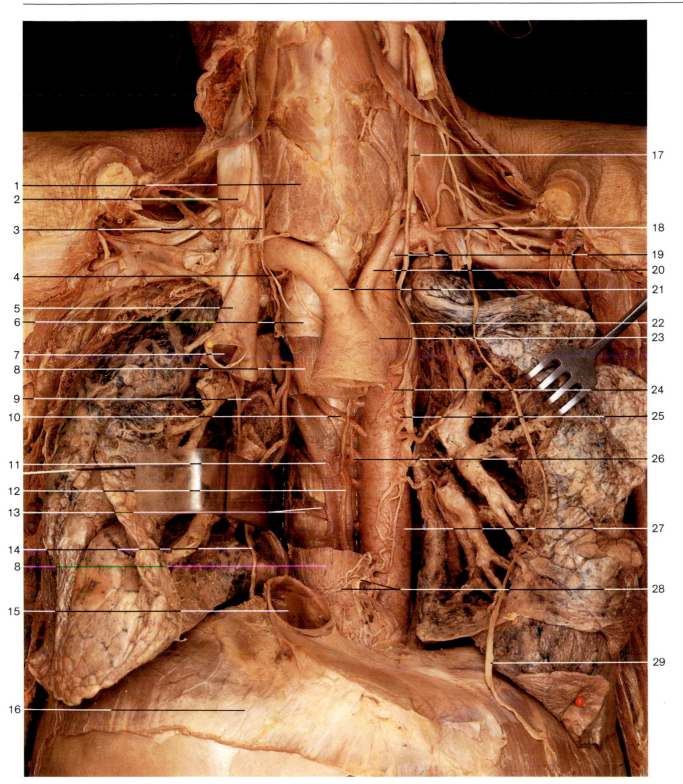

Mediastinal organs (ventral aspect). Heart and distal part of esophagus have been removed to display the vessels and nerves of the posterior mediastinum.

1 Thyroid gland	11 **Azygos vein**	20 Left common carotid artery
2 Right internal jugular vein	12 **Thoracic duct**	21 Brachiocephalic trunk
3 Right vagus nerve	13 Intercostal artery and vein	22 Left vagus nerve
4 Right recurrent laryngeal nerve	(in front of the vertebral column)	23 Aortic arch
5 Right brachiocephalic vein	14 Right phrenic nerve	24 Left recurrent laryngeal nerve
6 Trachea	15 Inferior vena cava	25 Left bronchial artery
7 Left brachiocephalic vein (reflected)	16 Diaphragm	26 Lymph node
8 Esophagus	17 Left vagus nerve	27 Thoracic aorta
9 Right bronchial artery	18 Thyrocervical trunk	28 Esophageal plexus
10 Intercostal artery	19 Left subclavian artery	29 Left phrenic nerve

251

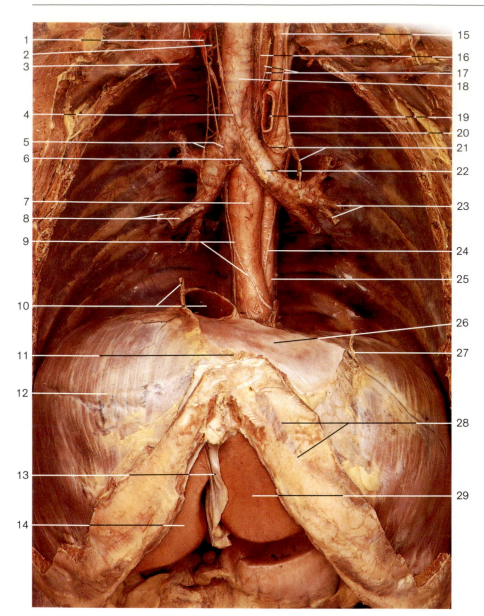

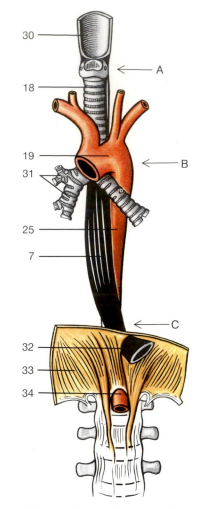

Diaphragm and organs of mediastinum (anterior aspect). Heart and lungs have been removed; the costal margin remains in place. Note the different courses of left and right vagus.

Organs of posterior mediastinum (ventral aspect). (Schematic drawing) (W.). Three regions in which the esophagus is narrowed are shown:

A at the level of the cricoid cartilage;

B at the level of the aortic arch;

C at the level of the diaphragm.

1	Right subclavian artery
2	Right recurrent laryngeal nerve
3	Right brachiocephalic vein
4	Superior cervical cardiac nerve
5	Inferior cervical cardiac nerves and pulmonary branches
6	Bifurcation of trachea
7	Esophagus (thoracic part)
8	Bronchi of lateral and medial segments of middle lobe
9	Esophageal plexus of vagus nerve
10	Inferior vena cava, right phrenic nerve (cut)
11	Sternal part of diaphragm
12	Costal part of diaphragm
13	Falciform ligament of liver
14	Right lobe of liver

15	Left common carotid artery
16	Left recurrent laryngeal nerve
17	Esophageal branches of vagus nerve, esohagus
18	Trachea
19	Aortic arch
20	Left vagus nerve
21	Left recurrent laryngeal nerve with inferior cardiac nerve
22	Left primary pulmonary bronchus
23	Superior and inferior lingular bronchi
24	Esophageal plexus of vagus nerve
25	Descending aorta
26	Central tendon of diaphragm covered with pericardium
27	Left phrenic nerve (divided)
28	Costal margin

29	Liver, left lobe
30	Pharynx
31	Bronchi
32	Esophagus (abdominal part)
33	Diaphragm
34	Abdominal aorta

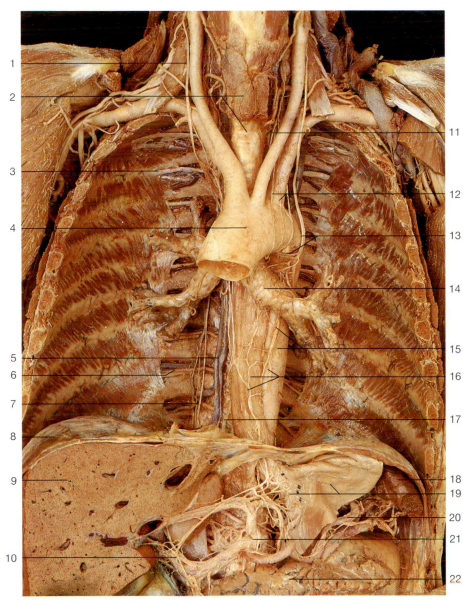

Organs of posterior mediastinum (anterior aspect).

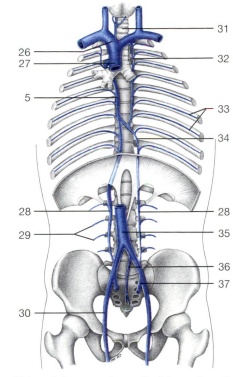

Veins of the posterior wall of thoracic and abdominal cavity. (Schematic drawing) (O.).

1 Right vagus nerve
2 Thyroid gland, trachea
3 Intercostal nerve
4 Aortic arch
5 **Azygos vein**
6 Posterior intercostal artery
7 **Greater splanchnic nerve**
8 Diaphragm
9 Liver
10 Proper hepatic artery, hepatic plexus
11 Recurrent laryngeal nerve
12 Inferior cervical cardiac nerves
13 Left vagus nerve, recurrent laryngeal nerve
14 Left main bronchus
15 Thoracic aorta, left vagus nerve
16 Esophagus, esophageal plexus
17 **Thoracic duct**
18 Spleen
19 Anterior gastric plexus, stomach (divided)
20 Splenic artery, splenic plexus
21 **Celiac trunk, celiac plexus**
22 Pancreas
23 Ramus communicans
24 **Sympathetic trunk, sympathetic ganglion**
25 **Intercostal vein, artery and nerve**
    (from above)
26 Right brachiocephalic vein
27 Superior vena cava
28 Ascending lumbar vein
29 Lumbar veins
30 Right external iliac vein
31 Trachea
32 Accessory hemiazygos vein
33 Intercostal veins
34 Hemiazygos vein
35 Inferior vena cava
36 Median sacral vein
37 Internal iliac vein

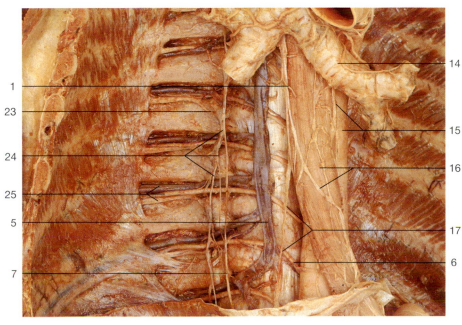

Inferior segment of posterior mediastinum (anterior aspect).

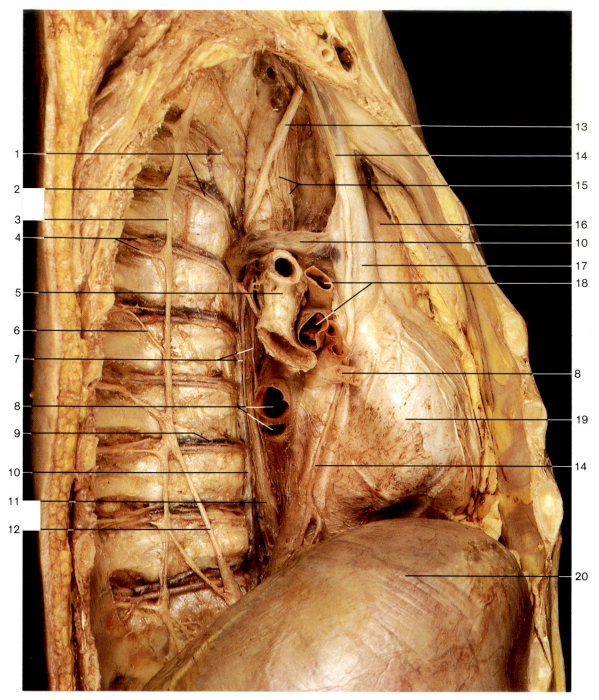

Mediastinal organs (right lateral aspect). Right lung and pleura of right half of the thorax have been removed.

1 Intercostal arteries	7 Esophageal plexus (branches of right vagus nerve)	14 Right phrenic nerve
2 Ganglion of sympathetic trunk		15 Inferior cervical cardiac branches of vagus nerve
3 Sympathetic trunk	8 Pulmonary veins	
4 Vessels and nerves of the intercostal space (from above: Intercostal vein, artery and nerve)	9 Intercostal vein	16 Aortic arch
	10 Azygos vein	17 Superior vena cava
	11 Esophagus	18 Right pulmonary artery
5 Right primary bronchus	12 Greater splanchnic nerve	19 Heart with pericardium
6 Ramus communicans of sympathetic trunk	13 Vagus nerve	20 Diaphragm

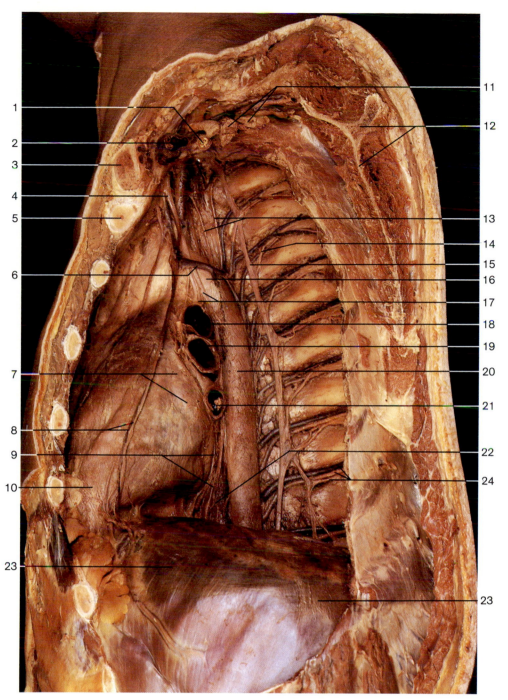

Organs of posterior and superior mediastinum (left lateral aspect).

1 Subclavian artery
2 Subclavian vein
3 Clavicle (divided)
4 Left vagus nerve
5 First rib (divided)
6 Accessory hemiazygos vein
7 Left atrium with pericardium
8 Left phrenic nerve, pericardiacophrenic artery and vein
9 Esophageal plexus, branches derived from left vagus nerve

10 Apex of heart with pericardium
11 Brachial plexus
12 Scapula (divided)
13 Posterior intercostal arteries
14 Ramus communicans of sympathetic trunk
15 Sympathetic trunk
16 Aortic arch
17 Left vagus nerve, recurrent laryngeal nerve
18 Left pulmonary artery

19 Left primary bronchus
20 Thoracic aorta
21 Pulmonary vein
22 Esophagus (thoracic part)
23 Diaphragm
24 Posterior intercostal artery and vein, intercostal nerve

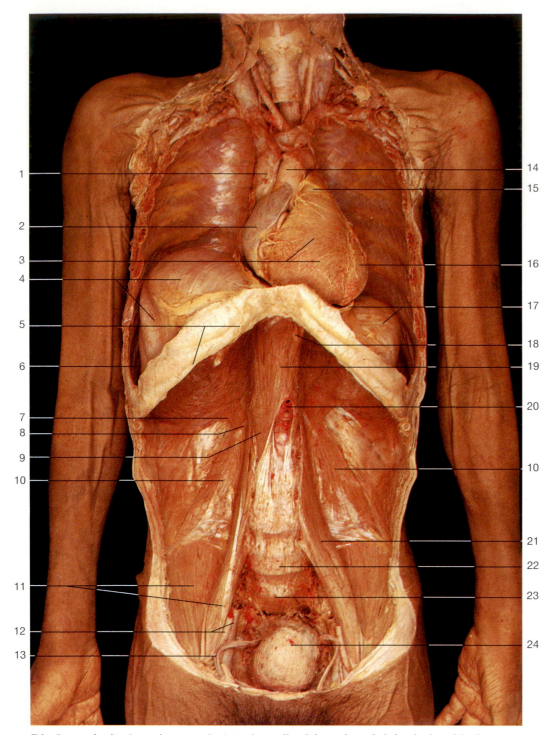

Diaphragm in situ (anterior aspect). Anterior walls of thoracic and abdominal cavities have been removed. Natural position of the heart above the central tendon on the diaphragm is shown.

1 Superior vena cava
2 Right atrium
3 Right ventricle
4 **Costal part of diaphragm**
5 Costal margin
6 Position of costodiaphragmatic recess
7 **Lateral arcuate ligament**
8 **Medial arcuate ligament**
9 Right crus of lumbar part of diaphragm
10 Quadratus lumborum
11 Iliopsoas muscle
12 Right external iliac artery and vein

13 Ductus deferens
14 Ascending aorta
15 Pulmonary trunk
16 Left ventricle
17 Pericardium, diaphragm
18 Esophageal hiatus
19 **Lumbar part of diaphragm**
20 Aortic hiatus
21 Psoas major muscle
22 Intervertebral disc of lumbar vertebra
23 Promontory
24 Urinary bladder

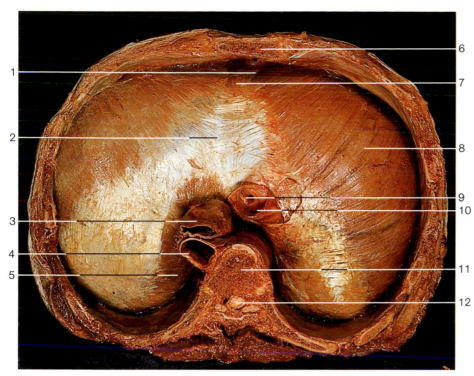

1	Sternocostal triangle
2	Central tendon (from above)
3	Esophagus
4	Aorta
5	Lumbar part of diaphragm
6	Sternum
7	Sternal part of diaphragm
8	Costal part of diaphragm
9	Entrance of hepatic veins
10	Inferior vena cava
11	Body of 9th thoracic vertebra
12	Spinal cord

Diaphragm (superior aspect). The pleura and thoracic wall have been removed.

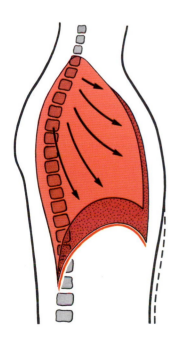

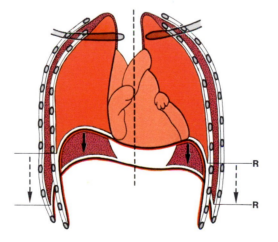

Changes in the position of the diaphragm and thoracic cage during respiration (W.). Left: lateral aspect; right: anterior aspect. During inspiration the diaphragm moves downwards and the lower part of the thoracic cage expands forward and laterally, causing the costodiaphragmatic recess (R) to enlarge (cf. dotted arrows).

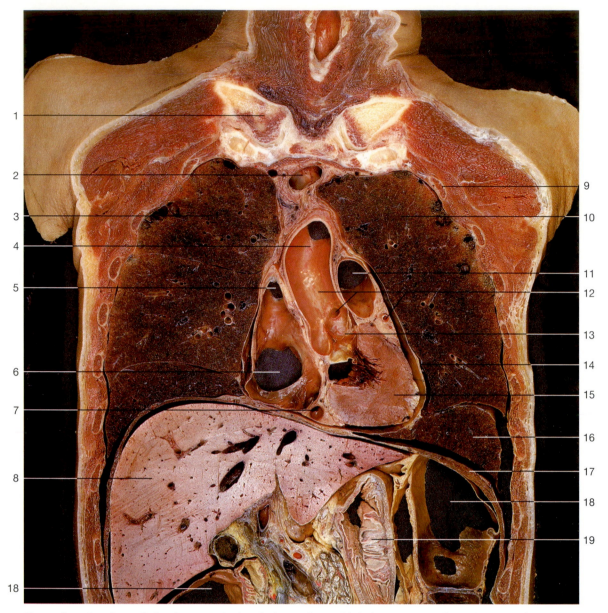

Coronal section through the thorax at the level of superior and inferior vena cava (anterior aspect).

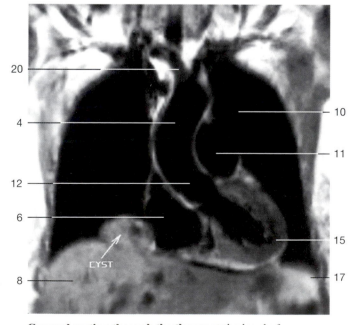

Coronal section through the thorax at the level of superior vena cava. MR-Scan.

1   Clavicle
2   Brachiocephalic vein
3   Superior lobe of right lung
4   Aortic arch
5   Superior vena cava
6   Right atrium (entrance of inferior vena cava)
7   Coronary sinus
8   Liver
9   Second rib
10 Superior lobe of left lung
11 Pulmonary trunk
12 Ascending aorta, left coronary artery
13 Aortic valve
14 Pericardium
15 Left ventricle
16 Inferior lobe of left lung
17 Diaphragm
18 Left colic flexure
19 Stomach
20 Brachiocephalic trunk

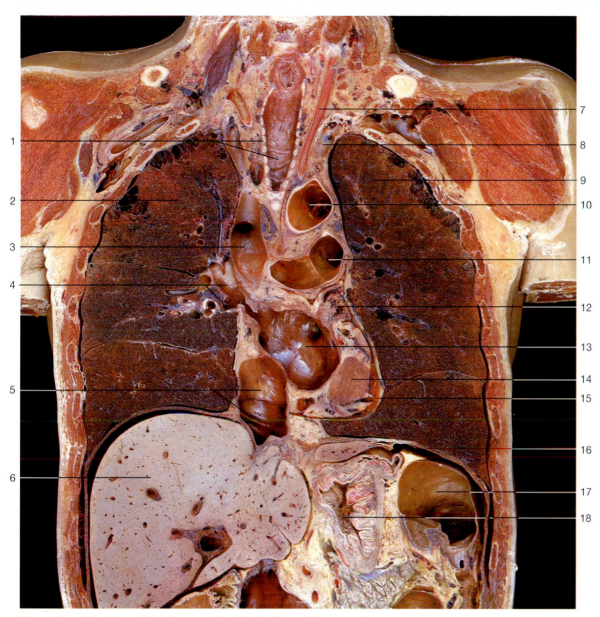

Coronal section through the thorax at the level of ascending aorta (anterior aspect).

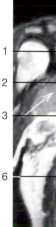

Coronal section through the thorax at the level of ascending aorta. MR-Scan.

1 Trachea
2 Superior lobe of lung
3 Superior vena cava
4 Right pulmonary veins
5 Inferior vena cava, right atrium
6 Liver
7 Left common carotid artery
8 Left subclavian vein
9 Superior lobe of left lung
10 Aortic arch
11 Left pulmonary artery
12 Left auricle
13 Left atrium with orifices
   of pulmonary veins
14 Left ventricle (myocardium)
15 Pericardium
16 Diaphragm
17 Left colic flexure
18 Stomach
19 Left subclavian artery

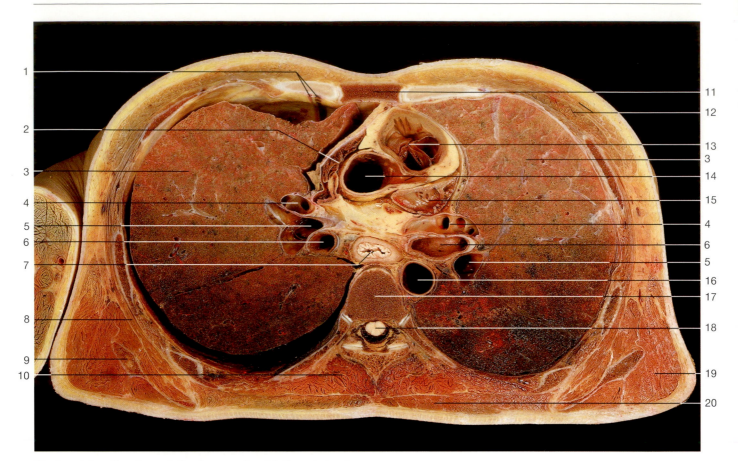

Horizontal section through the thorax at level 1 (from below).

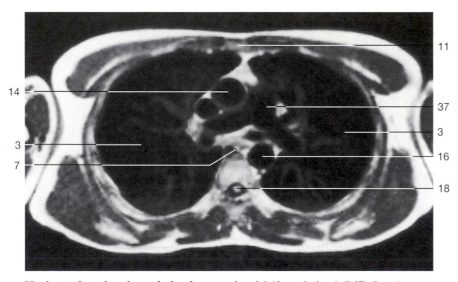

Horizontal section through the thorax at level 1 (from below) (MR-Scan).

1 Internal thoracic artery and vein	12 Pectoralis major and minor
2 Right atrium	13 Conus arteriosus (right ventricle), pulmonary valve
3 Lung	
4 Pulmonary artery	14 Ascending aorta, left coronary artery only in upper figure
5 Pulmonary vein	
6 Primary bronchus	15 **Left atrium**
7 Esophagus	16 **Descending aorta**
8 Serratus anterior	17 Thoracic vertebra
9 Scapula	18 Spinal cord
10 Longissimus thoracis	19 Latissimus dorsi
11 Sternum	20 Trapezius

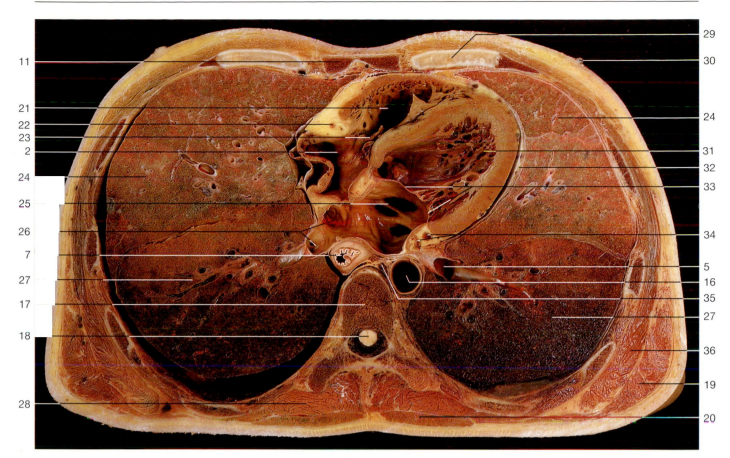

Horizontal section through the thorax at level 2 (from below).

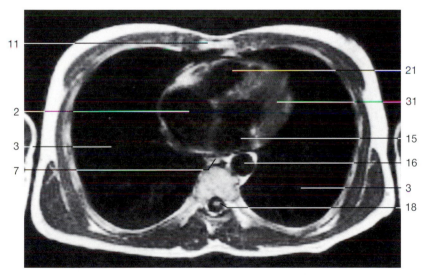

Horizontal section through the thorax at level 2 (from below) (MR-Scan).

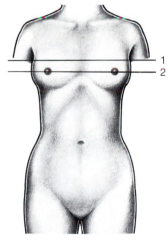

Levels of sections.

21	**Right ventricle**	31	**Left ventricle**
22	Right coronary artery	32	Pericardium
23	Right atrioventricular valve	33	Left atrioventricular valve
24	Lung, superior lobe	34	Left coronary artery, coronary sinus
25	**Left atrium**	35	Accessory hemiazygos vein
26	Pulmonary veins	36	Serratus anterior
27	Lung, inferior lobe	37	Pulmonary trunk
28	Erector muscle of spine		
29	Third costal cartilage		
30	Nipple		

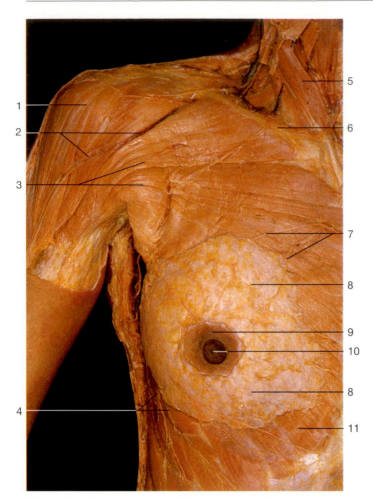

1 Deltoid muscle
2 Deltopectoral groove, cephalic vein
3 Pectoralis major
4 Lateral mammary branches of intercostal arteries
5 Sternocleidomastoid
6 Clavicle
7 Medial mammary branches of intercostal arteries
8 Breast tissue
9 Areola
10 Nipple
11 Abdominal part of pectoralis major
12 Pectoral fascia
13 Mammary gland
14 Serratus anterior
15 Lactiferous sinus
16 Lactiferous ducts

Dissection of mammary gland (anterior aspect).

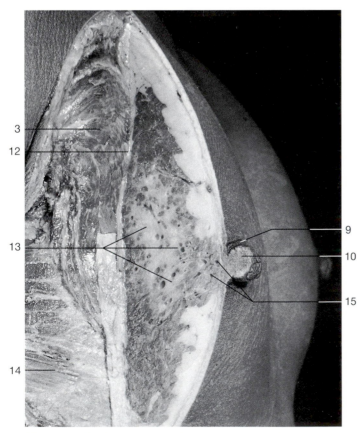

Mammary gland (sagittal section; pregnant female).

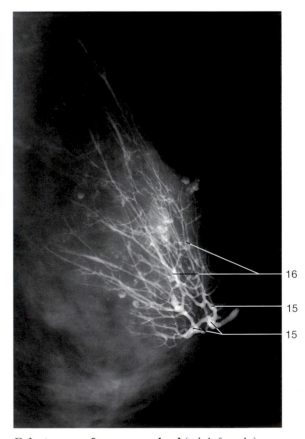

Galactogram of mammary gland (adult female).
Notice multiple duct cysts.

Chapter VI
Abdominal Organs

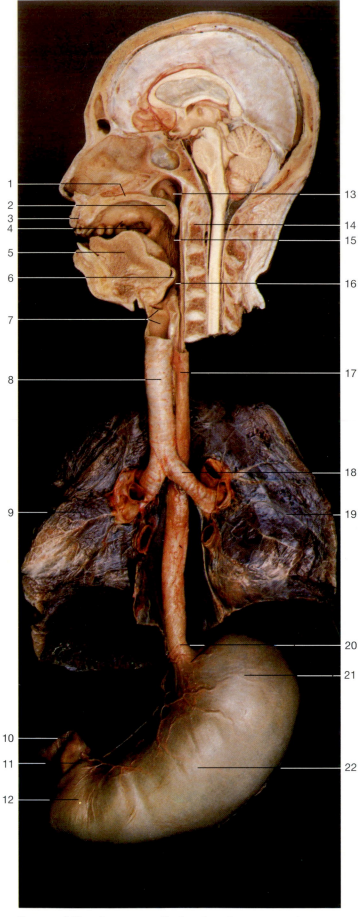

Survey of digestive system. Oral cavity, pharynx, esophagus and stomach.

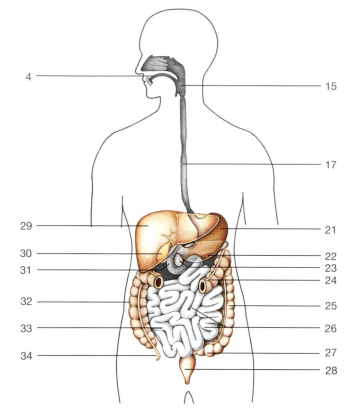

Organization of digestive system. Position of abdominal organs (O.).

1 Hard palate
2 Soft palate with uvula
3 Vestibule of the mouth
4 Oral cavity proper
5 Tongue
6 Epiglottis
7 Vocal ligament, larynx
8 Trachea
9 Right lung
10 Superior part of duodenum
11 Pylorus
12 Pyloric antrum
13 Nasopharynx
14 Dens of axis
15 Oropharynx
16 Laryngopharynx
17 Esophagus (thoracic part)
18 Left main bronchus
19 Left lung
20 Abdominal part of esophagus, cardia
21 Fundus of stomach
22 Body of stomach
23 Pancreas
24 Transverse colon (divided)
25 Descending colon
26 Jejunum
27 Sigmoid colon
28 Rectum
29 Liver
30 Gall bladder
31 Duodenum
32 Ascending colon
33 Ileum
34 Vermiform appendix

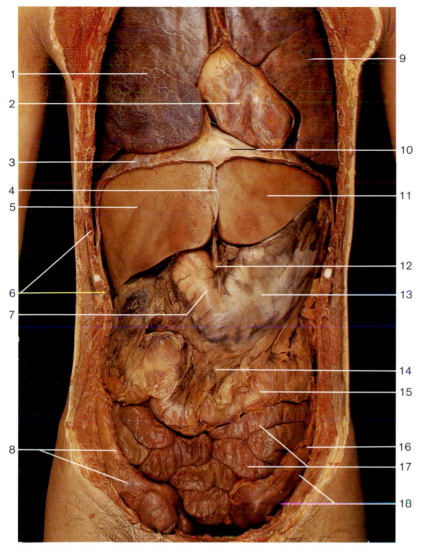

1 Right lung (middle lobe)
2 Heart (right ventricle)
3 Diaphragm (costal part)
4 Falciform ligament of liver
5 Right lobe of liver
6 Ribs of costal arch (cut)
7 Stomach (pyloric part)
8 Ascending colon
9 Left lung (upper lobe)
10 Central tendon of diaphragm
11 Left lobe of liver
12 Ligamentum teres
13 Stomach
14 Gastrocolic ligament
15 Transverse colon
16 Descending colon
17 Small intestine (jejunum)
18 Sigmoid colon
19 Rectus abdominis
20 Costal cartilage (cut)
21 Small intestine (section)
22 Splenic artery
23 Descending colon (section)
24 Pancreas
25 Left suprarenal gland
26 Abdominal aorta
27 Spleen
28 Kidney
29 Diaphragm
30 Linea alba
31 Transverse colon (cut)
32 Stomach
33 Gallbladder
34 Portal vein
35 Inferior vena cava
36 Right suprarenal gland
37 Intervertebral disc of lumbar vertebra
38 Retroperitoneal fatty tissue
39 Spinal cord
40 Intrinsic muscles of back

Abdominal organs in situ. The thoracic and abdominal walls have been removed. Note that the upper abdominal organs are located within the lower third of the thorax. The liver is enlarged.

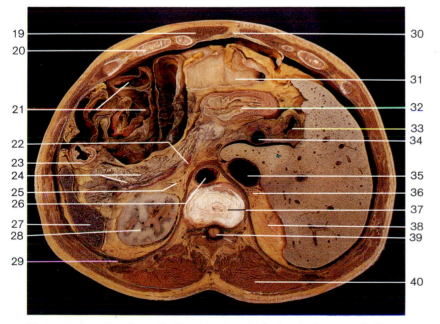

Horizontal section through abdominal cavity (at level of pancreas) (from above).

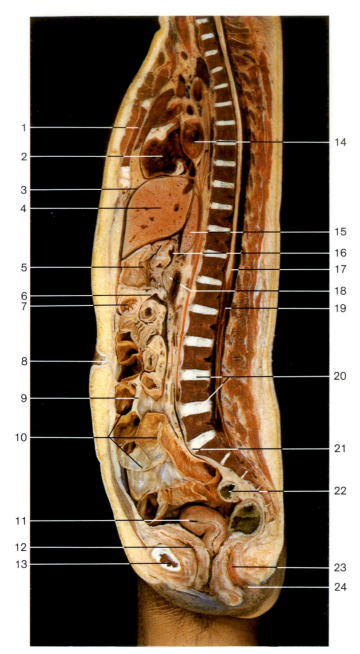

Median section through the trunk (female).

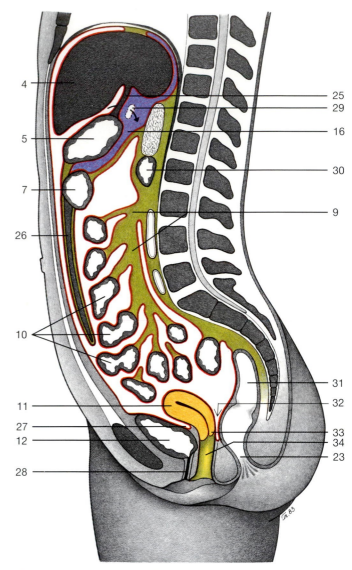

Median section through the female trunk. (Schematic drawing)
(Tr.). Blue = omental bursa; red = peritoneum.

1 Sternum	13 Pubic symphysis	24 Anus
2 Right ventricle of heart	14 Left atrium of heart	25 Lesser omentum
3 Diaphragm	15 Caudate lobe of liver	26 Greater omentum
4 Liver	16 Omental bursa or lesser sac	27 Vesicouterine pouch
5 Stomach	17 Conus medullaris	28 Urethra
6 Transverse mesocolon	18 Pancreas	29 Epiploic foramen
7 Transverse colon	19 Cauda equina	30 Duodenum
8 Umbilicus	20 Intervertebral discs	31 Rectum
9 Mesentery	(lumbar vertebral column)	32 Rectouterine pouch
10 Small intestine	21 Promontory	33 Vaginal part of
11 Uterus	22 Sigmoid colon	cervix of uterus
12 Urinary bladder	23 Anal canal	34 Vagina

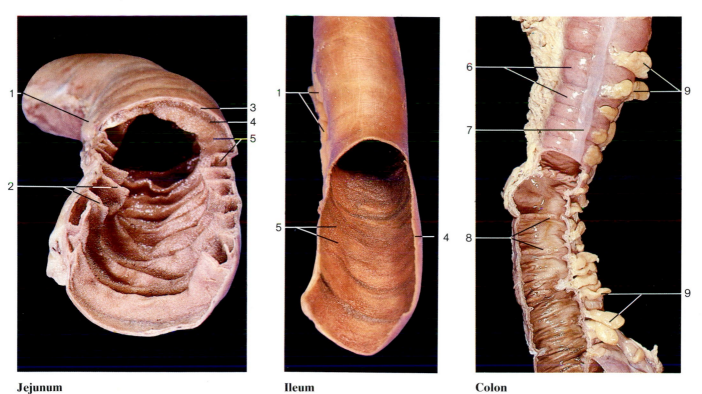

Jejunum   **Ileum**   **Colon**

The intestine has been partly opened to show the different patterns of the mucous membranes.

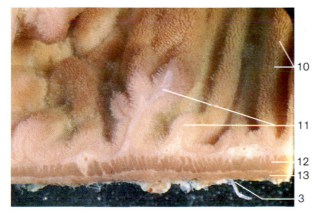

1	Line of attachment of mesentery	9	Appendices epiploicae
2	Plicae circulares	10	Intestinal villi
3	Serosa	11	Plicae circulares (cut edges)
4	Muscular coat	12	Circular muscle layer
5	Mucosa	13	Longitudinal muscle layer
6	Haustra of colon	14	Submucosa
7	Free taenia	15	Muscularis mucosae
8	Semilunar folds	16	Peritoneum
		17	Mesentery with vessels and nerves

Folds and villi of intestinal mucosa.

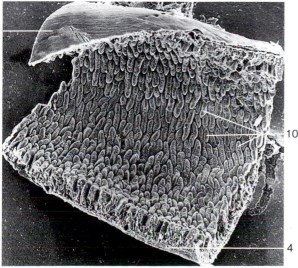

Ileum, intestinal villi (scanning-electron micrograph).

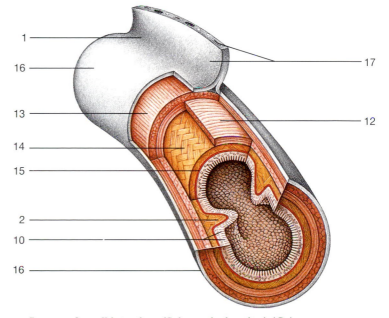

Layers of small intestine. (Schematic drawing) (O.).

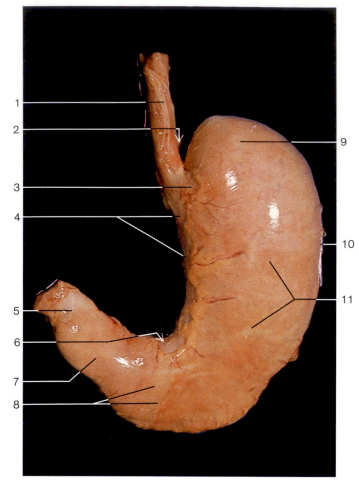

Stomach (ventral aspect).

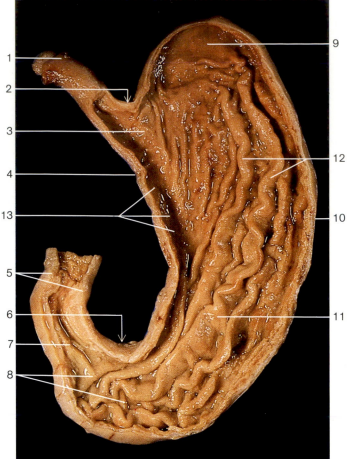

Mucosa of posterior wall of stomach (ventral aspect).

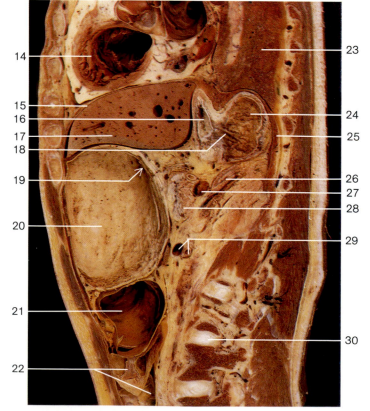

Paramedian section through upper part of left abdominal cavity 3.5 cm lateral to median plane.

1 Esophagus
2 Cardiac notch
3 Cardiac part of stomach
4 Lesser curvature of stomach
5 Pyloric sphincter
6 Angular notch (incisura angularis)
7 Pyloric antrum
8 Pyloric part of stomach
9 Fundus of stomach
10 Greater curvature of stomach
11 Body of stomach
12 Folds of mucous membrane
13 Gastric canal
14 Right ventricle of heart
15 Diaphragm (cut edge)
16 Abdominal portion of esophagus
17 Liver
18 Cardiac part of stomach (cut edge)
19 Position of pyloric canal
20 Body of stomach
21 Transverse colon
22 Small intestine
23 Lung (cut edge)
24 Fundus of stomach (section)
25 Lumbar portion of diaphragm (cut edge)
26 Suprarenal gland
27 Splenic vein
28 Pancreas
29 Superior mesenteric artery and vein
30 Intervertebral disc

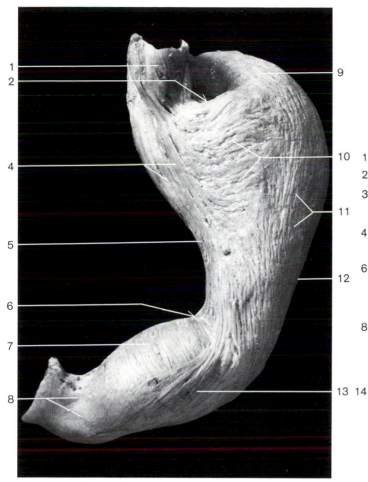

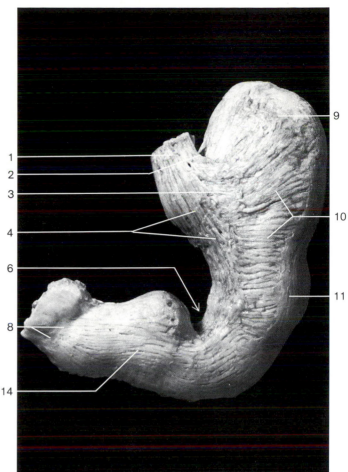

Muscular coat of stomach, outer layer (ventral aspect).

Muscular coat of stomach, middle layer (ventral aspect).

1 Esophagus (abdominal part)
2 Cardiac notch
3 Cardiac part of stomach
4 Longitudinal muscle layer at lesser curvature of stomach
5 Lesser curvature
6 Incisura angularis
7 Circular muscle layer of pyloric part of stomach
8 Pyloric sphincter
9 Fundus of stomach
10 Circular muscle layer of fundus of stomach
11 Longitudinal muscle layer of greater curvature of stomach
12 Greater curvature of stomach
13 Longitudinal muscle layer, transition from body to pyloric part of stomach
14 Pyloric part of stomach
15 Oblique muscle fibers

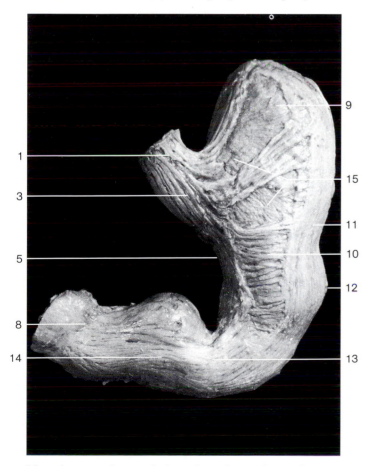

Muscular coat of stomach, inner layer (ventral aspect).

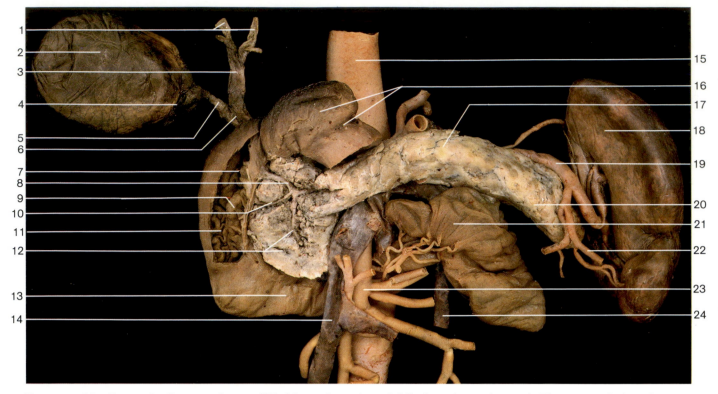

Pancreas with adjacent duodenum, spleen, gallbladder and extrahepatic bile ducts (ventral aspect). The pancreatic ducts have been partly dissected and the duodenum has been opened.

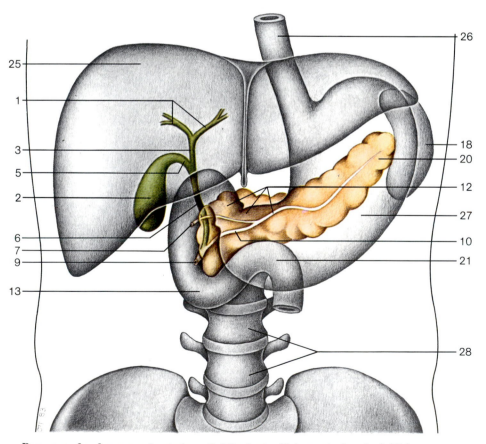

1 Right and left hepatic duct
2 Fundus of gallbladder
3 Common hepatic duct
4 Neck of gallbladder
5 Cystic duct
6 Common bile duct
7 Lesser duodenal papilla (probe)
8 **Accessory pancreatic duct**
9 Greater duodenal papilla (probe)
10 **Pancreatic duct** (probe)
11 Descending part of duodenum
12 Head of pancreas with pancreatic duct
13 Horizontal part of duodenum
14 Superior mesenteric vein
15 Aorta
16 Superior part of duodenum and pyloric sphincter
17 Body of pancreas
18 Spleen
19 Splenic artery
20 Tail of pancreas
21 Duodenojejunal flexure
22 Left gastroepiploic artery
23 Superior mesenteric artery
24 Inferior mesenteric vein
25 Liver
26 Esophagus
27 Stomach
28 Vertebral column

Pancreas, duodenum and extrahepatic bile ducts. (Schematic drawing) (O.).

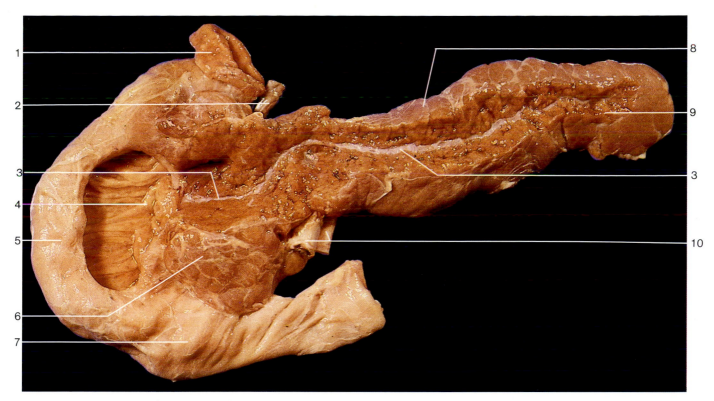

Pancreas and duodenum (ventral aspect). Anterior wall of duodenum has been removed and the pancreatic duct dissected.

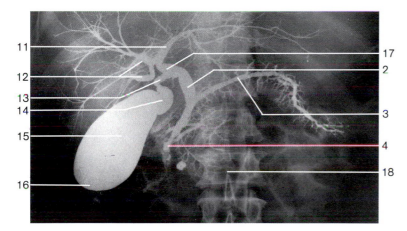

Radiograph of biliary ducts, gallbladder and pancreatic duct (anterior-posterior view).

1 Pyloric part of stomach
2 **Common bile duct**
3 **Pancreatic duct**
4 Greater duodenal papilla
5 Descending part of duodenum
6 Head of pancreas
7 Horizontal part of duodenum
8 Body of pancreas
9 Tail of pancreas
10 Superior mesenteric artery and vein
11 **Left hepatic duct**
12 **Right hepatic duct**
13 Cystic duct
14 Neck of gallbladder
15 Body of gallbladder
16 Fundus of gallbladder
17 Common hepatic duct
18 Second lumbar vertebra
19 Folds of mucous membrane of gallbladder
20 Muscular coat of gallbladder
21 Neck of gallbladder (opened)
22 Cystic duct with spiral fold

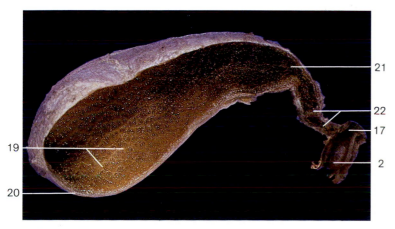

Isolated gallbladder and cystic duct (anterior aspect).
The gallbladder has been opened to display the mucous membrane.

The Liver

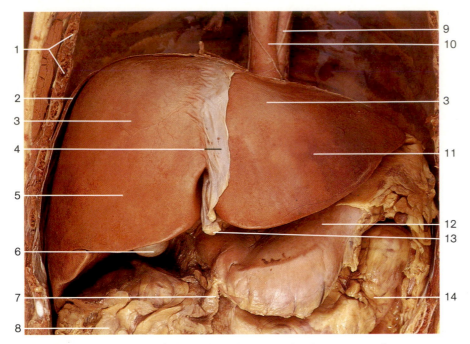

Liver in situ (ventral aspect). Part of the diaphragm has been removed.

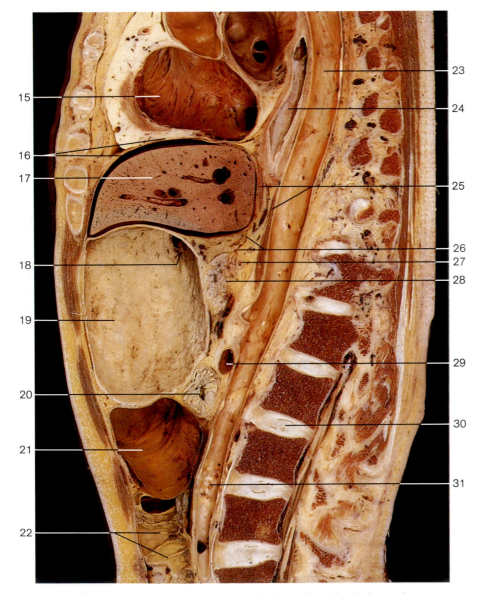

Liver in situ. Longitudinal section through the left side of the abdomen 2 cm lateral to median plane.

1 Ribs (cut edges)
2 Diaphragm
3 Diaphragmatic surface of liver
4 Falciform ligament of liver
5 Right lobe of liver
6 Fundus of gallbladder
7 Gastrocolic ligament
8 Greater omentum
9 Aorta
10 Esophagus
11 Left lobe of liver
12 Stomach
13 Ligamentum teres
14 Transverse colon
15 Right ventricle of heart
16 Central tendon and sternal portion of diaphragm
17 Liver (cut edge)
18 Entrance to duodenum (pylorus)
19 Stomach
20 Duodenum
21 Transverse colon (divided, dilated)
22 Small intestine
23 Thoracic aorta (longitudinally divided)
24 Esophagus (longitudinally divided)
25 Esophageal hiatus of diaphragm
26 Omental bursa
27 Splenic artery
28 Pancreas
29 Superior mesenteric vein
30 Intervertebral disc
31 Abdominal aorta (longitudinally divided)

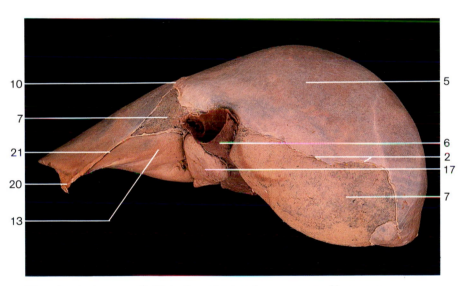

1	Fundus of gallbladder
2	Peritoneum (cut edges)
3	Cystic artery
4	Cystic duct
5	Right lobe of liver
6	Inferior vena cava
7	Bare area of liver
8	Notch for ligamentum teres
9	Ligamentum teres
10	Falciform ligament of liver
11	Quadrate lobe of liver
12	Common hepatic duct
13	Left lobe of liver
14	Hepatic artery proper
15	Common bile duct } Porta hepatis
16	Portal vein
17	Caudate lobe of liver
18	Ligamentum venosum
19	Ligament of inferior vena cava
20	Appendix fibrosa
21	Coronary ligament of liver
22	Hepatic veins
23	Porta hepatis

Liver (inferior aspect). Dissection of porta hepatis. Gallbladder partly collapsed. Ventral margin of liver above.

Liver (posterior aspect). Note the extent and appearance of bare area.

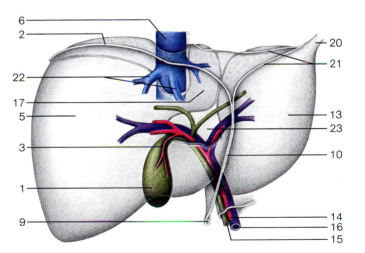

Liver (ventral aspect) (transparent drawing illustrating margins of peritoneal folds) (O.).

It should be noted that the anatomical left and right lobes of the liver do not reflect the internal distribution of the hepatic artery, portal vein, and biliary ducts. Using these structures as criteria the left lobe includes both the caudate and quadrate lobes and thus the line dividing the liver into left and right functional lobes passes through the gallbladder and inferior vena cava. The three main hepatic veins drain segments of the liver which have no visible external markings.

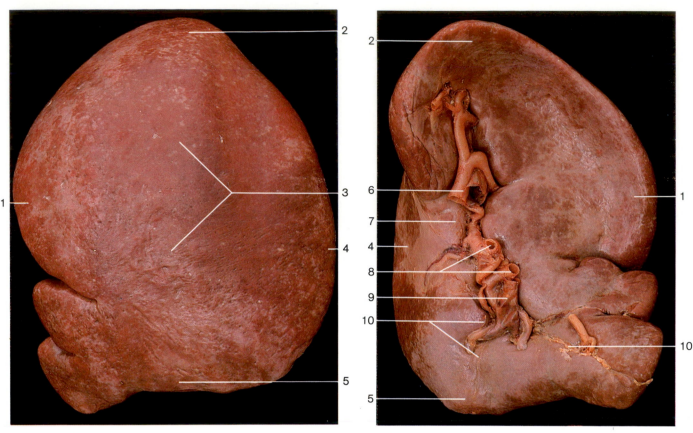

Spleen (diaphragmatic surface).

Spleen (visceral surface, hilum of spleen).

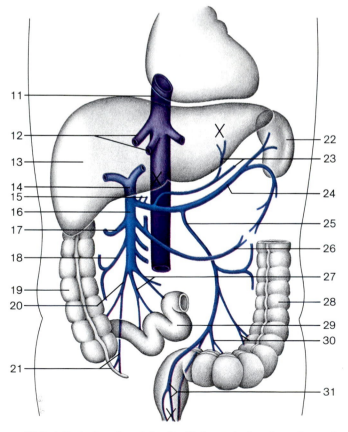

Main tributaries of portal vein. (Schematic drawing of portal circulation) (O.). X = sites of portocaval anastomoses.

1   Superior margin ⎫
2   Posterior extremity ⎪
3   Diaphragmatic surface ⎬ of spleen
4   Inferior margin ⎪
5   Anterior extremity ⎭
6   Posterior branch of splenic artery
7   Hilum of spleen
8   Anterior branches of splenic artery
9   Anterior tributary of splenic vein
10 Remnants of gastrosplenic ligament
11 Inferior vena cava
12 Hepatic veins
13 Liver
14 Portal vein
15 Paraumbilical veins within falciform ligament
16 Superior mesenteric vein
17 Middle colic vein
18 Right colic vein
19 Ascending colon
20 Ileocolic vein
21 Vermiform appendix and appendicular vein
22 Spleen
23 Gastric and esophageal veins
24 Splenic vein
25 Inferior mesenteric vein
26 Right gastroepiploic vein
27 Ileal veins
28 Descending colon
29 Ileum
30 Sigmoid veins
31 Superior rectal veins

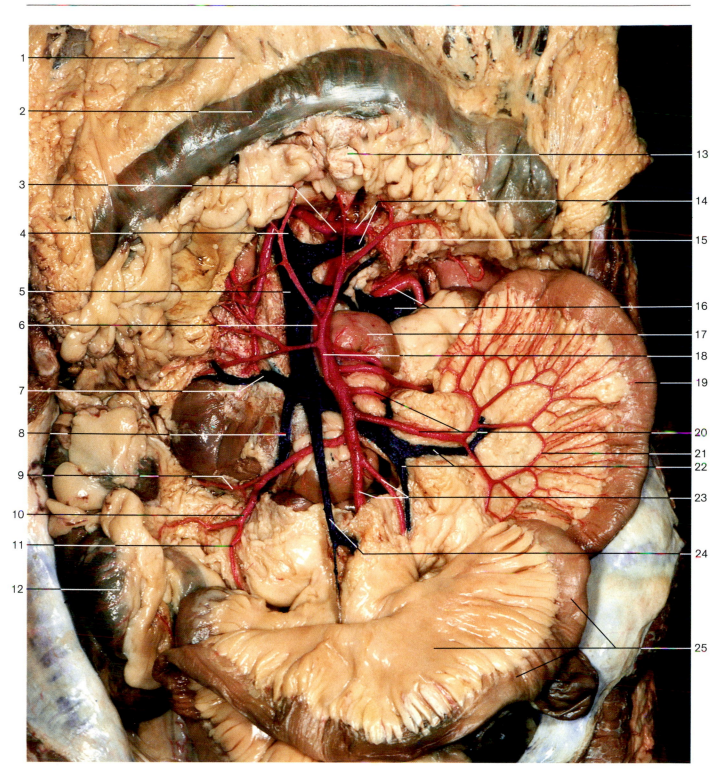

Tributaries of portal vein and branches of superior mesenteric artery (injected with colored solutions). Blue = veins; red = arteries. One layer of peritoneum has been removed to display the vascular arcades of the intestine. Part of the head of the pancreas and the mesocolon have also been removed to show the deeper vessels.

1 Greater omentum (reflected)	10 Ileocolic artery	19 Jejunum
2 Transverse colon (raised cranially)	11 Appendicular artery	20 Jejunal arteries
3 Celiac trunk	12 Cecum	21 Arterial arcades to intestine
4 **Portal vein**	13 Transverse mesocolon	22 Jejunal veins
5 Superior mesenteric vein	14 **Splenic artery and vein**	23 Ileal arteries
6 **Superior mesenteric artery**	15 Pancreas (divided)	24 Ileal vein
7 Right colic vein	16 Renal artery and vein	25 Ileum with mesentery
8 Ileocolic vein	17 Duodenojejunal flexure	
9 Right colic artery	18 Middle colic artery	

Arteries of the Abdominal Organs

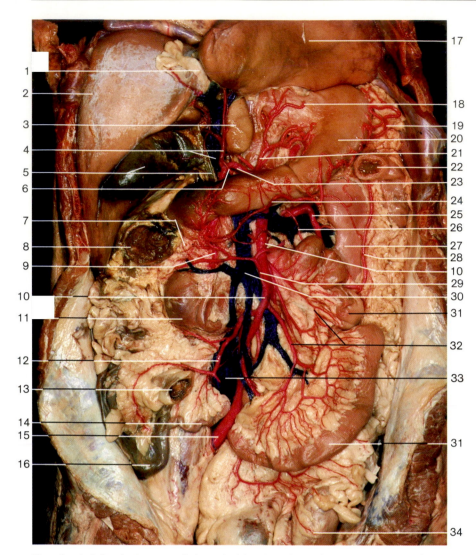

1   Ligamentum teres
2   Liver
3   Caudate lobe of liver
4   Proper hepatic artery, portal vein
5   Gallbladder and common bile duct
6   Right gastric artery
7   Pancreas
8   Right colic flexure
9   Gastroduodenal artery
10   Superior mesenteric artery
11   Duodenum
12   Ilecolic artery
13   Terminal part of ileum
14   Vermiform appendix
15   Right common iliac artery
16   Cecum
17   Left lobe of liver
18   Cardioesophageal branch of left gastric artery
19   Left gastroepiploic artery
20   Stomach
21   Left gastric artery
22   Left colic flexure
23   Common hepatic artery
24   Right gastroepiploic artery
25   Renal artery
26   Left testicular artery
27   Left kidney
28   Left colic artery
29   Middle colic artery
30   Superior mesenteric vein
31   Jejunum
32   Jejunal arteries
33   Inferior vena cava
34   Sigmoid colon
35   Right colic artery
36   Appendicular artery
37   Inferior mesenteric artery
38   Sigmoid arteries
39   Superior rectal artery
40   Fundus of gallbladder
41   Common bile duct
42   Portal vein
43   Beginning of jejunum
44   Duodenojejunal flexure
45   Ureter
46   Splenic artery
47   Celiac trunk
48   Renal vein
49   Abdominal aorta
50   Descending colon
51   Left common iliac artery
52   Transverse mesocolon

Vessels of abdominal organs (injected with colored solutions, ventral aspect). Red = arteries; blue = veins.
The transverse colon and parts of the small intestine and lesser omentum have been removed. The liver has been lifted.

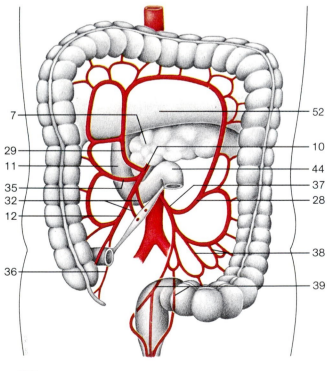

Main branches of superior and inferior mesenteric arteries. (Schematic drawing) (O.).

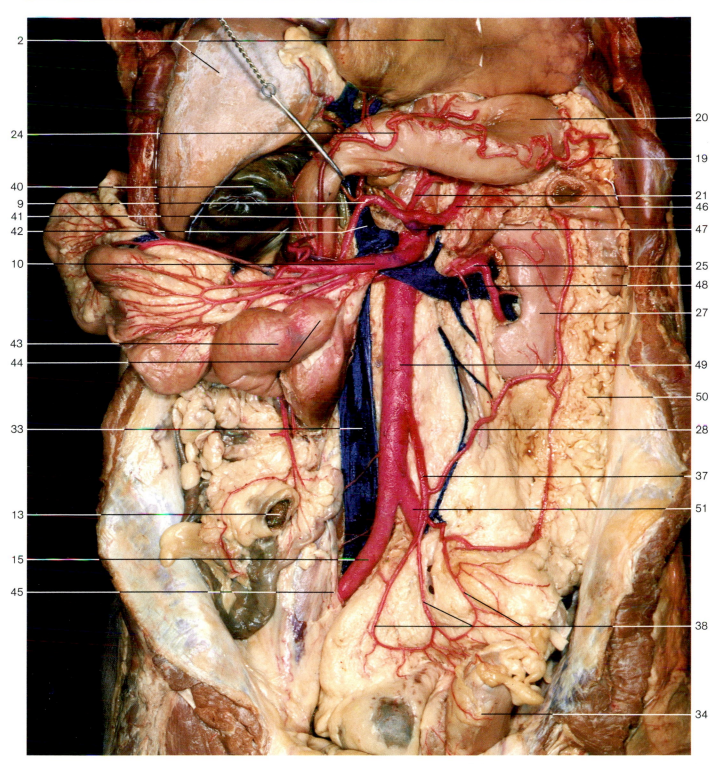

Vessels of abdominal organs; dissection of inferior mesenteric artery and celiac trunk (injected with colored solutions). Blue = veins; red = arteries.

The small intestine including the duodenojejunal flexure has been reflected laterally and the stomach and liver have been raised. The peritoneum of the posterior abdominal wall has been removed to display the inferior mesenteric artery and its branches to the colon.

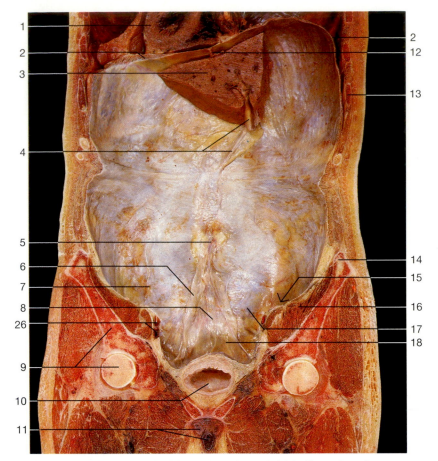

Anterior abdominal wall with pelvic cavity and thigh (frontal section, male) (internal aspect).

1 Left ventricle with pericardium
2 Diaphragm
3 Remnant of liver
4 Ligamentum teres
   (free margin of falciform ligament)
5 Site of umbilicus
6 **Medial umbilical fold**
   (containing the obliterated umbilical artery)
7 **Lateral umbilical fold** (containing inferior
   epigastric artery and vein)
8 **Median umbilical fold**
   (containing remnant of urachus)
9 Head of femur, pelvic bone
10 Urinary bladder
11 Root of penis
12 Falciform ligament of liver
13 Rib (divided)
14 Iliac crest (divided)
15 Site of **deep inguinal ring,**
   lateral inguinal fossa
16 Iliopsoas muscle (divided)
17 Medial inguinal fossa
18 Supravesical fossa
19 Posterior layer of rectus sheath
20 Transversus abdominis
21 Umbilicus and arcuate line
22 **Inferior epigastric artery**
23 Femoral nerve
24 Iliopsoas muscle
25 Remnant of umbilical artery
26 Femoral artery and vein
27 Tendinous intersection of rectus abdominis
28 Rectus abdominis muscle
29 Interfoveolar ligament
30 Pubic symphysis (divided)

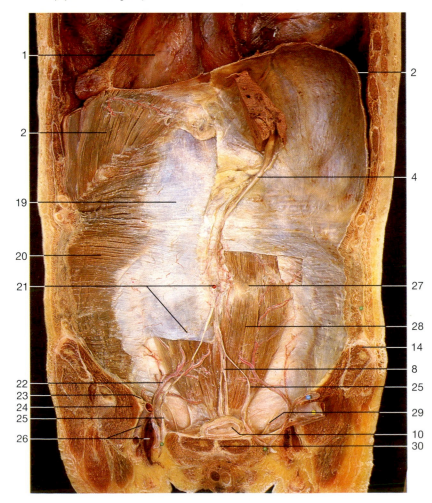

Anterior abdominal wall (male) (internal aspect). The peritoneum and parts of the posterior layer of rectus sheath have been removed. Dissection of inferior epigastric arteries and veins.

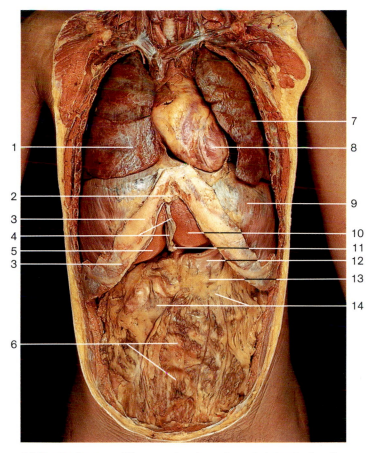

1 Middle lobe of right lung
2 Xiphoid process
3 Costal margin
4 Falciform ligament of liver
5 Right lobe of liver
6 Greater omentum
7 Left lung
8 Heart
9 Diaphragm
10 Left lobe of liver
11 Ligamentum teres
12 Stomach
13 Gastrocolic ligament
14 Transverse colon
15 Mesocolic taenia
16 Appendices epiploicae
17 Cecum
18 Free taenia
19 Ileum
20 Transverse mesocolon
21 Jejunum
22 Sigmoid colon
23 Position of root of mesentery
24 Vermiform appendix
25 Duodenojejunal flexure
26 Mesentery

Abdominal organs. The anterior thoracic and abdominal walls have been removed.

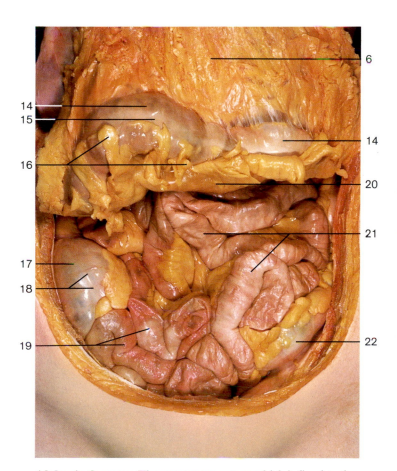

Abdominal organs. The greater omentum which is fixed to the transverse colon has been raised.

Abdominal organs (anterior aspect). The transverse colon has been reflected.

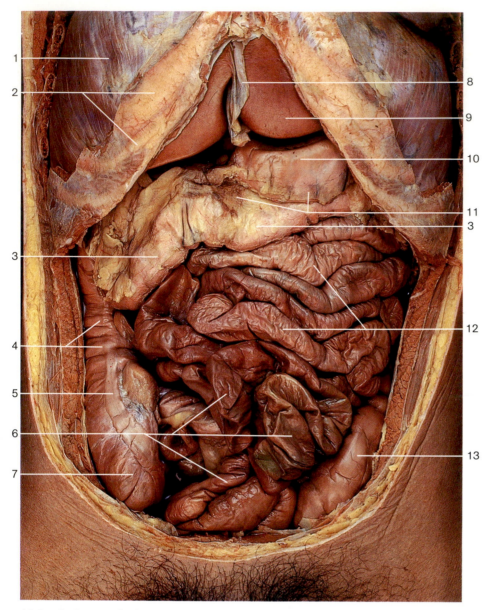

1	Diaphragm
2	Costal margin
3	Transverse colon
4	Ascending colon with haustra
5	Free taenia of cecum
6	**Ileum**
7	**Cecum**
8	**Falciform ligament of liver**
9	Liver
10	Stomach
11	Gastrocolic ligament
12	Jejunum
13	Sigmoid colon
14	**Vermiform appendix**
15	Terminal ileum
16	**Mesoappendix**
17	Mesentery

Abdominal organs in situ. The greater omentum has been removed.

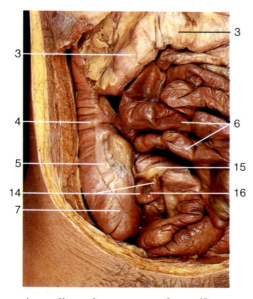

Ascending colon, cecum and vermiform appendix (detail of the preceding figure).

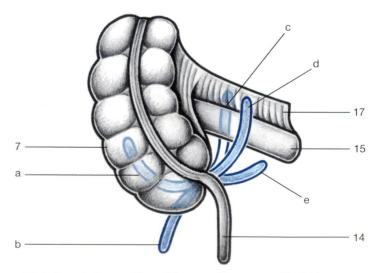

Variations in the position of the vermiform appendix (O.). a = retrocecal; b = paracolic; c = retroileal; d = pre-ileal; e = subcecal.

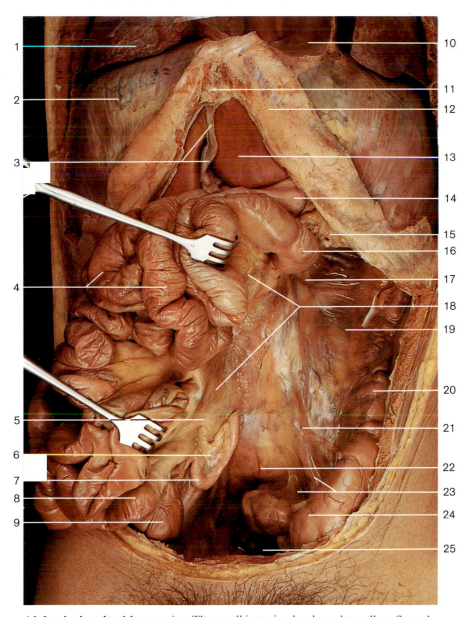

1	Lung
2	Diaphragm
3	Falciform ligament of liver
4	Jejunum
5	Ileocecal fold
6	Mesoappendix
7	Vermiform appendix
8	**Ileocecal junction**
9	**Cecum**
10	Pericardial sac
11	Xiphoid process
12	Costal margin
13	Liver
14	Stomach
15	Transverse colon
16	**Duodenojejunal flexure**
17	Inferior duodenal fold
18	Mesentery
19	Position of left kidney
20	Descending colon
21	Position of left common iliac artery
22	Promontory
23	Sigmoid mesocolon
24	Sigmoid colon
25	Rectum
26	Beginning of jejunum
27	Peritoneum of posterior abdominal wall
28	Transverse mesocolon
29	Superior duodenal fold
30	Superior duodenal recess
31	Retroduodenal recess
32	Free taenia of ascending colon
33	**Ileocecal valve**
34	Frenulum of ileocecal valve
35	Orifice of vermiform appendix (probe)
36	**Ileocolic artery**
37	Vermiform appendix with appendicular artery
38	Ascending colon

Abdominal cavity. Mesenteries. The small intestine has been laterally reflected to demonstrate the mesentery.

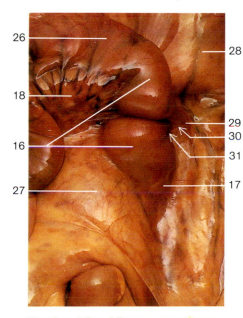

Duodenojejunal flexure (enlargement of preceding figure).

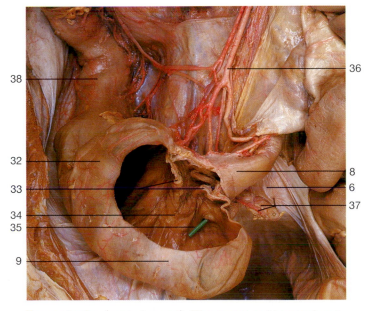

Ileocecal valve (ventral aspect). The cecum and terminal part of the ileum have been opened.

281

The Superior Mesenteric Vessels

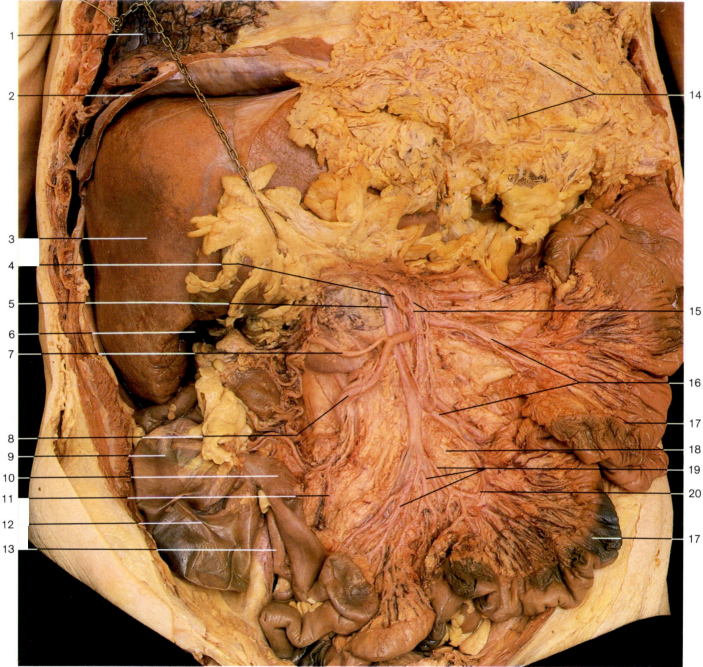

Dissection of superior mesenteric artery and vein (ventral aspect). The greater omentum has been raised.

1 Lung
2 Diaphragm (cut edge)
3 Liver
4 Middle colic artery
5 Superior mesenteric vein
6 Gallbladder
7 **Right colic artery**
8 **Ileocolic artery**
9 Free taenia of ascending colon
10 Terminal part of ileum
11 Appendicular artery
12 Cecum
13 Vermiform appendix
14 Greater omentum (reflected)
15 **Superior mesenteric artery and autonomic nerve plexus**
16 **Jejunal arteries**

17 Jejunum
18 Mesentery, posterior layer of peritoneum
19 **Ileal arteries**
20 Arterial arcades of small intestine
21 Horizontal part of duodenum (extended)
22 **Superior mesenteric artery and vein**
23 Ascending colon
24 Transverse colon
25 Transverse mesocolon
26 Duodenojejunal flexure
27 **Mesenteric nodes and lymph vessels**
28 Ileum
29 Autonomic nerves

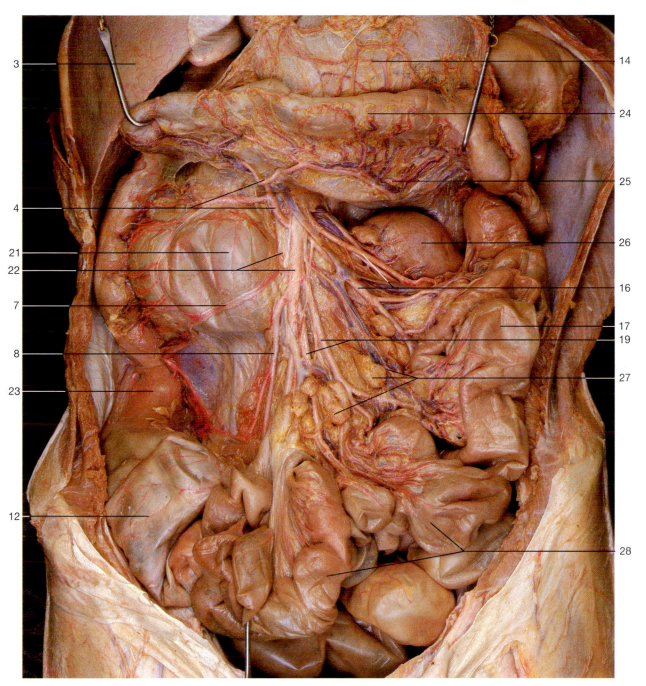

Abdominal organs. Superior mesenteric artery. Mesenteric nodes. Transverse colon reflected.

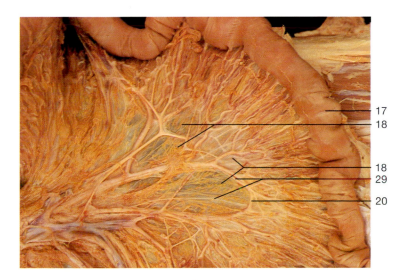

Dissection of arterial arcades of small intestine (higher magnification).

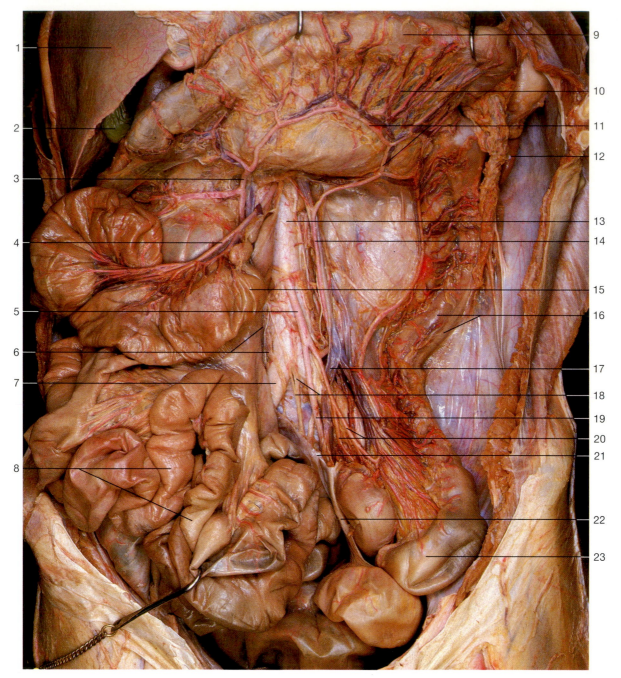

Abdominal organs. Retroperitoneal region. Dissection of inferior mesenteric artery and autonomic plexus.
Transverse colon with mesocolon has been raised, small intestine reflected.

1 Liver
2 Gallbladder
3 **Middle colic artery**
4 Jejunal artery
5 **Inferior mesenteric artery**
6 Sympathetic nerves and ganglia
7 Right common iliac artery
8 Small intestine (ileum)
9 Transverse colon (reflected)
10 Transverse mesocolon
11 Anastomosis between middle
     and left colic artery

12 Spleen
13 **Abdominal aorta**
14 **Left colic artery**
15 Duodenojejunal flexure
16 Descending colon, free taenia of colon
17 Inferior mesenteric vein
18 Superior hypogastric plexus
19 **Superior rectal artery**
20 Sigmoid arteries
21 Peritoneum (cut edge)
22 Sigmoid mesocolon
23 Sigmoid colon

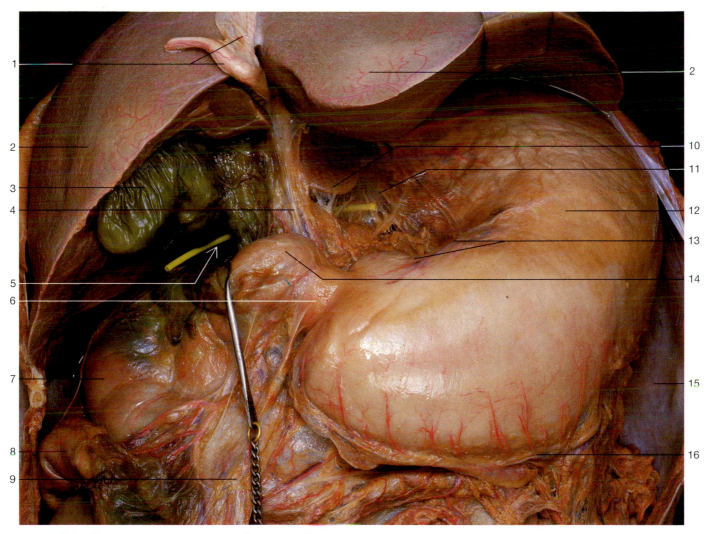

Upper abdominal organs. Thorax and anterior part of diaphragm have been removed and the liver raised to display the lesser omentum. A probe has been inserted into the epiploic foramen and lesser sac.

1 Falciform ligament and ligamentum teres
2 Liver
3 Gallbladder (fundus)
4 Hepatoduodenal ligament
5 **Epiploic foramen** (probe)
6 Pylorus
7 Descending part of duodenum
8 Right colic flexure
9 **Gastrocolic ligament**
10 Caudate lobe of liver (behind lesser omentum)
11 **Lesser omentum**
12 Stomach
13 Lesser curvature of stomach
14 Superior part of duodenum
15 Diaphragm
16 Greater curvature of stomach with gastroepiploic
   vessels
17 Twelfth thoracic vertebra
18 Right kidney
19 Right suprarenal gland
20 Inferior vena cava
21 Falciform ligament of liver
22 Abdominal aorta
23 Spleen
24 Phrenicolienal ligament (lienorenal)
25 Gastrosplenic ligament
26 Pancreas
27 Lesser sac

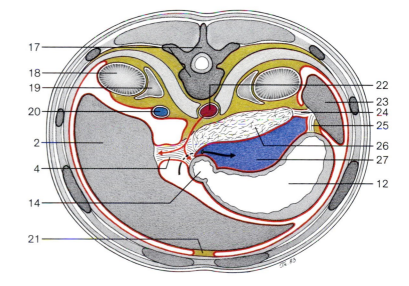

Horizontal section through omental bursa above the level of epiploic foramen (black arrow). Viewed from above. Red arrows: routes of the arterial branches of celiac trunk to liver, stomach, duodenum and pancreas. (Schematic drawing) (Tr.).

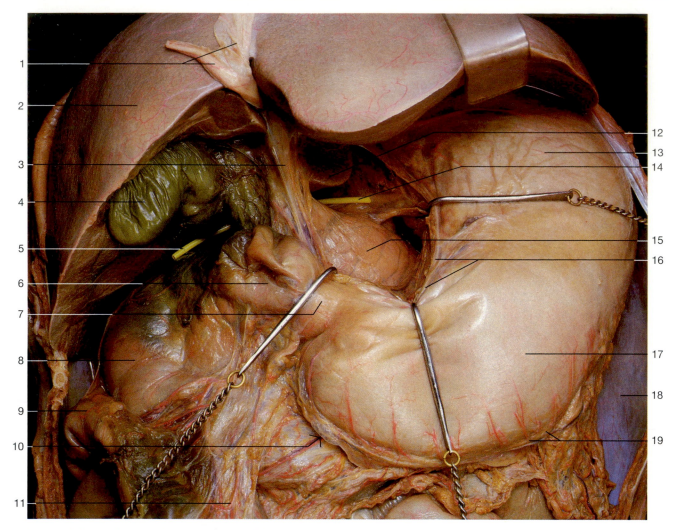

Upper abdominal organs, lesser sac (omental bursa) (anterior aspect). Lesser omentum partly removed, liver and stomach slightly reflected.

1 Falciform ligament and ligamentum teres
2 Liver
3 **Hepatoduodenal ligament**
4 Gallbladder
5 Probe within the epiploic foramen
6 Superior part of duodenum
7 Pylorus
8 Descending part of duodenum
9 Right colic flexure
10 Gastrocolic ligament
11 **Greater omentum**
12 Caudate lobe of liver
13 Fundus of stomach
14 Probe at the level of the vestibule of lesser sac
15 **Head of pancreas**
16 Lesser curvature of stomach
17 **Body of stomach**
18 Diaphragm

19 Greater curvature with gastroepiploic vessels
20 Head of pancreas, gastropancreatic fold
21 **Spleen**
22 **Tail of pancreas**
23 Left colic flexure
24 Root of transverse mesocolon
25 Transverse mesocolon
26 Gastrocolic ligament (cut edge)
27 **Transverse colon**
28 Umbilicus
29 Small intestine
30 Lesser omentum
31 Lesser sac (omental bursa)
32 Duodenum
33 Mesentery
34 Sigmoid colon

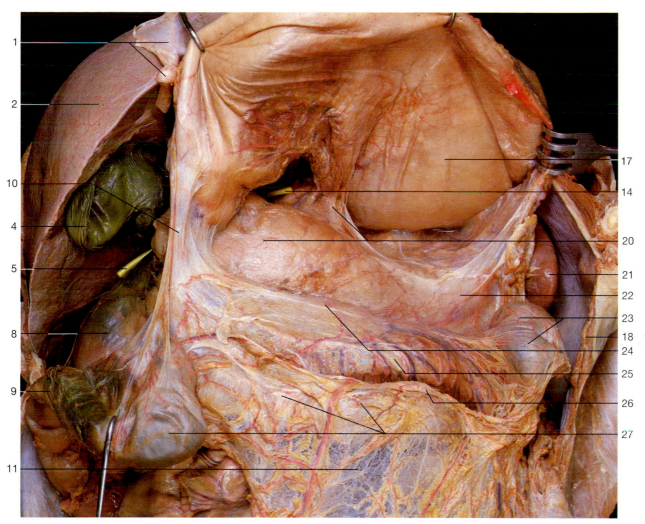

Upper abdominal organs, lesser sac (omental bursa) (anterior aspect). The gastrocolic ligament has been divided and the whole stomach raised to display the posterior wall of the lesser sac.

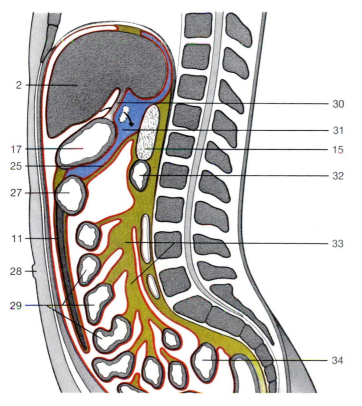

Median section through abdominal cavity demonstrating the site of lesser sac (blue). (Schematic drawing) (Tr.). The epiploic foramen, entrance to the lesser sac, is indicated by an arrow. Red = peritoneum.

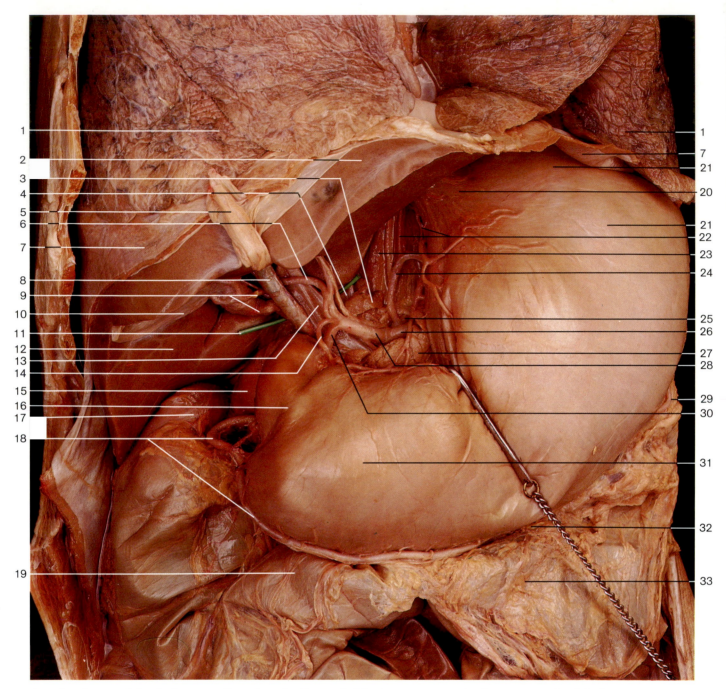

Arteries of upper abdominal organs; dissection of celiac trunk. The lesser omentum has been removed and the lesser curvature of the stomach reflected to display the branches of the celiac trunk.

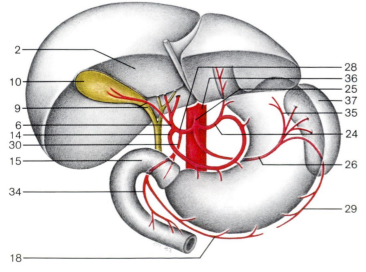

Branches of celiac trunk.
(Schematic drawing) (O.).

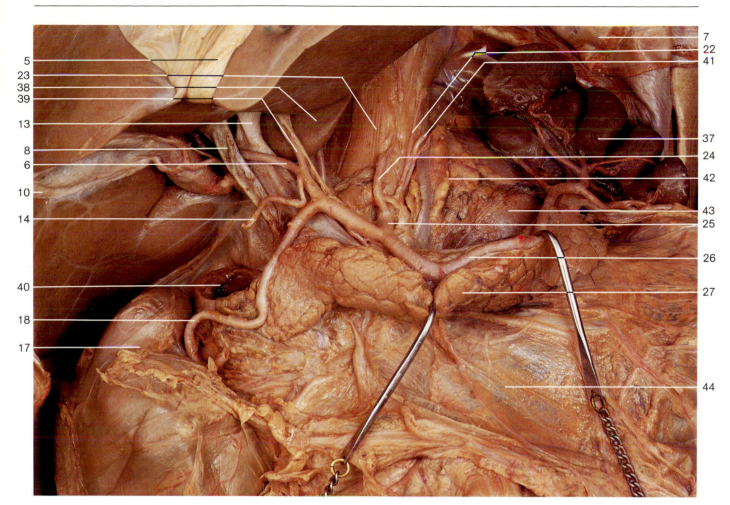

Branches of celiac trunk; blood supply of liver, pancreas and spleen. The stomach, superior part of duodenum and celiac ganglion have been removed to reveal the anterior aspect of the posterior wall of the lesser sac (omental bursa) and the vessels and ducts of the hepatoduodenal ligament. The pancreas has been slightly reflected anteriorly.

1	Lung	23	Lumbar part of diaphragm
2	Liver, visceral surface	24	Left gastric artery
3	Lymph node	25	**Celiac trunk**
4	Inferior vena cava	26	Splenic artery
5	Ligamentum teres (reflected)	27	Pancreas
6	Right branch of hepatic artery proper	28	Common hepatic artery
7	Diaphragm	29	Left gastroepiploic artery
8	Common hepatic duct (dilated)	30	Gastroduodenal artery
9	Cystic duct and artery	31	Pyloric part of stomach
10	Gallbladder	32	Greater curvature of stomach
11	Probe in epiploic foramen	33	Gastrocolic ligament
12	Right lobe of liver	34	Superior pancreaticoduodenal artery
13	Portal vein	35	Short gastric arteries
14	Right gastric artery	36	Aorta
15	Duodenum	37	Spleen
16	Pylorus	38	Caudate lobe of liver
17	Right colic flexure	39	Left branch of hepatic artery proper
18	Right gastroepiploic artery	40	Descending part of duodenum (cut)
19	Transverse colon	41	Left inferior phrenic artery
20	Abdominal part of esophagus, cardiac part of stomach	42	Suprarenal gland
21	Fundus of stomach	43	Kidney
22	Esophageal branches of left gastric artery	44	Transverse mesocolon

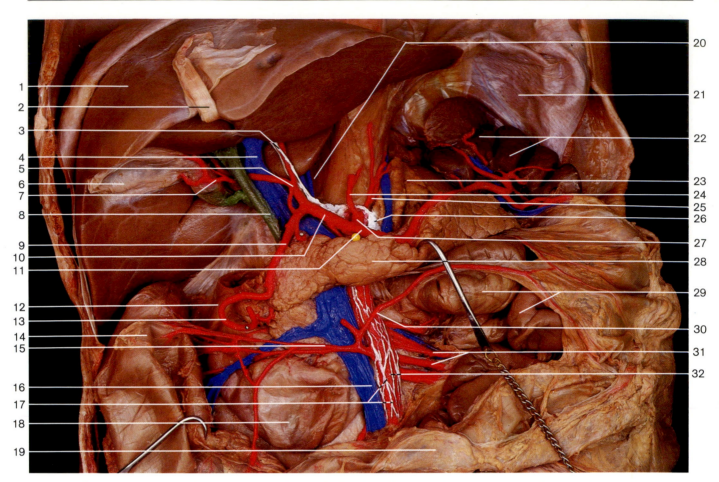

Vessels and autonomic nerves of the upper part of abdominal cavity. The stomach has been removed and the liver and pancreas have been slightly reflected. Part of the transverse mesocolon and the parietal layer of peritoneum have been removed to show the vessels and nerves on the posterior abdominal wall.

Green = bile ducts; red = arteries; blue = veins; white = autonomic nerves and plexus.

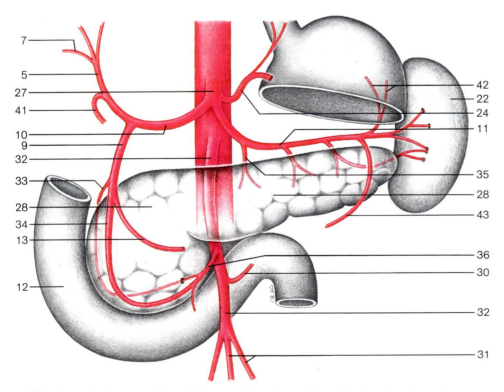

Blood supply of upper abdominal organs (branches of the celiac trunk and superior mesenteric artery). (Schematic drawing) (O.).

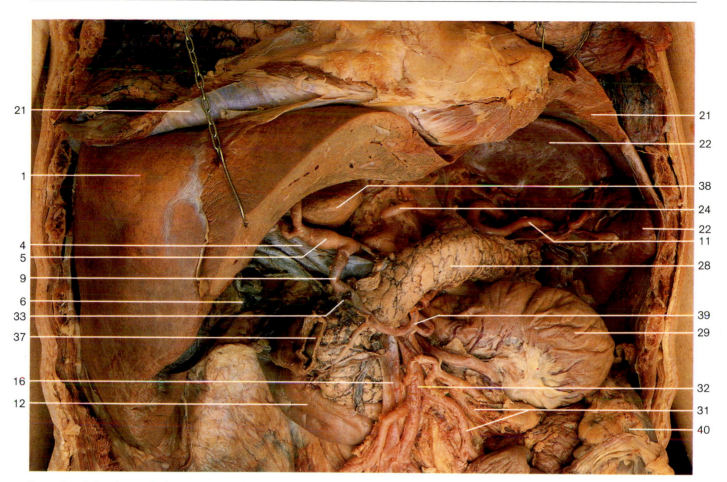

Posterior abdominal wall (anterior aspect). Part of the left lobe of the liver and the head of the pancreas and all of the stomach have been removed. In this specimen two hepatic arteries were found (variation).

1	Liver	23	Suprarenal gland
2	Ligamentum teres	24	Left gastric artery
3	Hepatic plexus	25	Inferior phrenic artery
4	Portal vein	26	Celiac ganglion (part of celiac plexus)
5	Hepatic artery proper with its branches	27	**Celiac trunk**
6	Gallbladder	28	Pancreas
7	Cystic artery	29	Jejunum
8	Common bile duct	30	Middle colic artery
9	Gastroduodenal artery	31	Jejunal arteries
10	**Common hepatic artery**	32	Superior mesenteric artery
11	**Splenic artery**	33	Retroduodenal artery
12	Descending part of duodenum	34	Superior pancreaticoduodenal artery
13	Right gastroepiploic artery	35	Dorsal pancreatic branch
14	Right colic flexure		of splenic artery
15	Right colic artery	36	Inferior pancreaticoduodenal artery
16	Superior mesenteric vein	37	Duodenum (cut edge)
17	Superior mesenteric plexus	38	Caudate lobe of liver
18	Horizontal part of duodenum (dilated)	39	Right gastroepiploic artery
19	Transverse colon	40	Descending colon
20	Inferior vena cava	41	Right gastric artery
21	Diaphragm	42	Short gastric arteries
22	Spleen	43	Left gastroepiploic artery

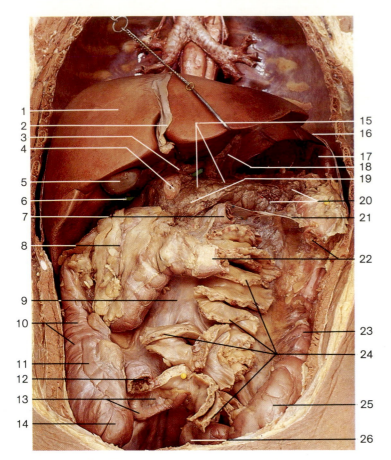

1 Liver
2 Falciform ligament
3 Hepatoduodenal ligament
4 Pylorus (divided)
5 Gallbladder
6 Probe within the epiploic foramen
7 Duodenojejunal flexure (divided)
8 Greater omentum
9 Root of mesentery
10 Ascending colon
11 Free colic taenia
12 End of ileum (divided)
13 Vermiform appendix with mesoappendix
14 Cecum
15 Lesser sac
16 Diaphragm
17 Spleen
18 Cardiac part of stomach (divided)
19 Head of pancreas
20 Body and tail of pancreas
21 Transverse mesocolon
22 Transverse colon (divided)
23 Descending colon
24 Cut edge of mesentery
25 Sigmoid colon
26 Rectum
27 Bare area of liver
28 Inferior vena cava
29 Kidney
30 Attachment of right colic flexure
31 Root of transverse mesocolon
32 Descending part of duodenum
33 Bare surface for ascending colon
34 Ileocecal recess
35 Retrocecal recess
36 Root of mesoappendix
37 Superior recess ⎫
38 Isthmus   ⎬ of lesser sac
39 Splenic recess ⎭
40 Superior duodenal recess
41 Inferior duodenal recess
42 Bare surface for descending colon
43 Paracolic recesses
44 Root of mesentery
45 Root of mesosigmoid
46 Intersigmoid recess
47 Hepatic veins
48 Duodenojejunal flexure
49 Attachment of left colic flexure

Abdominal cavity after removal of stomach, jejunum, ileum and part of the transverse colon. Liver has been slightly raised.

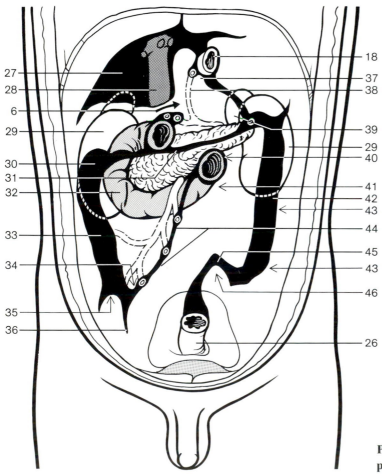

Position of root of mesentery and peritoneal recesses on the posterior abdominal wall. (Schematic drawing.)

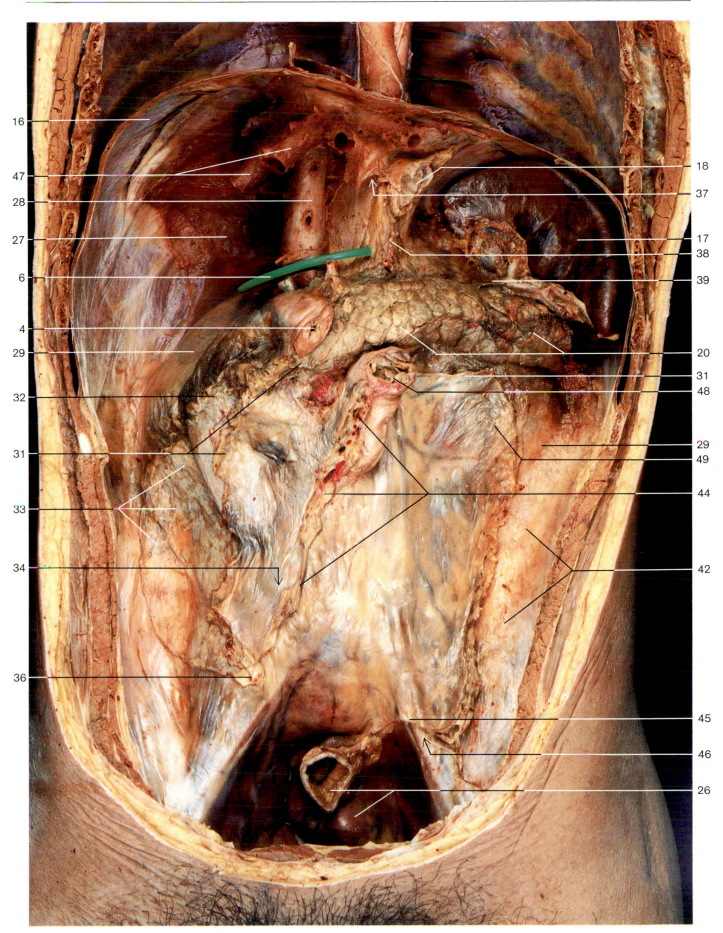

Peritoneal recesses on the posterior abdominal wall. The liver, stomach, jejunum, ileum, and colon have been removed. The duodenum, pancreas, and spleen have been left in place.

293

Sections through the Abdominal Cavity

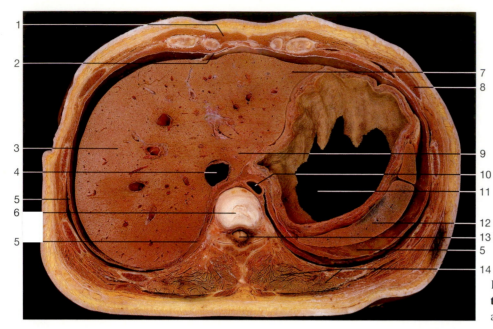

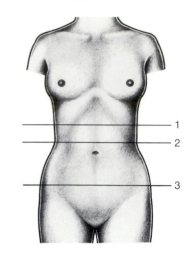

Horizontal section through the abdominal cavity at level 1 (from below).

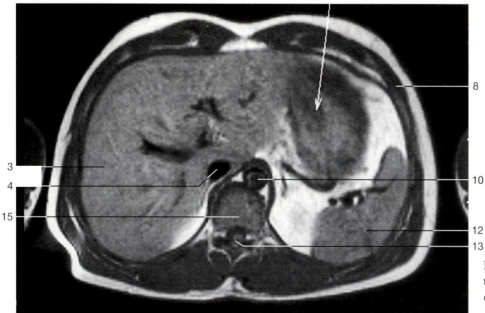

Horizontal section through the body. MR-Scan, corresponding to level 1. Arrow: stomach.

1	Rectus abdominis	20	Common bile duct
2	Falciform ligament	21	Duodenum
3	**Liver,** right lobe	22	Renal artery and vein
4	Inferior vena cava	23	**Kidney**
5	Diaphragm	24	Duodenojejunal flexure
6	Intervertebral disc	25	Superior mesenteric artery and vein
7	Liver, left lobe	26	Tail of pancreas
8	Rib	27	Descending colon
9	Liver, caudate lobe	28	Psoas major, quadratus lumborum
10	Abdominal (descending) aorta	29	Cauda equina
11	**Stomach**	30	Right renal vein
12	**Spleen**	31	**Small intestine**
13	Spinal cord	32	Mesentery
14	Longissimus, iliocostalis	33	Common iliac artery and vein
15	Body of vertebra	34	Sacroiliac joint
16	Transverse colon	35	Ureter
17	Gastroduodenal artery and vein	36	Left psoas major
18	Ascending colon	37	Interosseous sacroiliac ligaments
19	Head of **pancreas**		

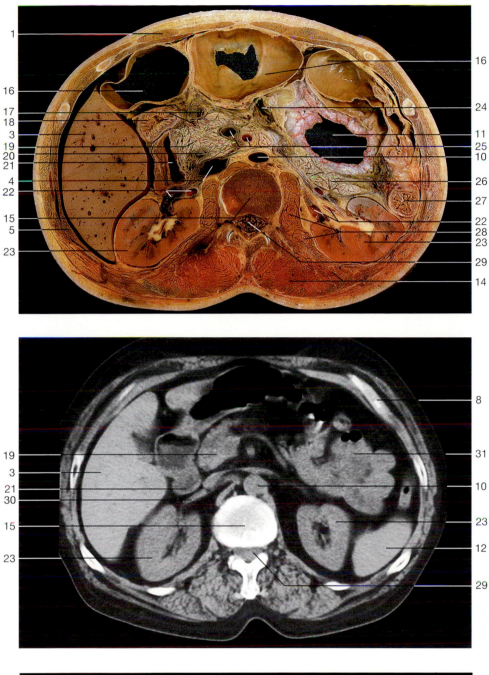

1

16

17
18
3
19
20
21

4
22

15
5

23

16

24

11
25
10

26

27

22
28
23

29

14 **Horizontal section through
    the abdominal cavity**
    at level 2 (from below).

19

3

21
30

15

23

8

31

10

23

12

29

**Horizontal section through
the body.** CT-Scan,
corresponding to level 2.

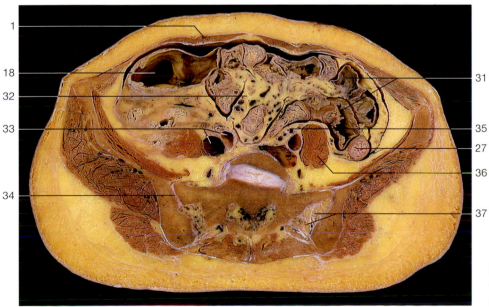

1

18

32

33

34

31

35

27

36

37

**Horizontal section through
the abdominal cavity**
at level 3 (from below).

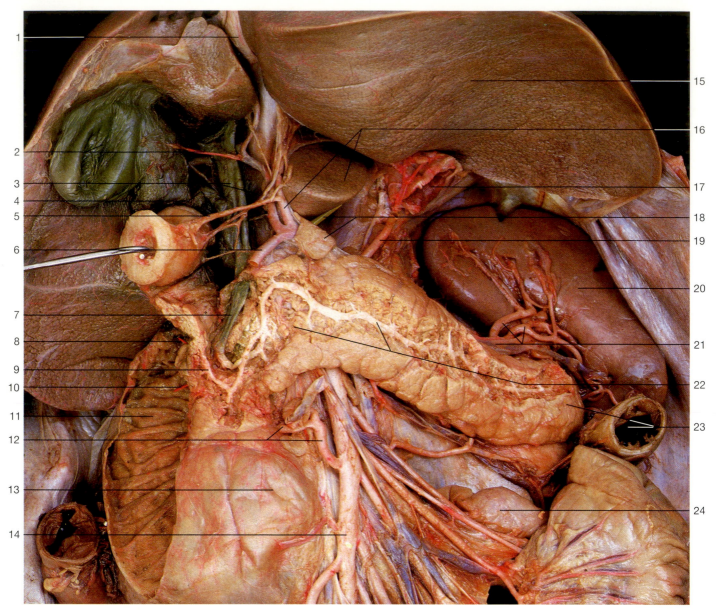

Posterior abdominal wall with duodenum, pancreas and spleen (anterior aspect). Dissection of pancreatic and common bile duct. The stomach has been removed, the liver raised and the duodenum partly fenestrated.

1 Ligamentum teres
2 Gallbladder, cystic artery
3 Common hepatic duct, portal vein
4 Cystic duct
5 Right gastric artery (pylorus with superior part of duodenum divided and reflected)
6 Gastroduodenal artery
7 **Common bile duct**
8 Probe within the minor duodenal papilla
9 **Accessory pancreatic duct**
10 Probe within the major duodenal papilla
11 Descending part of duodenum (fenestrated)
12 Middle colic artery, inferior pancreaticoduodenal artery

13 Horizontal part of duodenum (extended)
14 **Superior mesenteric artery**
15 Liver, left lobe
16 Caudate lobe of liver, hepatic artery proper
17 Abdominal part of esophagus (divided)
18 Probe in epiploic foramen, lymph node
19 Left gastric artery
20 **Spleen**
21 Splenic vein, branches of splenic artery
22 **Pancreatic duct, head of pancreas**
23 Left colic flexure, tail of pancreas
24 Duodenojejunal flexure

Chapter VII

Urogenital System
Retroperitoneal Organs

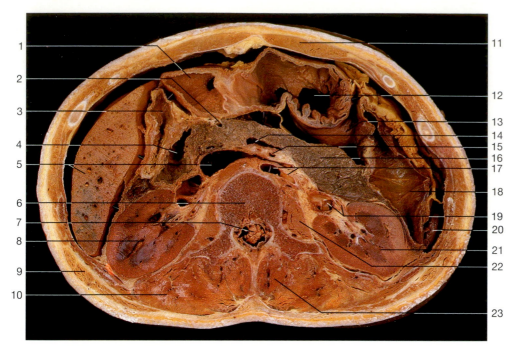

1	Pyloric antrum
2	Gastroduodenal artery
3	Descending part of duodenum
4	Vestibule of lesser sac
5	Inferior vena cava, liver
6	Body of first lumbar vertebra
7	Cauda equina
8	**Right kidney**
9	Latissimus dorsi
10	Iliocostalis
11	Rectus abdominis
12	Stomach
13	Lesser sac
14	Splenic vein
15	Superior mesenteric artery
16	Pancreas
17	Aorta, left renal artery
18	Transverse colon
19	Renal artery and vein
20	Spleen
21	**Left kidney**
22	Psoas major
23	Multifidus
24	Margin of lung
25	Margin of pleura
26	Renal pelvis
27	**Left ureter**
28	Descending colon
29	Rectum
30	Right suprarenal gland
31	12th rib
32	Ascending colon
33	**Right ureter**
34	Cecum
35	Vermiform appendix
36	Urinary bladder
37	Liver
38	Anterior layer of renal fascia
39	Duodenum
40	Perirenal fatty tissue
41	Posterior layer of renal fascia
42	Abdominal cavity

Horizontal section through the abdominal cavity at the level of the first lumbar vertebra (from below).

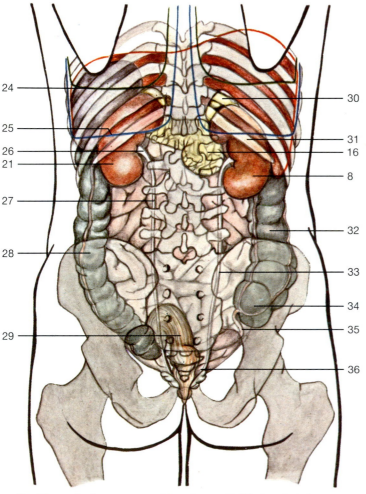

Positions of urinary organs (dorsal aspect). Notice that the upper part of the kidney reaches the level of the margin of pleura and lung.

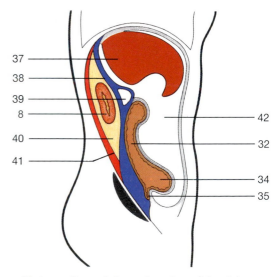

Retroperitoneal tissue, location of the right kidney. (Schematic drawing) (W.). Yellow = adipose capsule of kidney.

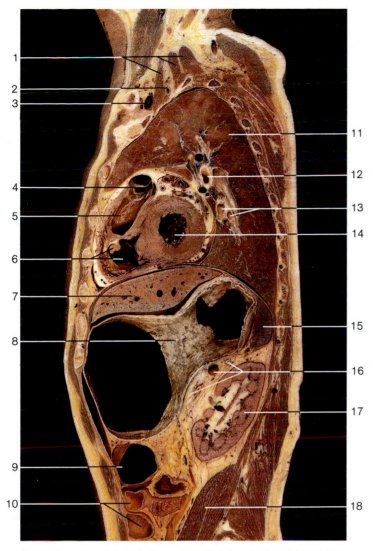

1	Anterior, middle and posterior scalene muscles
2	Left subclavian artery
3	Left subclavian vein
4	Pulmonary valve
5	Arterial cone
6	Right ventricle of heart
7	Liver
8	Stomach
9	Transverse colon
10	Small intestine
11	Left lung
12	Left main bronchus
13	Branches of pulmonary vein
14	Left ventricle of heart
15	Spleen
16	Splenic artery and vein, pancreas
17	Left kidney
18	Psoas major
19	Inferior vena cava
20	Renal vein
21	Body of 12th thoracic vertebra, vertebral canal
22	Right kidney
23	Superior mesenteric artery
24	Superior mesenteric vein
25	Pancreas
26	Abdominal aorta
27	Left psoas major, quadratus lumborum
28	Anterior layer of renal fascia
29	Posterior layer of renal fascia
30	Perirenal fatty tissue
31	Abdominal cavity
32	Descending and sigmoid colon

Sagittal section through thoracic and abdominal cavities at the level of the left kidney (5.5 cm left of median plane).

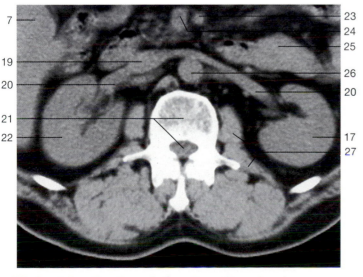

Horizontal section through the retroperitoneal region at level of 12th thoracic vertebra. CT-Scan (from below).

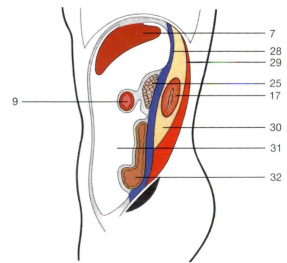

Retroperitoneal tissue, position of left kidney. (Schematic drawing) (W.).

The Kidney

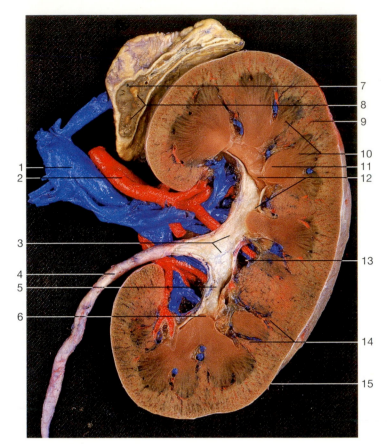

1 Renal vein
2 Renal artery
3 Renal pelvis
4 Abdominal part of ureter
5 Major calyx
6 Cribriform area of renal papilla
7 Cortex of suprarenal gland
8 Medulla of suprarenal gland
9 Cortex of kidney
10 Medulla of kidney
11 Renal papilla
12 Minor calyx
13 Renal sinus
14 Renal columns
15 Fibrous capsule of kidney
16 11th rib
17 Left kidney
18 Pelvic part of ureter
19 Urinary bladder
20 Male urethra

Longitudinal section through right kidney and suprarenal gland
(posterior aspect). The renal pelvis has been opened and the
fatty tissue removed to display the renal vessels.

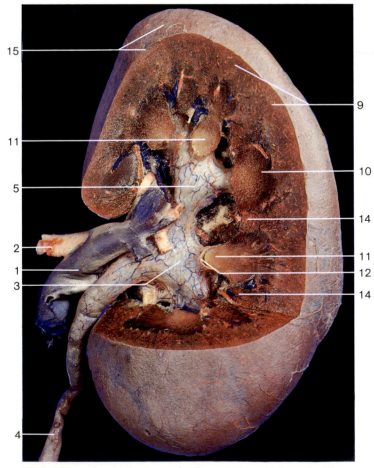

Right kidney (posterior aspect). The vessels are injected with
colored solutions.

Position of kidneys and urinary system (ventral aspect).
The excursions of the kidneys with the respiratory
movements of the diaphragm are indicated.
(Schematic drawing) (W.).

1 Minor calices
2 Subcortical or arcuate vein
3 Subcortical or arcuate artery
4 Radiating cortical arteries
5 Interlobular vein
6 Interlobular artery
7 Venous system of renal cortex
8 Anterior branch of renal artery
9 Posterior branch of renal artery
10 Anterior branch of renal vein
11 Posterior branch of renal vein
12 Renal pelvis
13 Interlobar artery and vein
14 Arterial system of renal cortex
15 Afferent arteriole of glomerulus
16 Glomeruli
17 Efferent arteriole of glomerulus
18 Vessels of renal capsule
19 Vasa recta of medulla
20 Spiral arteries of renal pelvis

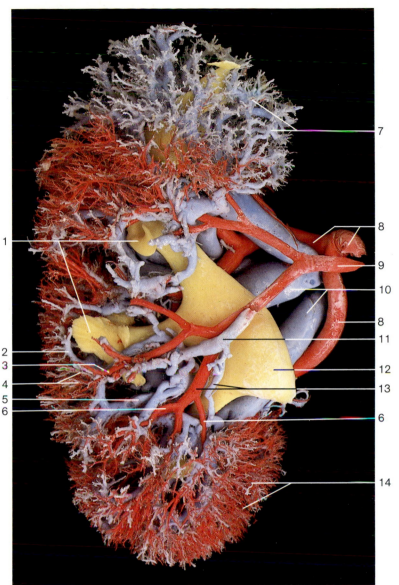

Cast of vessels of kidney (left side, dorsal aspect).
Red = arteries; blue = veins; yellow = calices and renal pelvis.

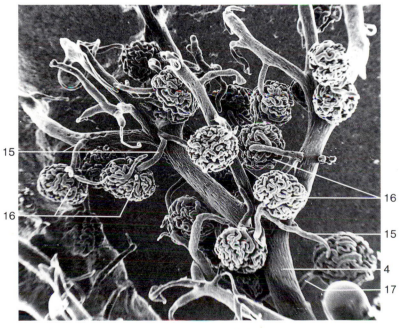

Scanning electron micrograph of glomeruli (210×).

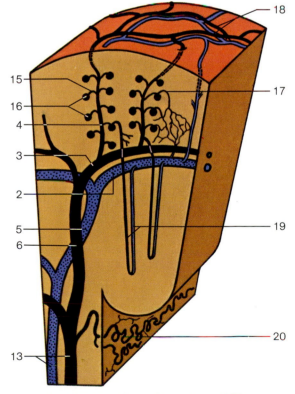

Architecture of vascular system of kidney.
(Schematic drawing) (W.).

301

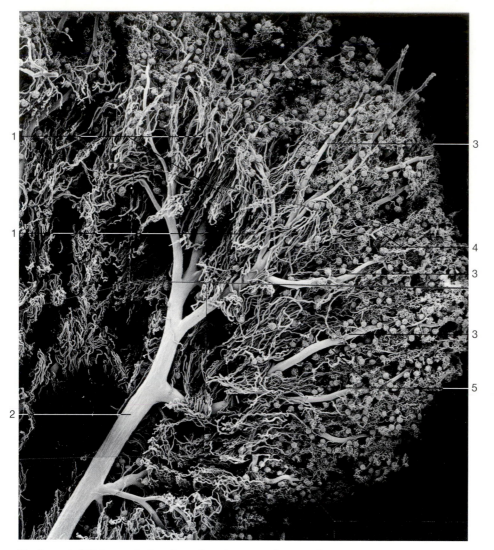

1 Arteriolae rectae of renal medulla
2 Interlobar artery
3 Interlobular arteries
4 Cortical glomeruli
5 Juxtamedullary glomeruli
6 Body of first lumbar vertebra
7 Left renal artery
8 Abdominal aorta with catheter
9 Upper pole of kidney
10 Anterior branch } of renal
11 Posterior branch } artery
12 Anterior inferior segmental artery
13 Lower pole of kidney
14 Celiac trunk
15 Superior mesenteric artery
16 Middle colic artery
17 Splenic artery

Resin cast of kidney arteries. Scanning electron micrograph.

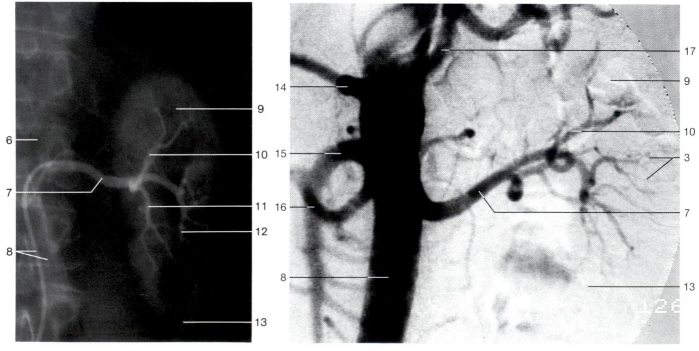

Arteriogram of left kidney.

Abdominal aorta. Subtraction angiograph.

1 Right common carotid artery
2 Right subclavian artery
3 Brachiocephalic trunk
4 Thoracic aorta
5 Diaphragm
6 Celiac trunk
7 Right renal artery
8 Superior mesenteric artery
9 Lumbar arteries
10 Right common iliac artery
11 Internal iliac artery
12 External iliac artery
13 Left common carotid artery
14 Left subclavian artery
15 Highest intercostal artery
16 Aortic arch
17 Intercostal arteries
18 Left renal artery
19 Left testicular (or ovarian) artery
20 Inferior mesenteric artery
21 Median sacral artery
22 Superior suprarenal artery
23 Upper capsular artery
24 Anterior branch of renal artery
25 Perforating artery
26 Lower capsular artery
27 Ureter
28 Right inferior phrenic artery
29 Left inferior phrenic artery
30 Middle suprarenal artery
31 Inferior suprarenal artery
32 Posterior branch of renal artery

Main branches of descending aorta. (Schematic drawing) (O.).

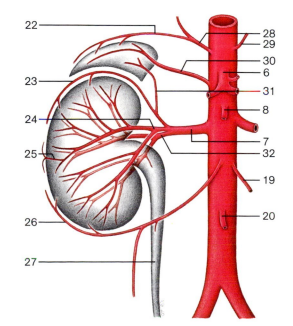

Arteries of kidney and suprarenal gland. (Schematic drawing) (O.).

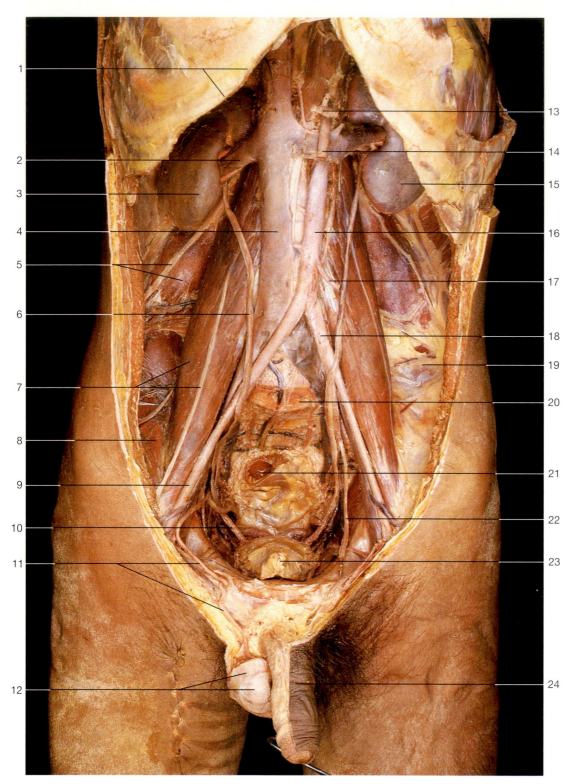

Retroperitoneal organs, urinary system in the male (ventral aspect). The peritoneum has been removed.

1 Costal arch	9 External iliac artery	18 Common iliac artery
2 Right renal vein	10 **Ureter,** pelvic part	19 Iliac crest
3 **Right kidney**	11 Ductus deferens	20 Promontory
4 Inferior vena cava	12 Testis, epididymis	21 Rectum (divided)
5 Iliohypogastric nerve, quadratus lumborum	13 Celiac trunk	22 Testicular artery
	14 Superior mesenteric artery	23 **Urinary bladder**
6 **Ureter,** abdominal part	15 **Left kidney**	24 Penis
7 Psoas major, genitofemoral nerve	16 Abdominal aorta	
8 Iliacus	17 Inferior mesenteric artery	

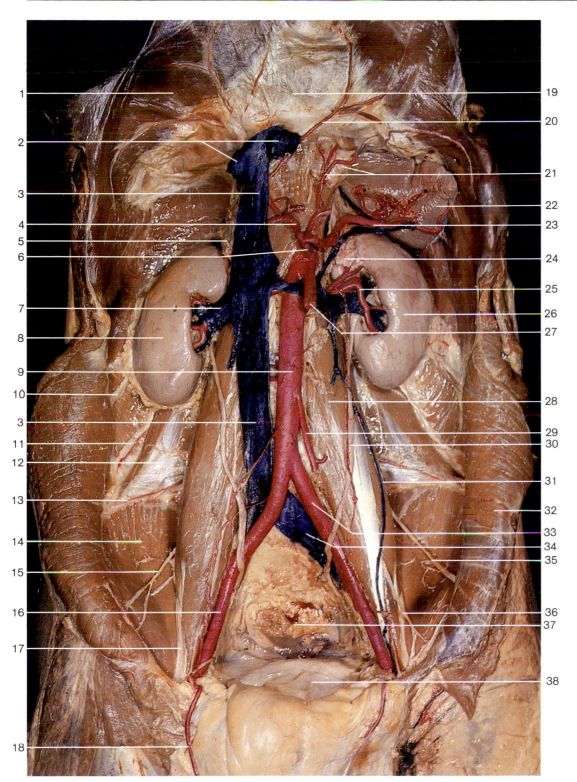

Retroperitoneal organs, urinary system in situ (ventral aspect). The peritoneum has been removed. Red = arteries; blue = veins.

1 Diaphragm	12 Quadratus lumborum	esophageal branches of	31 Testicular artery and vein
2 Hepatic veins	13 Iliac crest	left gastric artery	32 Transversus abdominis
3 Inferior vena cava	14 Iliacus	22 Spleen	33 Left common iliac artery
4 Common hepatic artery	15 Right lateral femoral	23 Splenic artery	34 Left common iliac vein
5 Right suprarenal gland	cutaneous nerve	24 Left suprarenal gland	35 Lateral femoral cutaneous
6 Celiac trunk	16 External iliac artery	25 Left renal artery	nerve
7 Right renal vein	17 Femoral nerve	26 Left kidney	36 Genitofemoral nerve
8 Right kidney	18 Right inferior epigastric artery	27 Superior mesenteric artery	37 Rectum (divided)
9 Abdominal aorta	19 Central tendon of diaphragm	28 Psoas major	38 Urinary bladder
10 Subcostal nerve	20 Inferior phrenic artery	29 Inferior mesenteric artery	
11 Iliohypogastric nerve	21 Cardiac part of stomach,	30 Ureter	

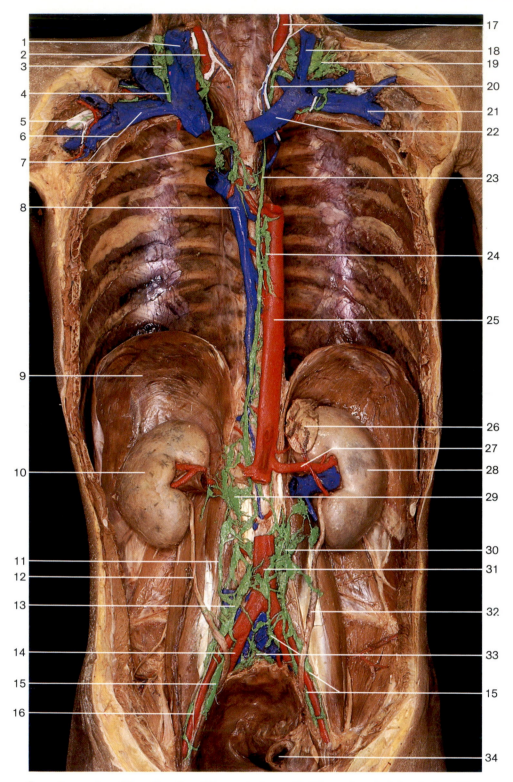

1 Internal jugular vein
2 Right common carotid artery and right vagus nerve
3 Jugulo-omohyoid lymph node
4 Right lymphatic duct
5 Subclavian trunk
6 Right subclavian vein
7 Bronchomediastinal trunk
8 Azygos vein
9 Diaphragm
10 Right kidney
11 Right lumbar trunk
12 Right ureter
13 Common iliac lymph nodes
14 Right internal iliac artery
15 External iliac lymph nodes
16 Right external iliac artery
17 Left common carotid artery, left vagus nerve
18 Internal jugular vein
19 Deep cervical lymph nodes
20 Thoracic duct entering left jugular angle
21 Left subclavian vein
22 Left brachiocephalic trunk
23 Thoracic duct
24 Mediastinal lymph nodes
25 Thoracic aorta
26 Left suprarenal gland
27 Left renal artery
28 Left kidney
29 Cisterna chyli
30 Lumbar lymph nodes
31 Abdominal aorta
32 Left ureter
33 Sacral lymph nodes
34 Rectum (cut edge)

Lymph vessels and lymph nodes of the posterior wall of thoracic and abdominal cavities (ventral aspect). Green = lymph vessels and nodes; blue = veins; red = arteries; white = nerves.

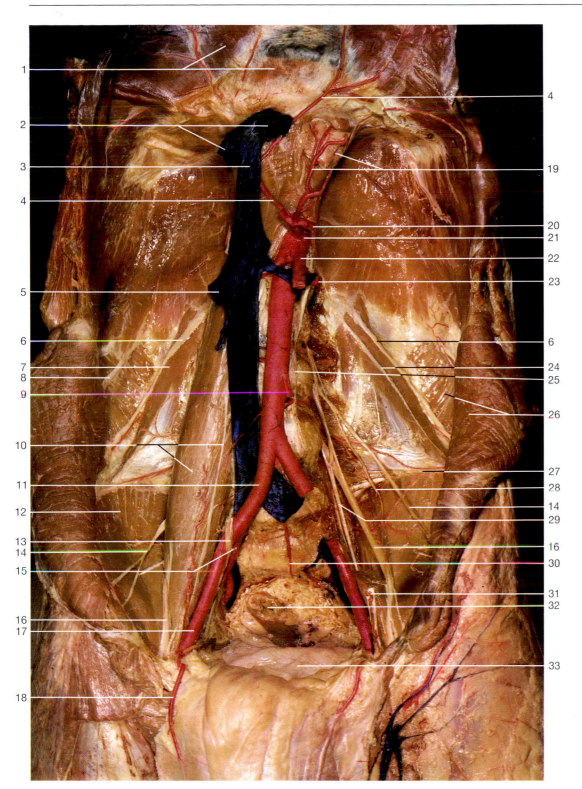

Vessels and nerves of posterior abdominal wall (ventral aspect). Part of the left psoas major has been removed to display the lumbar plexus. Red = arteries; blue = veins.

1 Diaphragm	11 Common iliac artery	20 Splenic artery	31 Psoas major (divided)
2 Hepatic veins	12 Iliacus	21 Celiac trunk	with supplying artery
3 Inferior vena cava	13 Right ureter (divided)	22 Superior mesenteric artery	32 Rectum (divided)
4 Inferior phrenic artery	14 Lateral femoral cutaneous nerve	23 Left renal artery	33 Urinary bladder
5 Right renal vein	15 Internal iliac artery	24 Ilioinguinal nerve	
6 Iliohypogastric nerve	16 Femoral nerve	25 Sympathetic trunk	
7 Quadratus lumborum	17 External iliac artery	26 Transversus abdominis	
8 Subcostal nerve	18 Inferior epigastric artery	27 Iliac crest	
9 Inferior mesenteric artery	19 Cardiac part of stomach,	28 Left genitofemoral nerve	
10 Right genitofemoral nerve,	esophageal branches of left	29 Left obturator nerve	
psoas major muscle	gastric artery	30 Median sacral artery	

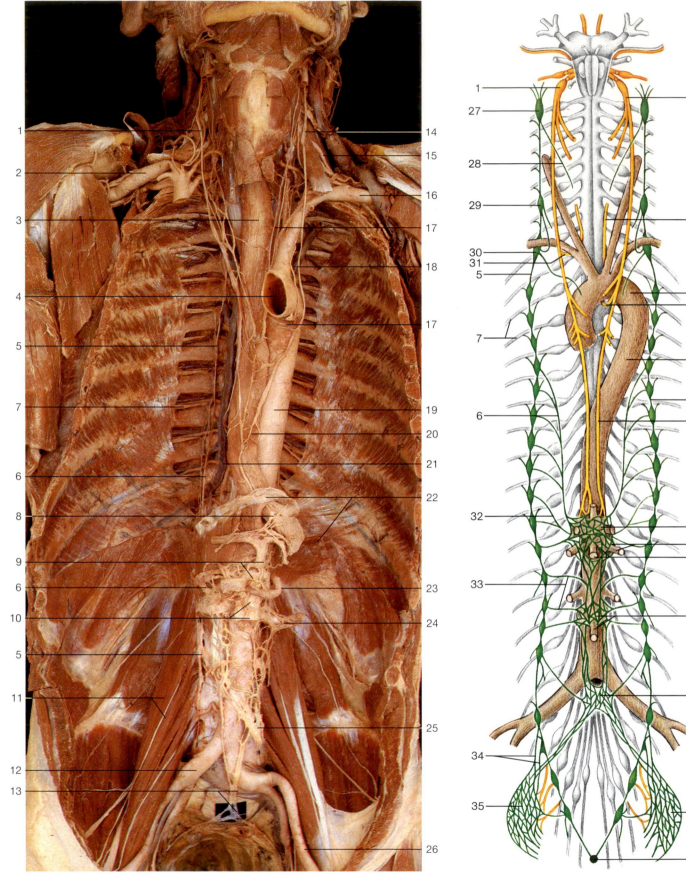

Posterior wall of thoracic and abdominal cavities with sympathetic trunk, vagus nerve and autonomic ganglia (anterior aspect). Thoracic and abdominal organs removed, except esophagus and aorta.

Organization of autonomic nervous system (after MATTUSCHKA). (Schematic drawing) (O.). Yellow = parasympathetic nerves; green = sympathetic nerves.

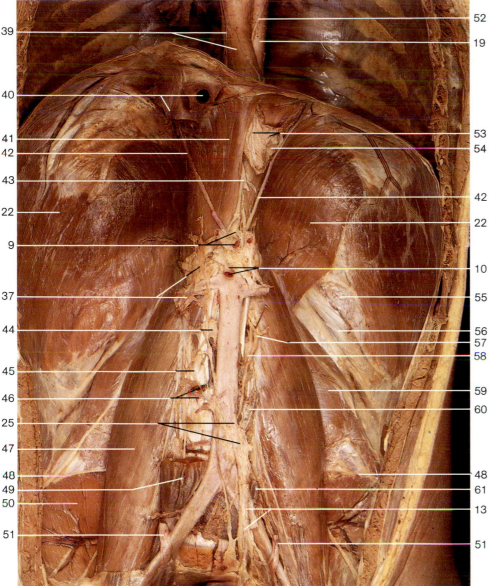

15 Brachial plexus
16 Left subclavian artery
17 Left recurrent laryngeal nerve
18 Inferior cervical cardiac nerve
19 Thoracic aorta
20 Esophageal plexus
21 Azygos vein
22 Diaphragm
23 Splenic artery
24 Left renal artery and plexus
25 **Inferior mesenteric ganglion and artery**
26 Left external iliac artery
27 **Superior cervical gangion** of sympathetic trunk
28 Superior cardiac branch of sympathetic trunk
29 Middle cervical ganglion of sympathetic trunk
30 **Inferior cervical ganglion** of sympathetic trunk
31 Right recurrent laryngeal nerve
32 Lesser splanchnic nerve
33 Lumbar splanchnic nerves
34 Sacral splanchnic nerves
35 **Inferior hypogastric ganglion and plexus**
36 Left recurrent laryngeal nerve
37 **Aorticorenal plexus** and renal artery
38 Ganglion impar
39 Esophagus with branches of vagus nerve
40 Hepatic veins
41 Right crus of diaphragm
42 Inferior phrenic artery
43 Right vagus nerve entering the celiac ganglion
44 Right lumbar lymph trunk
45 Lumbar part of right sympathetic trunk
46 Lumbar artery and vein
47 Psoas major
48 Iliac crest
49 Inferior vena cava
50 Iliacus
51 Ureter
52 Left vagus nerve forming the esophageal plexus
53 Left vagus nerve forming the gastric plexus
54 Esophagus continuing into the cardiac part of stomach
55 Lumbocostal triangle
56 Position of 12th rib
57 Left lumbar lymph trunk
58 Ganglion of sympathetic trunk
59 Quadratus lumborum
60 Lumbar part of left sympathetic trunk
61 Iliac lymph vessels

Ganglia and plexus of the autonomic nervous system within the retroperitoneal space (ventral aspect). The kidneys and the inferior vena cava with its tributaries have been removed.

1 **Right vagus nerve**
2 Right subclavian artery
3 Esophagus
4 Aortic arch
5 **Sympathetic trunk**
6 Greater splanchnic nerve
7 Intercostal nerve
8 Abdominal part of esophagus and vagal trunk
9 **Celiac trunk with celiac ganglion**
10 **Superior mesenteric artery and ganglion**
11 Psoas major muscle, genitofemoral nerve
12 Common iliac artery
13 **Superior hypogastric plexus and ganglion**
14 **Left vagus nerve**

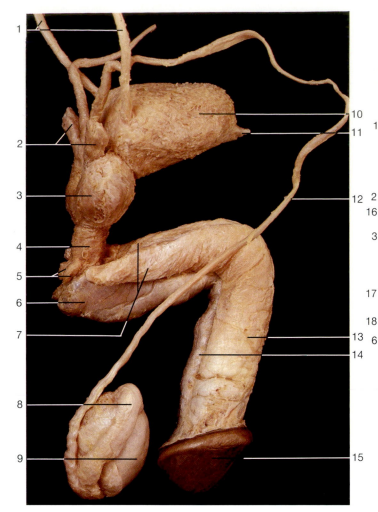

Male genital organs isolated (right lateral aspect).

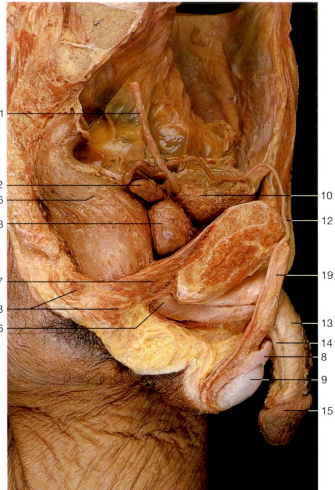

Male genital organs in situ (right lateral aspect).

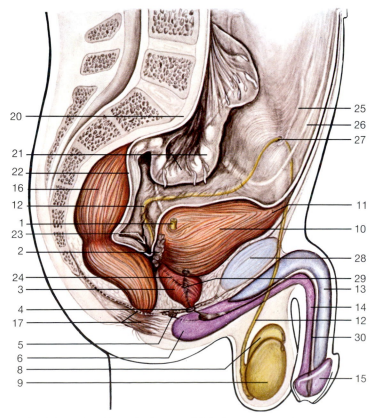

Positions of male genital organs (right lateral aspect).
(Schematic drawing) (W.).

1 Ureter
2 Seminal vesicle
3 Prostate gland
4 Urogenital diaphragm and membranous part of urethra
5 Bulbourethral or Cowper's gland
6 Bulb of penis
7 Left and right crus penis
8 Epididymis
9 Testis
10 Urinary bladder
11 Apex of urinary bladder
12 Ductus deferens
13 Corpus cavernosum of penis
14 Corpus spongiosum of penis
15 Glans penis
16 Ampulla of rectum
17 Levator ani muscle
18 Anal canal and sphincter ani externus
19 Spermatic cord (divided)
20 Promontory
21 Sigmoid colon
22 Peritoneum (cut edge)
23 Rectovesical pouch
24 Ejaculatory duct
25 Lateral umbilical fold
26 Medial umbilical fold
27 Deep inguinal ring, ductus deferens
28 Pubic symphysis
29 Prostatic part of urethra
30 Spongy urethra

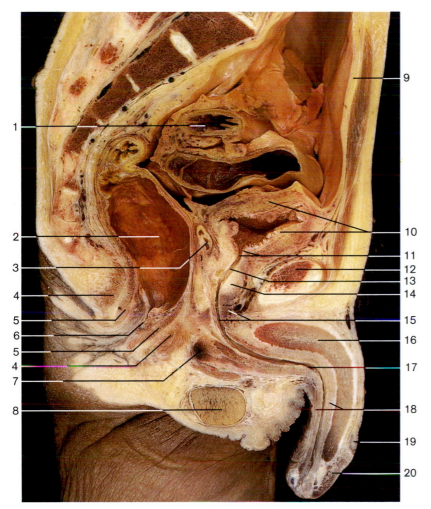

Sagittal section through the male pelvis.

1 Sigmoid colon
2 Ampulla of rectum
3 Ampulla of ductus deferens
4 Sphincter ani externus
5 Sphincter ani internus
6 Anal canal
7 Bulb of penis
8 Testis (cut surface)
9 Median umbilical ligament
10 Urinary bladder
11 Internal urethral orifice and sphincter
    (sphincter vesicae)
12 Pubic symphysis
13 Prostatic part of urethra
14 Prostate gland
15 Membranous urethra and external urethral
    sphincter (sphincter urethrae)
16 Corpus cavernosum of penis
17 Spongy urethra
18 Corpus spongiosum of penis
19 Foreskin or prepuce
20 Glans penis
21 Kidney
22 Renal pelvis
23 Abdominal part of ureter
24 Pelvic part of ureter
25 Seminal vesicle
26 Ejaculatory duct
27 Bulbourethral or Cowper's gland
28 Ductus deferens
29 Epididymis
30 Umbilicus
31 Trigone of bladder and ureteric orifice
32 Navicular fossa of urethra
33 External urethral orifice
34 Testis

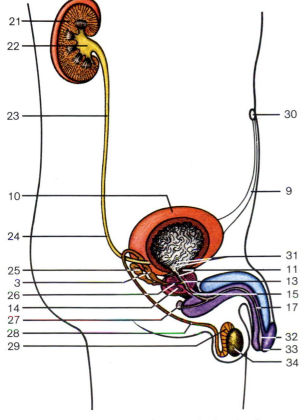

Male urogenital system. (Schematic drawing.)

The prostate is situated between bladder and urogenital diaphragm. The penis which corresponds to the female clitoris includes the urethra and thus serves for both ejaculation and micturition. The internal (involuntary) and external (voluntary) urethral sphincters are widely separated. The ureter having crossed the ductus deferens enters the urinary bladder at its base. The peritoneum is reflected off the base of the bladder onto the rectum thus forming the rectovesical pouch.

311

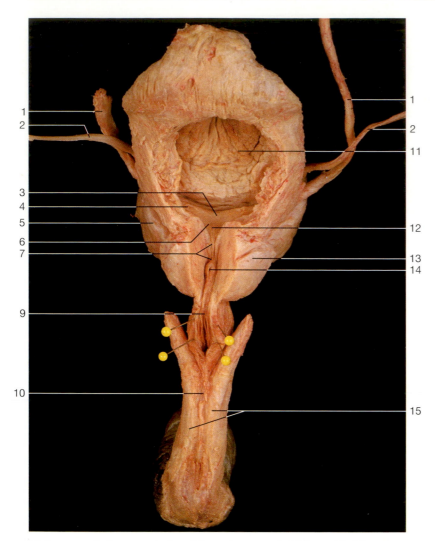

1 Ureter
2 Ductus deferens
3 Interureteric fold
4 Ureteric orifice
5 Seminal vesicle
6 Trigone of bladder
7 Prostatic urethra with seminal colliculus and urethral crest
8 Deep transverse perineal muscle
9 Membranous urethra
10 Spongy urethra
11 Mucous membrane of bladder
12 Internal urethral orifice and uvula of bladder
13 Prostate
14 Prostatic utricle
15 Right and left corpus cavernosum of penis
16 Ejaculatory duct
17 Sphincter urethrae
18 Medial umbilical fold
19 Lateral umbilical fold
20 Deep inguinal ring
21 Muscles of abdominal wall
22 Sigmoid mesocolon
23 Psoas major
24 Median umbilical fold
25 Urinary bladder
26 Rectovesical pouch
27 Rectum
28 Body of lumbar vertebra
29 Cauda equina within dural sac

Male urogenital organs; isolated (anterior aspect). Urinary bladder, prostate and urethra have been opened. The urinary bladder is contracted.

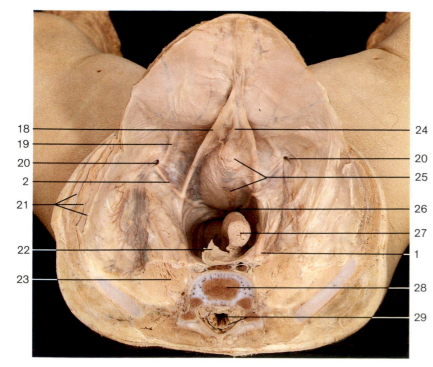

Urinary bladder of a newborn in situ (from above).

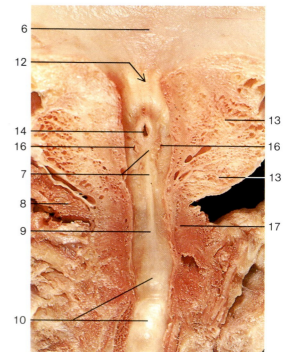

Dorsal half of male urethra and prostate in continuity with neck of bladder (ventral aspect).

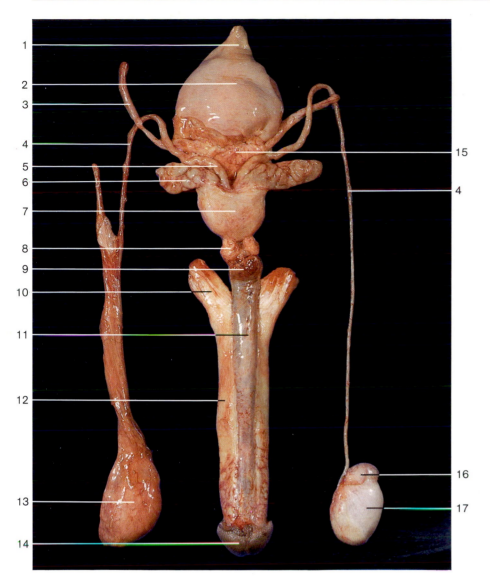

1 Apex of urinary bladder with
  urachus
2 Urinary bladder
3 Ureter
4 Ductus deferens
5 Ampulla of ductus deferens
6 Seminal vesicle
7 Prostate
8 Bulbourethral or Cowper's gland
9 Bulb of penis
10 Crus penis
11 Corpus spongiosum of penis
12 Corpus cavernosum of penis
13 Testis and epididymis with coverings
14 Glans penis
15 Fundus of bladder
16 Head of epididymis
17 Testis
18 Mucous membrane of bladder
19 Trigone of bladder
20 Ureteric orifice
21 Internal urethral orifice
22 Seminal colliculus
23 Prostate
24 Prostatic urethra
25 Membranous urethra
26 Spongy urethra
27 Skin of penis
28 Deep dorsal vein of penis (unpaired)
29 Dorsal artery of penis (paired)
30 Tunica albuginea of corpora
   cavernosa
31 Septum pectiniforme
32 Deep artery of penis
33 Tunica albuginea of corpus
   spongiosum
34 Deep fascia of penis

Male genital organs, isolated (dorsal aspect).

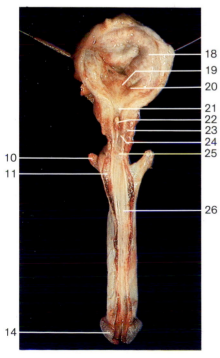

Urinary bladder, urethra and penis
(opened, ventral aspect).

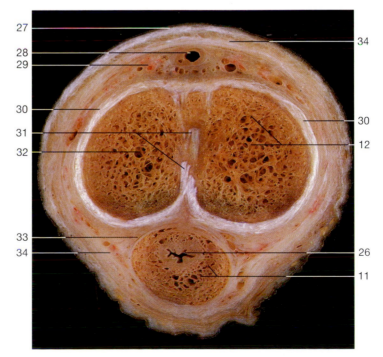

Cross-section of penis.

313

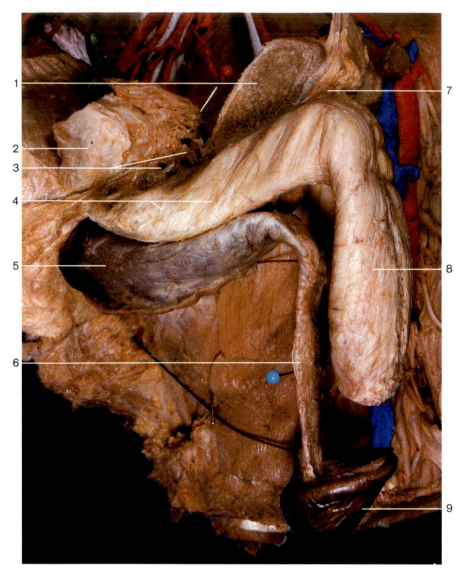

1	Pubic bone (cut edge)
2	Prostate
3	Venous plexus of prostate
4	Crus penis
5	Bulb of penis
6	Corpus spongiosum of penis
7	Suspensory ligament of penis
8	Corpus cavernosum of penis
9	Glans penis
10	Bulbourethral or Cowper's gland
11	Urinary bladder
12	Seminal vesicle
13	Ampulla of ductus deferens
14	Ductus deferens
15	Membranous urethra
16	Ureter
17	Deep dorsal vein of penis
18	Septum pectiniforme
19	Dorsal artery of penis

Male external genital organs (oblique lateral aspect). The corpus spongiosum of the penis with the glans penis has been isolated and reflected, the pubic symphysis divided and the urinary bladder removed.

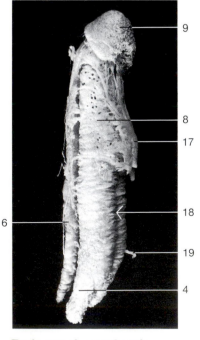

Resin cast of erected penis.

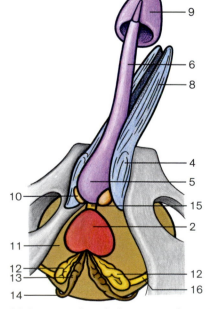

Male external genital organs and accessory glands. (Schematic drawing) (W.).

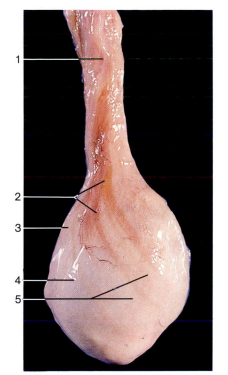

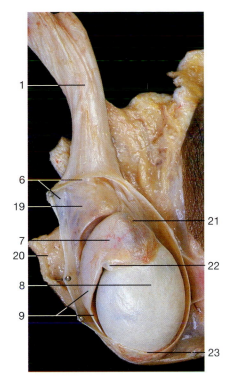

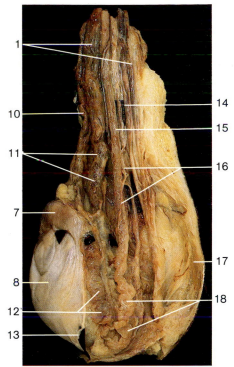

Testis and epididymis with investing layers (lateral aspect).

Testis and epididymis (lateral aspect). The tunica vaginalis has been opened.

Testis, epididymis and spermatic cord. Dissection of spermatic cord and ductus deferens (left side, dorsolateral aspect).

1 Spermatic cord covered with cremasteric fascia
2 Cremaster
3 Position of epididymis
4 Internal spermatic fascia
5 Position of testis
6 Internal spermatic fascia with adjacent investing layers of testis (cut surface)

7 Head of epididymis
8 Testis with tunica vaginalis (visceral layer)
9 Tail of epididymis
10 Testicular artery
11 Pampiniform plexus
12 Tail of epididymis

13 Tunica vaginalis (cut edge)
14 Artery of the ductus deferens
15 Ductus deferens
16 Autonomic plexus on artery to ductus deferens
17 Scrotum (reflected)
18 Transition of epididymidal duct to ductus deferens
19 Parietal layer of tunica vaginalis
20 Skin, dartos muscle
21 Appendix of epididymis
22 Appendix of testis
23 Gubernaculum testis

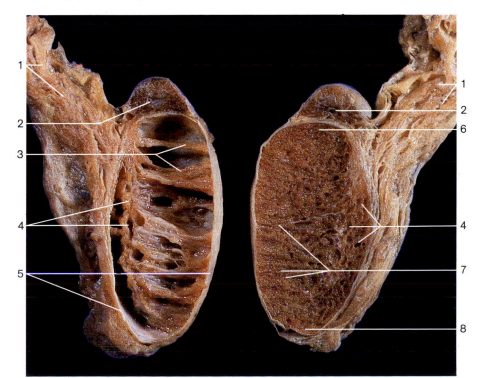

Longitudinal section through testis and epididymis. The left figure shows the testicular septa after removal of the seminiferous tubules.

1 Spermatic cord (cut surface)
2 Head of epididymis (cut surface)
3 Septa of testis
4 Mediastinum testis
5 Tunica albuginea
6 Superior pole of testis
7 Convoluted seminiferous tubules
8 Inferior pole of testis

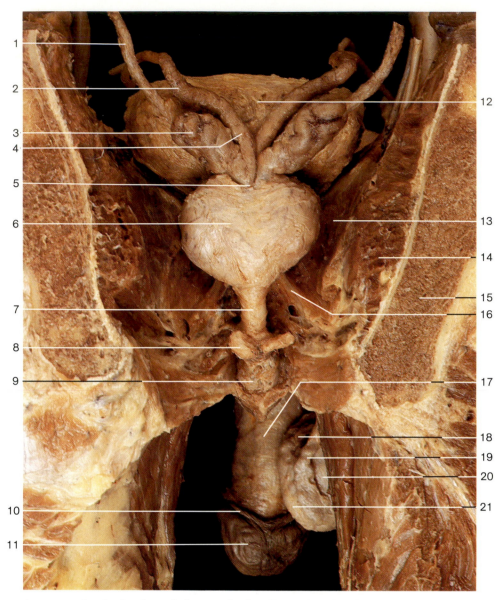

1   Ureter
2   Ductus deferens
3   Seminal vesicle
4   Ampulla of ductus deferens
5   Ejaculatory duct
6   Prostate
7   Membranous urethra
8   Bulbourethral or Cowper's
    gland
9   Bulb of penis
10 Penis
11 Glans penis
12 Urinary bladder
13 Levator ani
14 Obturator internus
15 Pelvic bone (cut edge)
16 Puboprostatic ligament
17 Corpus spongiosum
    of penis
18 Head of epididymis
19 End of ductus deferens
20 Testis
21 Tail of epididymis
22 Corpus cavernosum of penis
23 Spermatic cord
24 Adductor muscles
25 Pubic bone
26 Prostatic part of urethra
    (seminal colliculus)
27 Rectum
28 Sciatic nerve
29 Great saphenous vein
30 Sartorius
31 Femoral artery and vein
32 Rectus femoris
33 Tensor fasciae latae
34 Pectineus
35 Iliopsoas
36 Vastus lateralis
37 Obturator externus
38 Greater trochanter
39 Ischial tuberosity
40 Gluteus maximus

Accessory glands of male genital organs in situ. Coronal section through the pelvic cavity. Posterior aspect of urinary bladder, prostate and seminal vesicles.

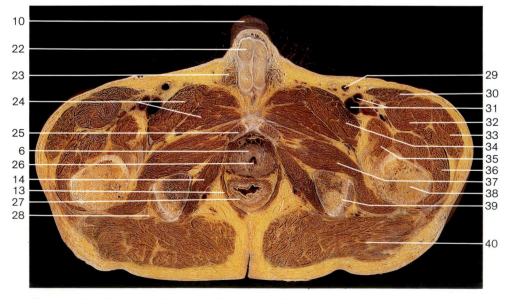

Horizontal section through pelvic cavity at level of prostate.

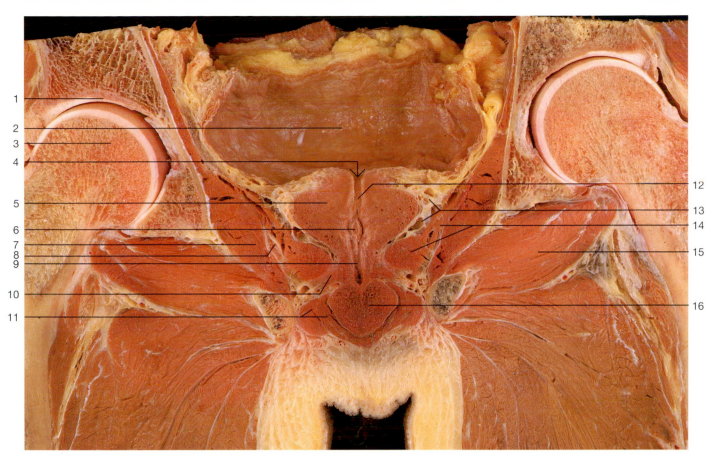

Coronal section through pelvic cavity at the level of prostate and hip joint (anterior aspect).

1	Acetabulum of hip joint	10	Deep transverse perineal muscle	19	Seminal vesicle
2	Urinary bladder	11	Crus penis, ischiocavernosus muscle	20	Sphincter ani internus
3	Head of femur	12	Prostatic part of urethra	21	Sphincter ani externus
4	Internal urethral orifice	13	Prostatic plexus	22	Anus
5	Prostate	14	Levator ani	23	Psoas major
6	Seminal colliculus	15	Obturator externus muscle	24	Intervertebral disc
7	Obturator internus muscle	16	Bulb of penis	25	Ilium
8	Ischiorectal fossa	17	Ampulla of rectum	26	Ligament of the head of the femur
9	Membranous urethra	18	Anal canal	27	Promontory

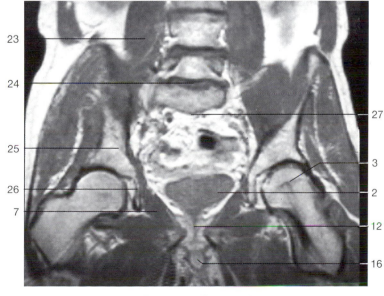

Coronal section through pelvic cavity. MR-Scan.

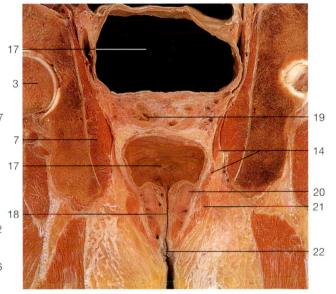

Coronal section through anal canal.

317

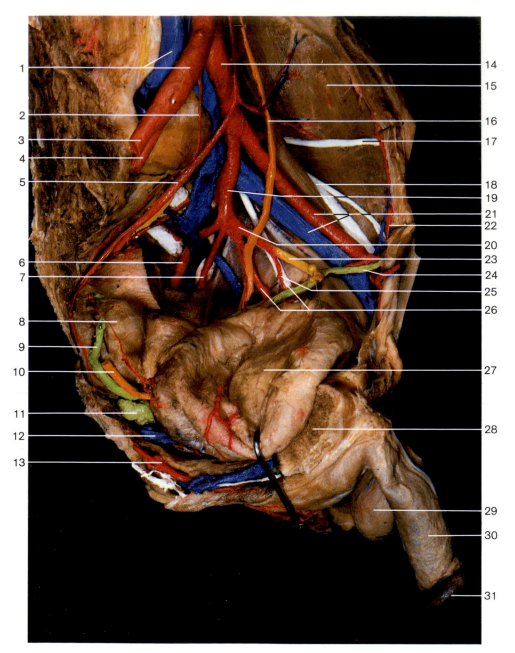

Pelvic cavity in the male with vessels and nerves (left half, medial aspect). The urinary bladder has been reflected and the parietal layer of peritoneum has been removed. Red = arteries; blue = veins; orange = ureter; green = ductus deferens and seminal vesicle; white = nerves.

1	Right common iliac artery and vein	17	Lateral femoral cutaneous nerve
2	Median sacral artery	18	Femoral nerve
3	Right external iliac artery (divided)	19	**Left internal iliac artery**
4	Right internal iliac artery (divided)	20	Umbilical artery
5	Superior rectal artery	21	Left external iliac artery and vein
6	Inferior gluteal artery	22	Inferior epigastric artery and vein
7	Internal pudendal artery	23	Medial umbilical ligament (yellow)
8	Rectum	24	Left ductus deferens
9	Right ductus deferens	25	Superior vesical artery
10	Right ureter	26	Obturator artery and nerve
11	Seminal vesicle	27	Urinary bladder
12	Vesicoprostatic venous plexus	28	Pubic bone (cut surface)
13	Levator ani (cut edge)	29	Left testis
14	Left common iliac artery	30	Penis
15	Iliacus	31	Glans penis
16	Left ureter		

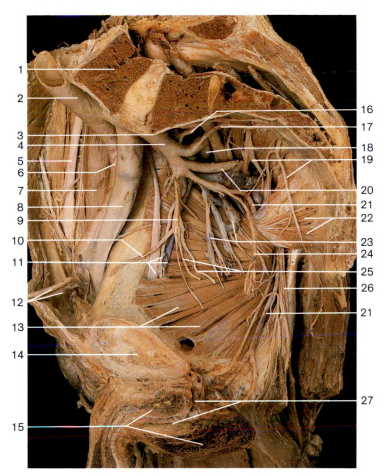

1	5th lumbar vertebra
2	Right common iliac artery
3	Promontory
4	Right internal iliac artery
5	Femoral nerve
6	Right external iliac artery
7	Iliopsoas muscle
8	Right external iliac vein
9	Umbilical artery
10	Medial umbilical ligament with obliterated umbilical artery
11	Obturator nerve, artery and vein
12	Inferior epigastric artery and vein
13	Obturator internus
14	Pubic symphysis
15	Root of penis (cut surface)
16	Iliolumbar artery
17	Lateral sacral artery
18	Superior gluteal artery
19	Pudendal and coccygeal plexus
20	Inferior gluteal artery
21	Internal pudendal artery
22	Coccygeus muscle
23	Tributaries of internal iliac vein (middle rectal vein, inferior vesical vein, etc.)
24	Middle rectal artery
25	Superior vesical artery and branch to the ductus deferens
26	Pudendal nerve
27	Membranous and spongy urethra
28	Right ureter
29	Right ductus deferens
30	Left ureter
31	Urinary bladder
32	Prostate
33	Urogenital diaphragm
34	Deep artery of penis
35	Dorsal artery of penis
36	Penis
37	Testis
38	Left common iliac artery
39	Obturator artery
40	Inferior vesical artery
41	Levator ani
42	Inferior rectal artery

Vessels of pelvic cavity in the male (sagittal section, right side, medial aspect). Urinary bladder, prostate, rectum, etc. have been removed.

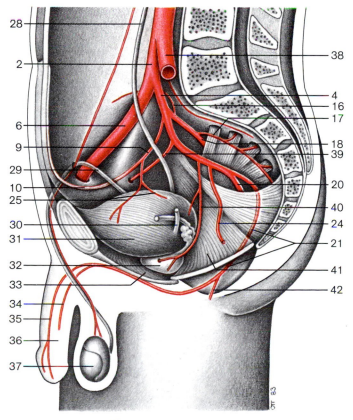

Main branches of internal iliac artery in the male.
(Schematic drawing) (O.).

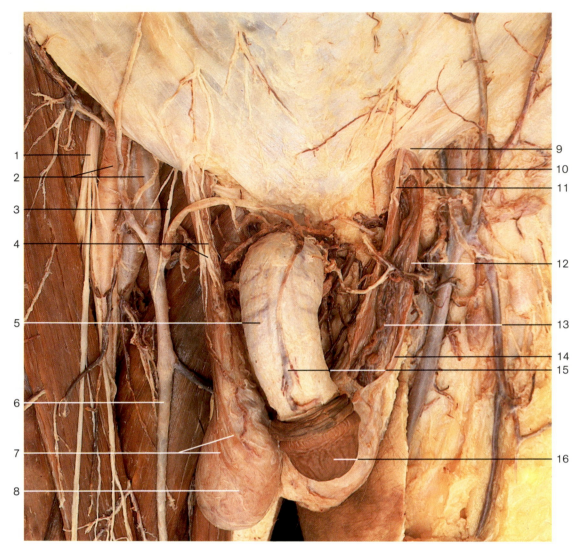

1
2
3
4
5
6
7
8

9
10
11
12
13
14
15
16

Male external genital organs with penis, testis and spermatic cord, superficial layers (ventral aspect).

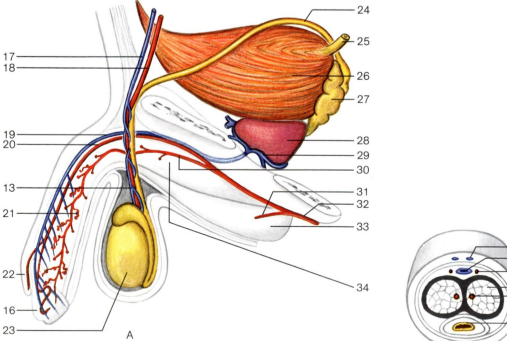

17
18
19
20
13
21
22
16
23

24
25
26
27
28
29
30
31
32
33
34

A

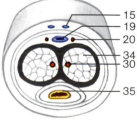

15
19
20
34
30
35

B

Vessels of male genital organs. (Schematic drawing) (W.).
A = lateral aspect; B = cross-section of penis.

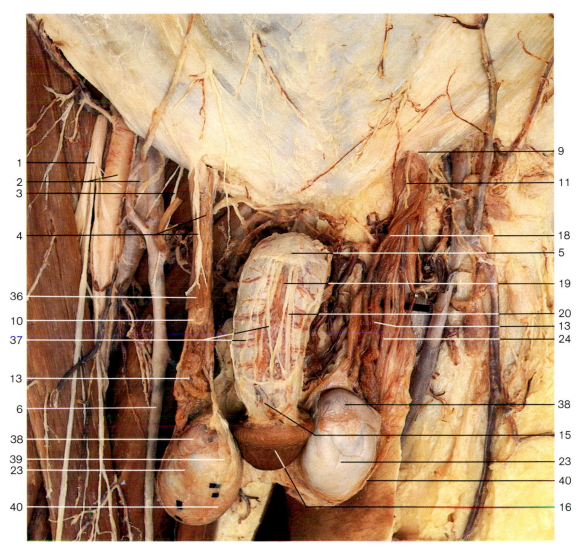

Male external genital organs with penis, testis and spermatic cord, deeper layers (ventral aspect).
The deep fascia of the penis has been opened to display the dorsal nerves and vessels.

1	Femoral nerve	21	Helicine arteries
2	Femoral artery and vein	22	Prepuce
3	Femoral branch of genitofemoral nerve	23	Testis with tunica albuginea
4	Spermatic cord with genital branch of genitofemoral nerve	24	Ductus deferens
		25	Ureter
5	Penis with deep fascia	26	Urinary bladder
6	Great saphenous vein	27	Seminal vesicle
7	Cremaster	28	Prostate
8	Testis with cremaster muscle	29	Vesicoprostatic venous plexus
9	Superficial inguinal ring	30	Deep artery of penis
10	Internal spermatic fascia (cut edge)	31	Artery of bulb of penis
11	Ilioinguinal nerve	32	Internal pudendal artery
12	Left spermatic cord	33	Corpus spongiosum of penis
13	Pampiniform plexus	34	Corpus cavernosum of penis
14	External spermatic fascia	35	Urethra
15	Superficial dorsal vein of penis	36	Cremasteric fascia with cremaster
16	Glans penis	37	Dorsal nerve of penis
17	Testicular vein	38	Epididymis
18	Testicular artery	39	Tunica vaginalis, visceral layer
19	Deep dorsal vein of penis	40	Tunica vaginalis, parietal layer
20	Dorsal artery of penis		

321

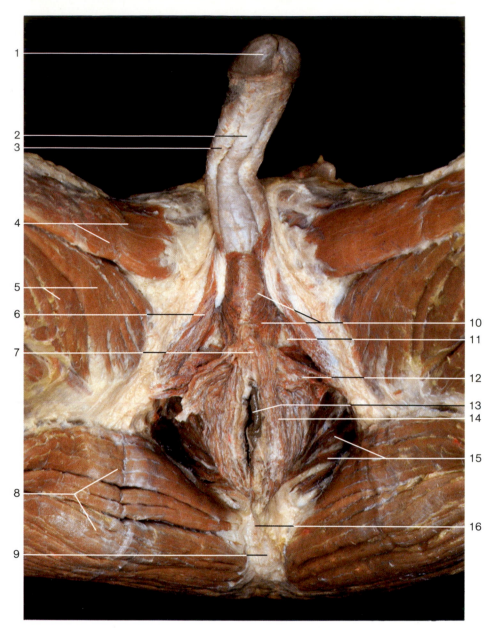

1 Glans penis
2 Corpus spongiosum of penis
3 Corpus cavernosum of penis
4 Gracilis
5 Adductor muscles
6 Ischiocavernosus muscle with crus penis
7 Perineum
8 Gluteus maximus
9 Coccyx
10 Bulbospongiosus muscle
11 Deep transverse perineal muscle with inferior fascia of urogenital diaphragm
12 Superficial transverse perineal muscle
13 Anus
14 Sphincter ani externus
15 Levator ani
16 Anococcygeal ligament
18 Obturator internus
19 Urethra
20 Deep transverse perineal muscle

Muscles of urogenital and pelvic diaphragms in the male (from below).

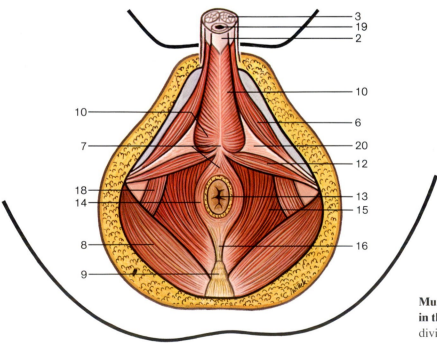

Muscles of urogenital and pelvic diaphragms in the male (from below). The penis has been divided. (Schematic drawing) (W.).

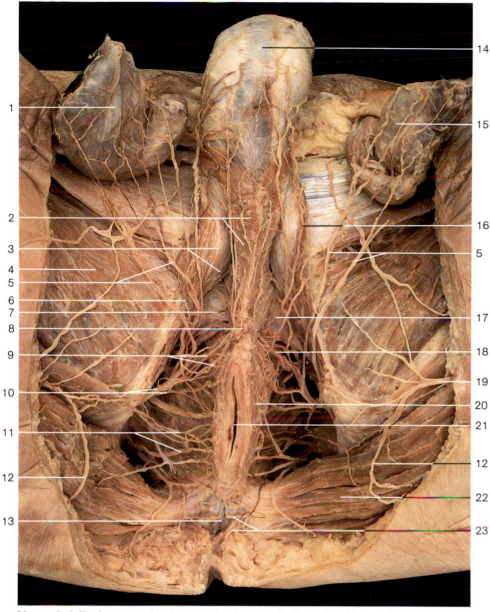

1	Right testis (reflected laterally and upward)
2	Bulbocavernosus muscle
3	Ischiocavernosus muscle
4	Adductor magnus
5	Posterior scrotal nerves
6	Right dorsal artery of penis
7	Right artery of bulb of penis
8	Perineum
9	Perineal branches of pudendal nerve
10	Pudendal nerve and internal pudendal artery
11	Inferior rectal arteries and nerves
12	Inferior clunial nerve
13	Coccyx
14	Penis
15	Left testis (reflected laterally)
16	Left dorsal artery of penis
17	Deep transverse perineal muscle
18	Left artery of bulb of penis
19	Posterior femoral cutaneous nerve
20	Sphincter ani externus
21	Anus
22	Gluteus maximus
23	Anococcygeal nerves
24	Sacrotuberous ligament (fenestrated)
25	Perforating cutaneous nerve
26	Inferior gluteal artery and nerve
27	Sciatic nerve
28	Piriformis

Urogenital diaphragm and external genital organs in the male with vessels and nerves (from below). The testes have been reflected laterally.

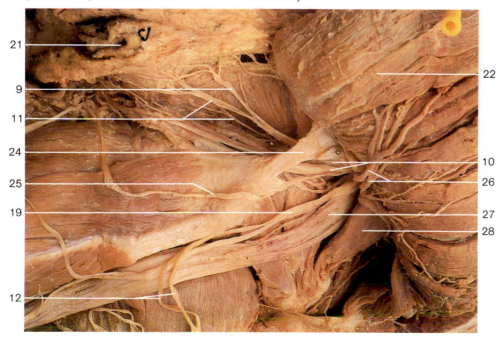

Gluteal region and pelvic diaphragm (right side, lateral aspect). The gluteus maximus has been cut and reflected. The sacrotuberous ligament has been fenestrated to display the pudendal arteries and nerves.

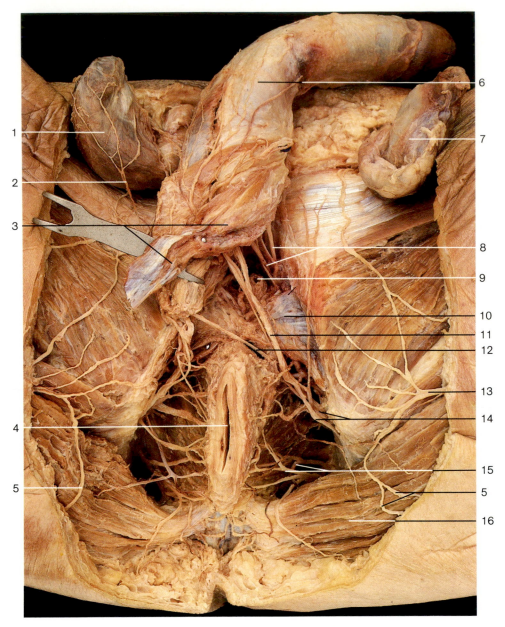

Urogenital diaphragm and external genital organs in the male (from below).
The left crus penis has been isolated and reflected laterally together with the bulb of the
penis. The urethra has been cut.

1 Right testis (reflected)
2 Posterior scrotal nerves
3 Left crus penis with ischiocavernosus muscle (laterally reflected)
4 Anus
5 Inferior clunial nerves
6 Penis
7 Left testis (reflected)
8 Dorsal artery and nerve of penis
9 Urethra
10 Deep transverse perineal muscle
11 Perineal branch of pudendal nerve
12 Artery of bulb of penis
13 Branch of posterior femoral cutaneous nerve
14 Internal pudendal artery, pudendal nerve
15 Inferior rectal arteries and nerves
16 Gluteus maximus

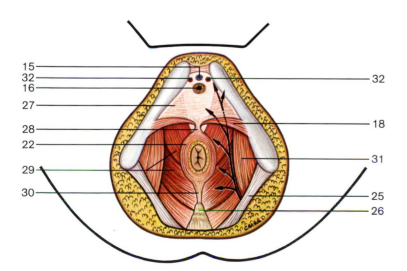
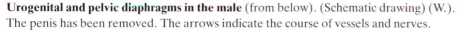

1	Right testis (reflected)
2	Corpus spongiosum of penis
3	Corpus cavernosum of penis
4	Perineal branch of posterior femoral cutaneous nerve
5	Posterior scrotal arteries and nerves
6	Deep artery of penis
7	Deep transverse perineal muscle
8	Right perineal nerves
9	Inferior rectal nerves
10	Inferior clunial nerve
11	Anococcygeal nerves
12	Left spermatic cord
13	Left testis (cut surface)
14	Dorsal artery and nerve of penis
15	Deep dorsal vein of penis
16	Urethra (cut)
17	Artery of bulb of penis
18	Superficial transverse perineal muscles
19	Left artery of bulb of penis
20	Perineal nerve of pudendal nerve
21	Anus
22	Sphincter ani externus
23	Gluteus maximus
24	Internal pudendal artery and pudendal nerve
25	Sacrotuberous ligament
26	Coccyx
27	Urogenital diaphragm (deep transverse perineal muscle)
28	Tendinous center of perineum (perineal body)
29	Levator ani
30	Anococcygeal ligament
31	Obturator internus
32	Dorsal artery of penis

Anal and urogenital region in the male (from below). The root of penis has been cut. Dissection of the urogenital diaphragm.

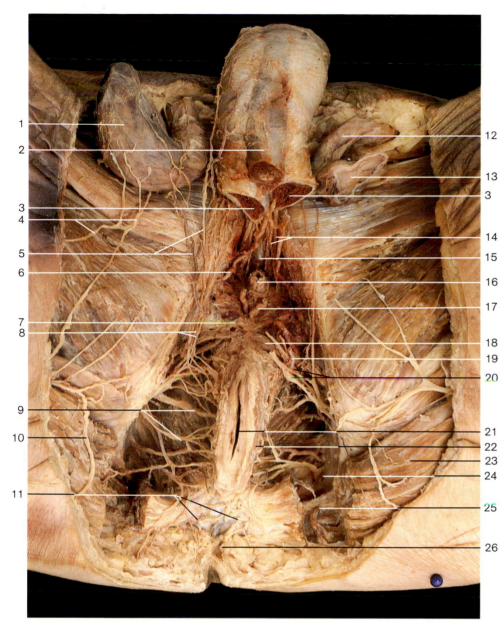

Urogenital and pelvic diaphragms in the male (from below). (Schematic drawing) (W.). The penis has been removed. The arrows indicate the course of vessels and nerves.

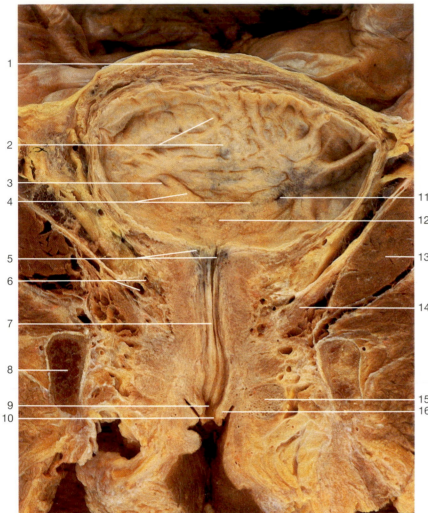

1 Muscular coat of urinary bladder
2 Folds of mucous membrane of urinary bladder
3 Right ureteric orifice
4 Interureteric fold
5 Internal urethral orifice
6 Vesicouterine venous plexus
7 Urethra
8 Pubic bone (cut edge)
9 External urethral orifice
10 Vestibule of vagina
11 Left ureteric orifice
12 Trigone of bladder
13 Obturator internus
14 Levator ani
15 Bulb of the vestibule
16 Left labium minus
17 Uterine tube
18 Mesosalpinx
19 Ovary
20 Sigmoid colon
21 Saphenous opening
22 Urinary bladder
23 Uterovesical pouch
24 Fundus of uterus
25 Rectouterine pouch
26 Ampulla of rectum
27 Kidney
28 Abdominal part of ureter
29 Pelvic part of ureter
30 Anal canal
31 Perineum
32 Umbilicus
33 Ampulla of uterine tube
34 Vaginal portion of cervix of uterus
35 Vagina
36 Pubic symphysis
37 Clitoris
38 Deep transverse perineal muscle

Coronal section through the female urinary bladder and urethra (ventral aspect).

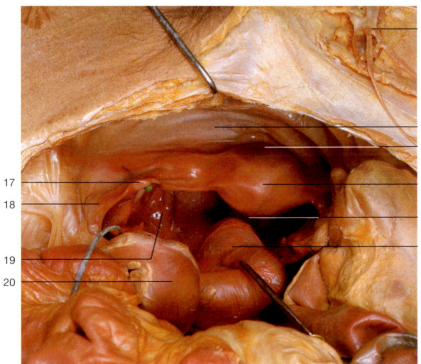

Femal internal genital organs. Pelvic cavity (from above).

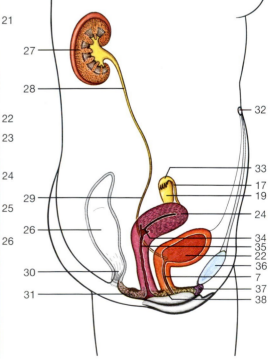

Female urogenital system (midsaggital section). (Schematic drawing) (W.).

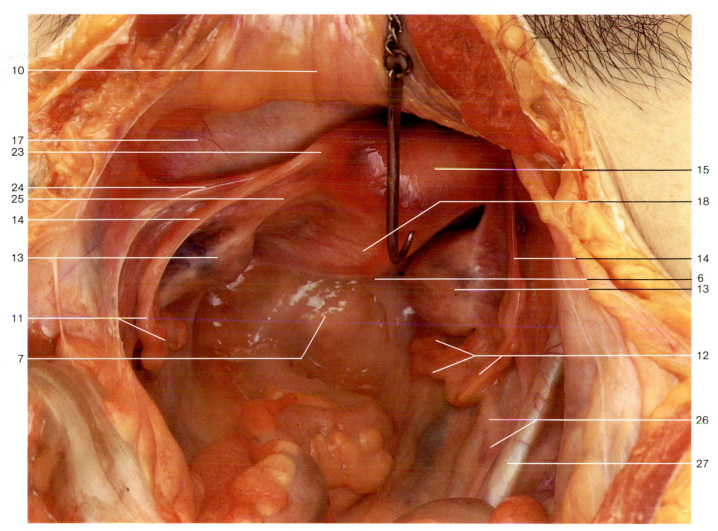

Female internal genital organs. Pelvic cavity, seen from above. The uterus has been reflected to the right.

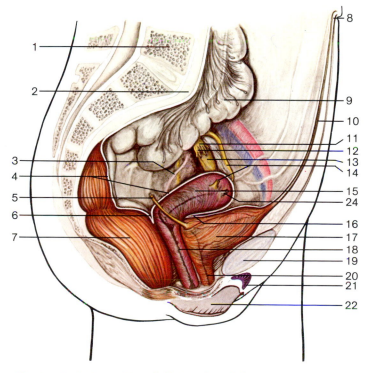

Regional relations of female internal genital organs (medial aspect). (Schematic drawing) (W.).

1   Body of 5th lumbar vertebra
2   Promontory
3   Left ureter
4   Peritoneum (cut edge)
5   Right ureter (divided)
6   Rectouterine pouch
7   Rectum
8   Umbilicus
9   Sigmoid colon
10 Median umbilical fold with urachus
11 Ampulla of uterine tube
12 Fimbriae of uterine tube
13 Ovary
14 Uterine tube
15 Uterus
16 Uterovesical pouch
17 Urinary bladder
18 Vagina
19 Pubic symphysis
20 Urethra
21 Clitoris
22 Labium minus
23 Insertion of uterine tube at fundus of uterus
24 Round ligament of uterus
25 Ligament of the ovary
26 Suspensory ligament of ovary
27 Right common iliac artery (covered by peritoneum)

327

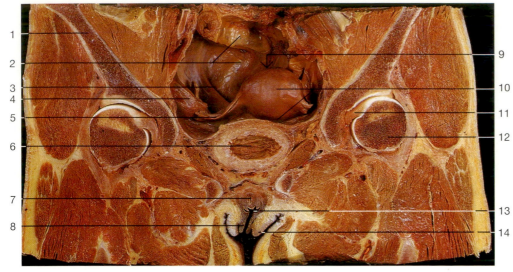

Coronal section through the pelvic cavity of the female (cf. MR-Scan on opposite page).

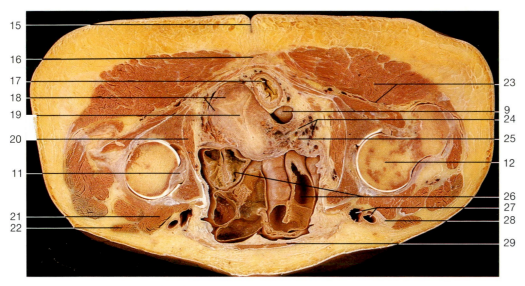

Horizontal section through pelvic cavity at level of uterus (from below). The uterus is retroverted to the left.

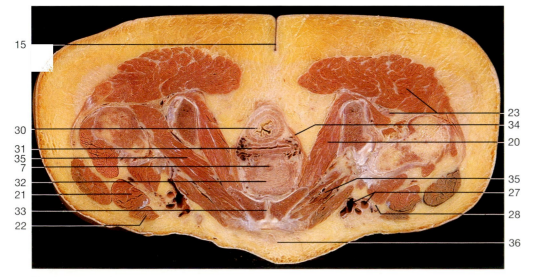

Horizontal section through the pelvic cavity at level of the urethral sphincter and vagina (from below).

1 Ilium
2 Rectum
3 Rectouterine fold
4 **Ovary**
5 **Uterine tube**
6 **Urinary bladder**
7 **Urethra**
8 Labium minus
9 Rectouterine pouch of Douglas
10 **Uterus,** uterovesical pouch
11 Ligament of the head of the femur
12 Head of femur
13 Vestibule of vagina
14 Labium majus
15 Anal cleft
16 Coccyx
17 Rectum
18 Myometrium of uterus
19 Uterine cavity
20 Obturator internus muscle
21 Iliopsoas muscle
22 Sartorius muscle
23 Sciatic nerve, gluteus maximus
24 Uterine venous plexus
25 Broad ligament
26 Small intestine
27 Femoral artery and vein
28 Femoral nerve
29 Pyramidalis muscle
30 Rectum, anal canal
31 Vagina
32 Urethral sphincter (urinary bladder)
33 Pubic symphysis
34 Levator ani
35 Obturator externus muscle
36 Mons pubis

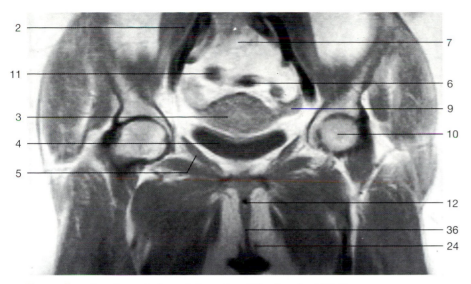

Coronal section through the pelvic cavity of the female. MR-Scan.

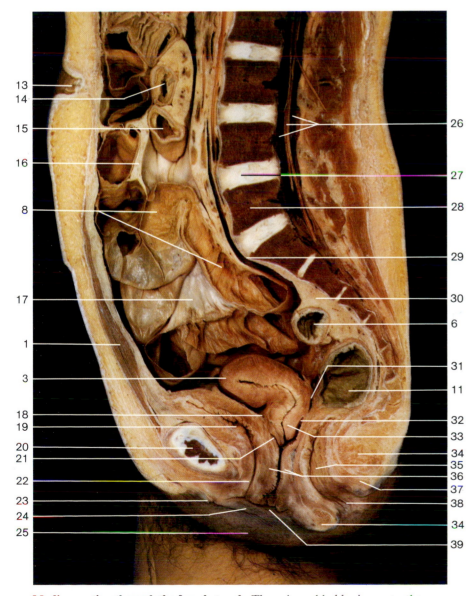

Median section through the female trunk. The urinary bladder is empty, the position and shape of the uterus are normal.

1   Rectus abdominis
2   Psoas major
3   **Uterus**
4   Urinary bladder
5   Obturator internus muscle
6   Sigmoid colon
7   Promontory
8   Small intestine
9   Uterine tube
10 Head of femur
11 Ampulla of rectum
12 Urethra
13 Umbilicus
14 Duodenum
15 Ascending part of duodenum
16 Root of mesentery
17 Mesentery
18 Uterovesical pouch
19 **Urinary bladder** (collapsed)
20 Pubic symphysis
21 Anterior fornix of vagina
22 Urethra
23 Clitoris
24 Labium minus
25 Labium majus
26 Vertebral canal with cauda equina
27 Intervertebral disc
28 Body of 5th lumbar vertebra
29 Promontory
30 Mesosigmoid
31 **Rectouterine pouch** of Douglas
32 Posterior fornix of vagina
33 Vaginal portion of the cervix of the uterus
34 Sphincter ani externus
35 Anal canal
36 **Vagina**
37 Sphincter ani internus
38 Anus
39 Hymen

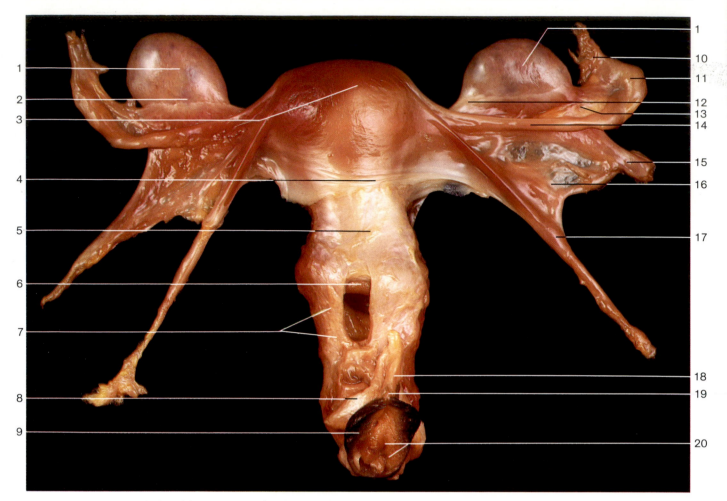

1
10
11
12
13
14
15
16
17
18
19
20

1
2
3
4
5
6
7
8
9

Female genital organs, isolated (ventral aspect). The anterior wall of the vagina has been opened to display the vaginal portion of the cervix.

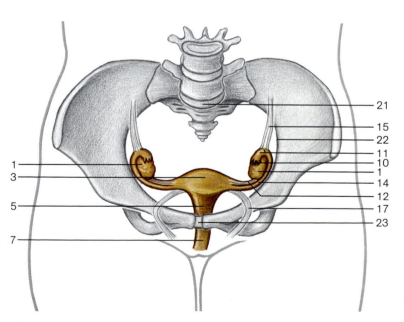

Female internal genital organs. (Schematic drawing) (W.).

1 Ovary
2 Mesovarium
3 Fundus of uterus
4 Uterovesical pouch
5 Cervix of uterus
6 Vaginal portion of cervix
7 Vagina
8 Crus of clitoris
9 Labium minus
10 Fimbriae of uterine tube
11 Ampulla of uterine tube
12 Ligament of the ovary
13 Mesosalpinx
14 Isthmus of uterine tube
15 Suspensory ligament of ovary
   (caudally displaced)
16 Broad ligament of uterus
17 Round ligament of uterus
18 Corpus cavernosum of clitoris
19 Glans of clitoris
20 Hymen, vaginal orifice
21 Promontory
22 Linea terminalis of pelvis
23 Pubic symphysis

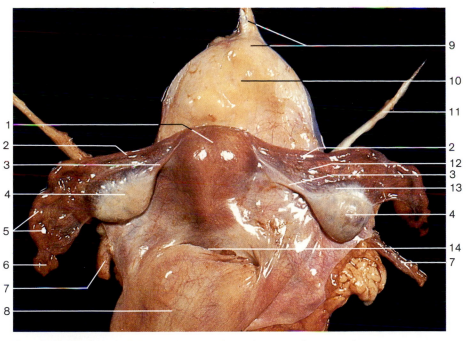

Female internal genital organs, isolated (superior-posterior aspect).

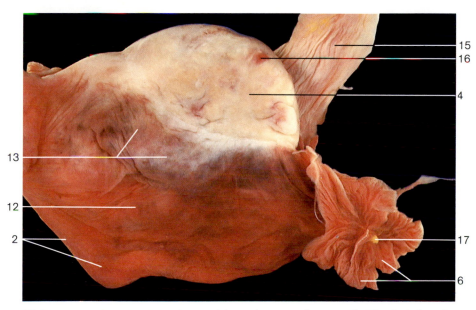

Right ovary and uterine tube, isolated (superior-posterior aspect). The fimbriae of the uterine tube have been reflected to show the abdominal ostium.

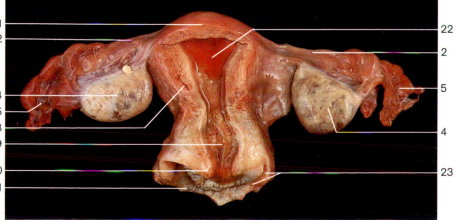

Uterus and related organs (dorsal aspect). The posterior wall of the uterus has been opened.

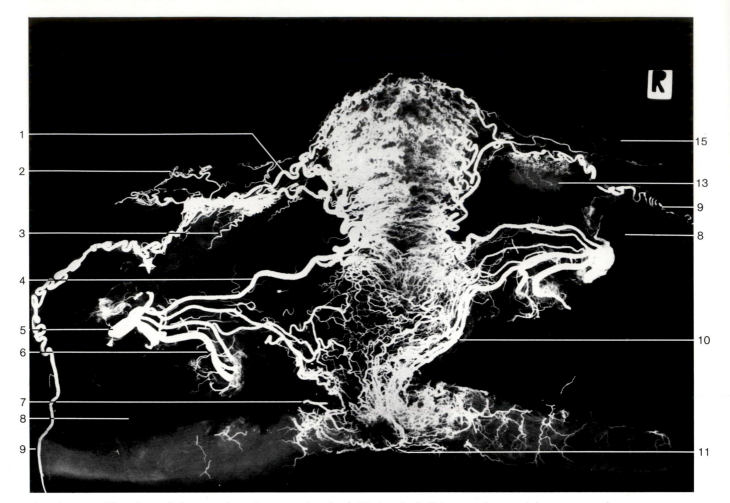

Arteriogram of female genital organs (anterior-posterior view). Notice the helicine arteries supplying uterus and ovary.

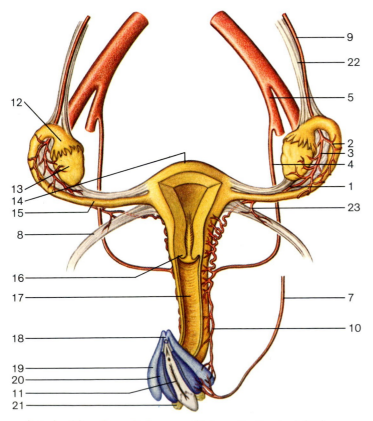

Arteris of female genital organs. (Schematic drawing) (W.).

1 Ovarian branch of uterine artery (anastomoses with ovarian artery)
2 Tubal branch of ovarian artery
3 Ovarian branch of ovarian artery
4 **Uterine artery**
5 Internal iliac artery
6 Inferior gluteal artery
7 **Internal pudendal artery**
8 Round ligament of uterus
9 **Ovarian artery**
10 Vaginal artery
11 Vaginal orifice
12 Ampulla of uterine tube
13 Ovary
14 Fundus of uterus
15 Isthmus of uterine tube
16 Vaginal portion of cervix of uterus
17 Vagina
18 Clitoris
19 Corpus cavernosum of clitoris
20 Bulb of vestibule
21 Greater vestibular gland
22 Suspensory ligament of ovary
23 Artery of round ligament

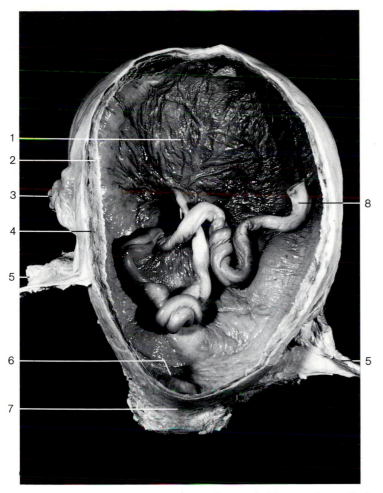

1 Placenta
2 Amnion and chorion
3 Adnexa of uterus (uterine tube and ovaries)
4 Myometrium
5 Round ligament of uterus
6 Internal os of uterus
7 Cervix of uterus
8 Umbilical cord
9 Lumbar lymph nodes
10 External iliac lymph nodes
11 Inguinal lymph nodes
12 Abdominal aorta
13 Suspensory ligament of ovary
14 External iliac artery
15 Sacral lymph nodes
16 Internal iliac artery
17 Ovary
18 Uterine tube
19 Internal iliac lymph nodes
20 External genital organs

Full term uterus with placenta (ventral aspect). The anterior wall of the uterus has been removed to show the location of the placenta.

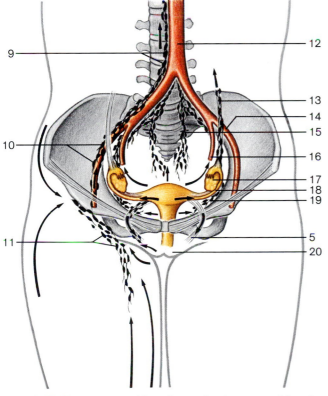

Main drainage routes of lymph vessels of uterus and its adnexa (indicated by arrows). (Schematic drawing) (W.).
Red = arteries; black = lymph vessels and nodes;
yellow = internal genital organs.

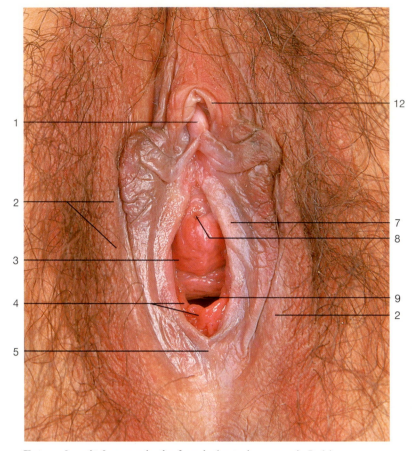

1. Glans clitoris
2. Labium majus
3. Vestibule of vagina
4. Hymen
5. Posterior labial commissure
6. Body of clitoris
7. Labium minus
8. External orifice of urethra
9. Vaginal orifice
10. Ureter
11. Adnexa of uterus
12. Prepuce of clitoris
13. Crus of clitoris
14. Greater vestibular glands
15. Anus and sphincter ani externus
16. Median umbilical ligament containing urachus
17. Urinary bladder
18. Ampulla of uterine tube
19. Ovary
20. Isthmus of uterine tube
21. Suspensory ligament of the ovary
22. Bulbocavernosus muscle and bulb of vestibule
23. Central tendon of perineum (perineal body)
24. Sphincter ani externus

External genital organs in the female (anterior aspect). Labia reflected.

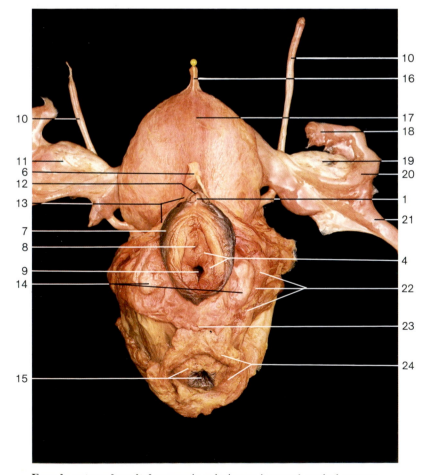

Female external genital organs in relation to internal genital organs and urinary system (isolated, anterior aspect).

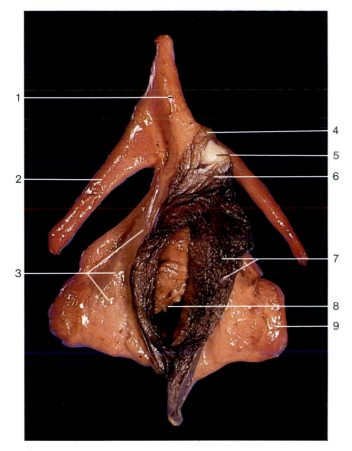

Cavernous tissue of female external genital organs, isolated (anterior aspect).

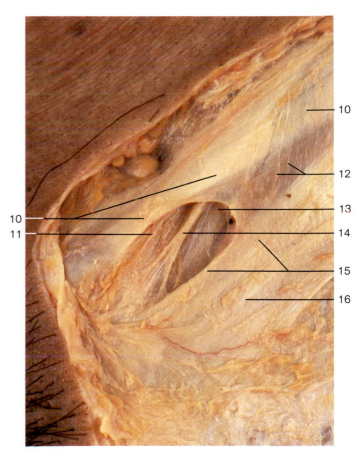

Inguinal canal and round ligament of uterus in situ (left side, ventral aspect).

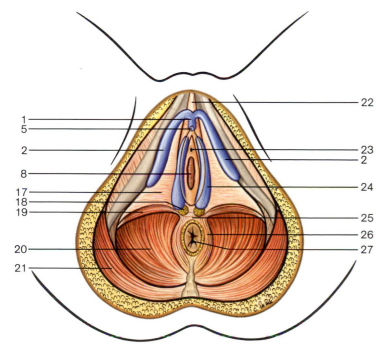

Urogenital and pelvic diaphragms (inferior aspect). (Schematic drawing) (W.).
Blue = cavernous tissue of clitoris and bulb of vestibule.

1 Body of clitoris
2 Crus of clitoris
3 Bulb of vestibule
4 Prepuce of clitoris
5 Glans of clitoris
6 Frenulum
7 Labium minus
8 Vaginal orifice
9 Greater vestibular gland
10 Medial crus of superficial inguinal ring
11 Ilioinguinal nerve
12 Intercrural fibers
13 Superficial inguinal ring
14 Round ligament of uterus
15 Lateral crus of superficial inguinal ring
16 Inguinal ligament
17 Deep transverse perineal muscle with fascia
18 Greater vestibular gland
19 Superficial transverse perineal muscle
20 Levator ani
21 Gluteus maximus
22 Suspensory ligament of clitoris
23 External orifice of urethra
24 Bulb of vestibule
25 Perineal body
26 Sphincter ani externus
27 Anus

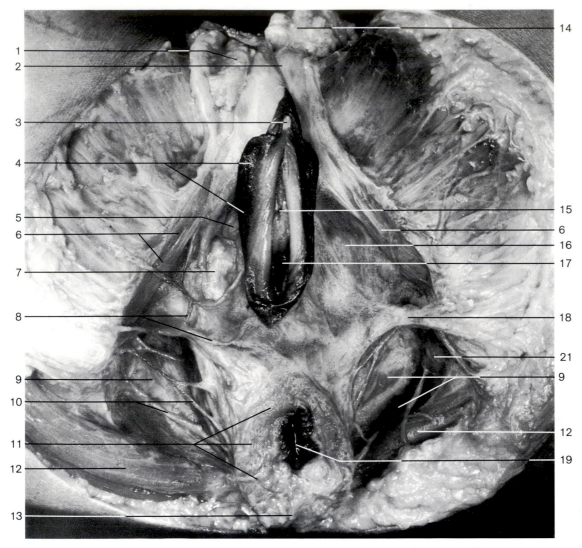

Female urogenital diaphragm and external genital organs, superficial layer (from below).

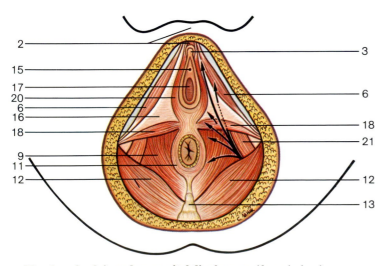

Muscles of pelvic and urogenital diaphragms (from below). (Schematic drawing) (W.).

1 Fatty tissue encasing round ligament
2 Position of pubic symphysis
3 Clitoris
4 Labium minus
5 Bulb of vestibule
6 Ischiocavernosus muscle
7 Greater vestibular gland
8 Perineal branches of pudendal nerve
9 Levator ani
10 Inferior rectal nerves
11 Sphincter ani externus
12 Gluteus maximus
13 Coccyx
14 Fatty tissue of mons pubis
15 External orifice of urethra
16 Urogenital diaphragm with fascia of deep transverse perineal muscle
17 Vaginal orifice
18 Superficial transverse perineal muscle
19 Anus
20 Bulbospongiosus muscle
21 Obturator internus

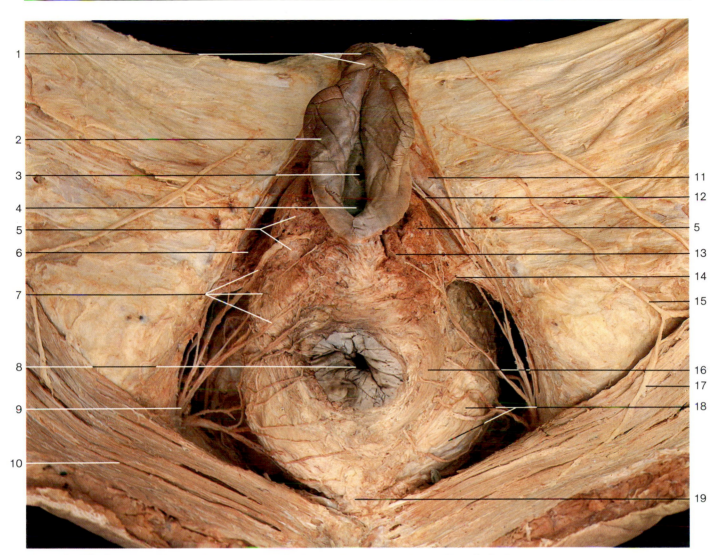

Urogenital diaphragm and external genital organs in the female, superficial layer (from below).

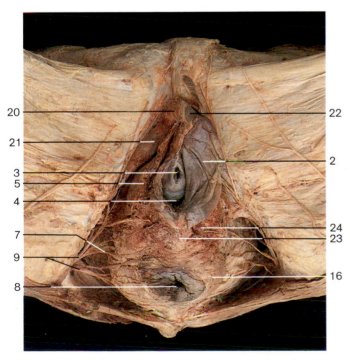

External genital organs, dissection of bulb of vestibule and body of clitoris (from below). The right labium minus has been removed.

1　Clitoris and prepuce of clitoris
2　Labium minus
3　External urethral orifice
4　Vaginal orifice
5　Bulb of vestibule
6　Urogenital diaphragm (deep transverse perineal muscle)
7　Perineal branches of pudendal nerve
8　Anus
9　Pudendal nerve and internal pudendal arteries and veins
10　Gluteus maximus
11　Crus of clitoris with ischiocavernosus muscle
12　Dorsal nerve and artery of clitoris and posterior labial nerves
13　Greater vestibular gland
14　Superficial transverse perineal muscle
15　Perineal branch of posterior femoral cutaneous nerve
16　Sphincter ani externus
17　Inferior clunial nerve
18　Levator ani
19　Anococcygeal ligament
20　Body of clitoris
21　Crus of clitoris
22　Glans of clitoris
23　Perineal body
24　Bulbospongiosus muscle

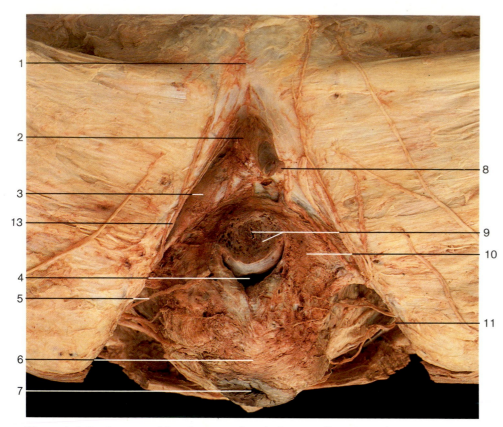

1   Position of pubic symphysis
2   Body of clitoris
3   Crus of clitoris
4   External orifice of vagina
5   Perineal branches of pudendal nerve
6   Perineum
7   Anus
8   Glans of clitoris
9   Urethra
10 Deep transverse perineal muscle
11 Pudendal nerve and artery
12 Dorsal vein of clitoris
13 Posterior labial nerves
14 Gluteus maximus
15 Anococcygeal ligament
16 Deep dorsal vein of clitoris
17 Dorsal nerve and artery of clitoris
18 Superficial transverse perineal muscle
19 Perineal and inferior rectal branches of pudendal nerve
20 Inferior clunial nerve
21 Sacrotuberous ligament
22 Coccyx

Urogenital diaphragm and female external genital organs (from below). Both labia and the left crus of clitoris have been removed.

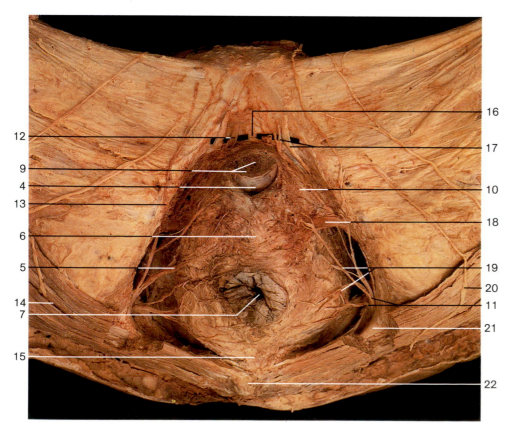

Urogenital diaphragm (from below). Both labia, the clitoris and the bulb of the vestibule have been removed.

Chapter VIII
Upper Limb

The Shoulder Girdle and Thorax

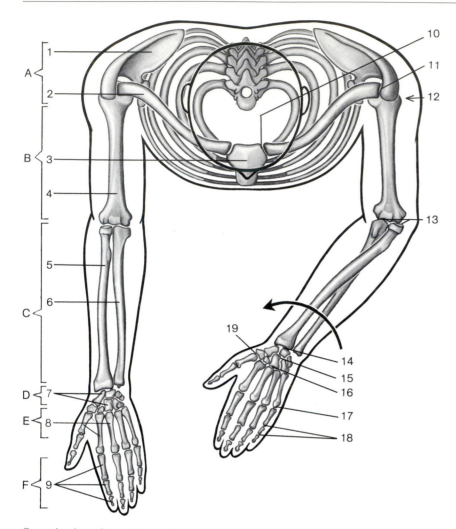

A   Pectoral girdle
B   Arm
C   Forearm
D   Wrist
E   Palm of hand
F   Finger

Bones
1   Scapula
2   Clavicle
3   Sternum
4   Humerus
5   Radius
6   Ulna
7   Carpal bones
8   Metacarpal bones
9   Phalanges

Joints
10   Sternoclavicular joint
11   Acromioclavicular joint
12   Shoulder joint
13   Elbow joint
14   Radiocarpal joint
15   Midcarpal joint
16   Carpometacarpal joint
17   Metacarpophalangeal joint
18   Interphalangeal joints of fingers
19   Carpometacarpal joint of thumb

Organization of shoulder girdle and upper limb (superior aspect). The two positions of the forearm essential to manual skills in the human, supination (right arm) and pronation (left arm) are shown.

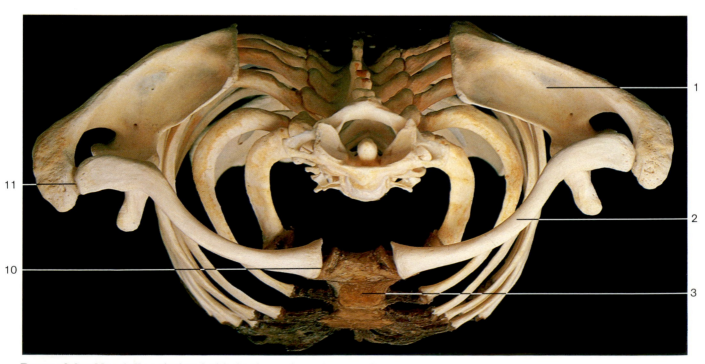

Bones of shoulder girdle articulated with the thorax (superior aspect).

340

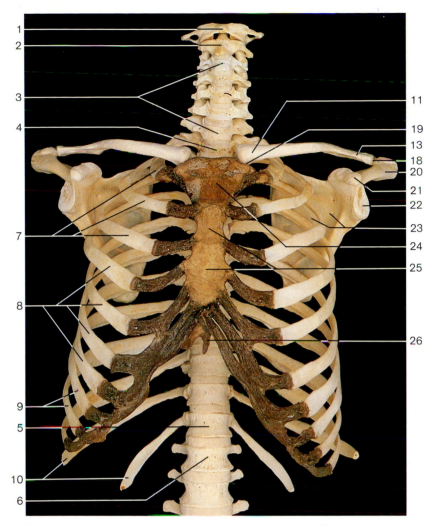

Skeleton of shoulder girdle and thorax (anterior aspect). The cartilaginous parts of the ribs appear dark brown.

Vertebral column
1 Atlas
2 Axis
3 3rd-7th cervical vertebrae
4 1st thoracic vertebra
5 12th thoracic vertebra
6 1st lumbar vertebra

Ribs
7 1st–3rd ribs ⎫
8 4th–7th ribs ⎬ True ribs
9 8th–10th ribs ⎫
10 11th and 12th ribs ⎬ False ribs
(floating ribs) ⎭

Clavicle
11 Sternal end
12 Articular facet for sternum
13 Acromial end
14 Articular facet for acromion
15 Impression for costoclavicular ligament
16 Conoid tubercle
17 Trapezoid line
18 Site of acromioclavicular joint
19 Site of sternoclavicular joint

Scapula
20 Acromion
21 Coracoid process
22 Glenoid cavity
23 Costal surface

Sternum
24 Manubrium
25 Body
26 Xiphoid process

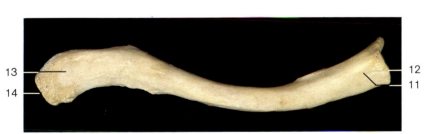

Right clavicle (superior aspect).

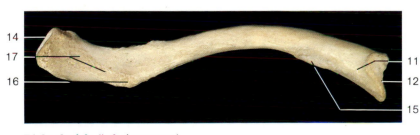

Right clavicle (inferior aspect).

Because of his upright posture, man's upper limb has developed a high degree of mobility. The shoulder girdle is to a great extent movable in the thorax and is connected with the trunk only by the sternoclavicular joint. A further characteristic of man's forearm is the capacity for rotation (i. e. pronation and supination).

341

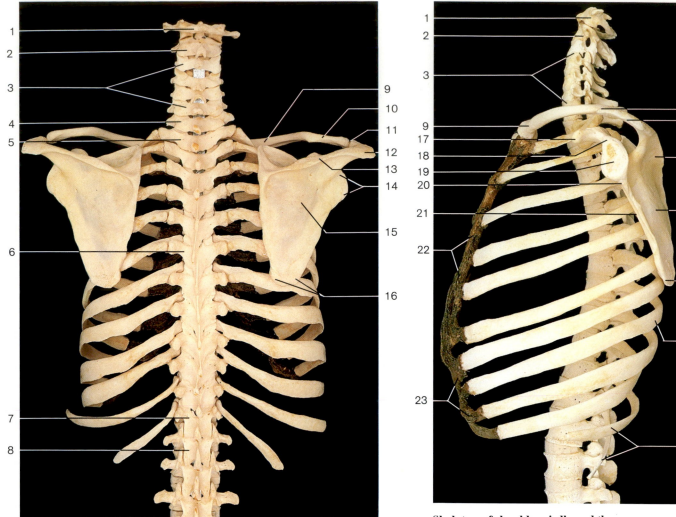

Skeleton of shoulder girdle and thorax (posterior aspect).

Skeleton of shoulder girdle and thorax (lateral aspect).

Vertebral column
1 Atlas
2 Axis
3 3rd–6th cervical vertebrae
4 7th vertebra (vertebra prominens)
5 1st thoracic vertebra
6 6th thoracic vertebra
7 12th thoracic vertebra
8 1st lumbar vertebra

Clavicle
9 Sternal end
10 Acromial end
11 Site of acromioclavicular joint

Scapula
12 Acromion
13 Spine of scapula
14 Lateral angle
15 Dorsal surface
16 Inferior angle
17 Coracoid process
18 Supraglenoid tubercle
19 Glenoid cavity
20 Infraglenoid tubercle
21 Lateral margin

Thorax
22 Body of sternum
23 Costal arch
24 Angle of ribs
25 Free ribs

342

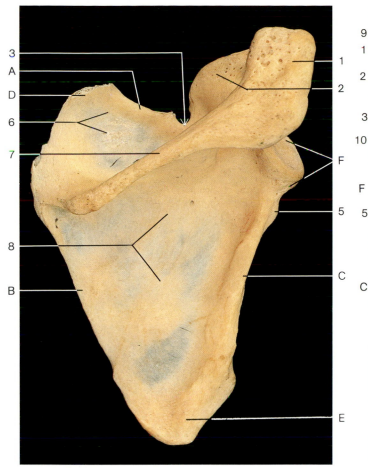

Right scapula (dorsal aspect).

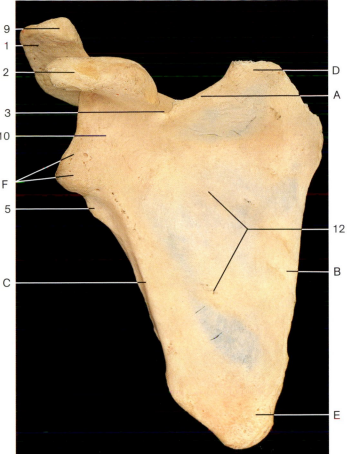

Right scapula (ventral aspect, costal surface).

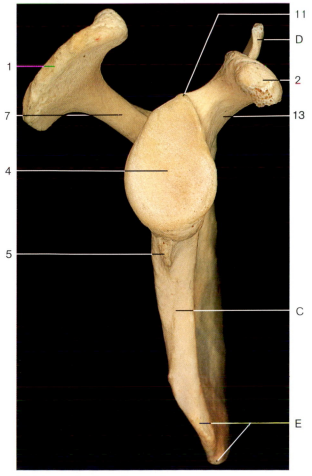

Right scapula (lateral aspect).

Scapula

A Superior border
B Medial border
C Lateral border
D Superior angle
E Inferior angle
F Lateral angle

1 Acromion
2 Coracoid process
3 Scapular notch
4 Glenoid cavity
5 Infraglenoid tubercle
6 Supraspinous fossa
7 Spine
8 Infraspinous fossa
9 Articular facet for acromion
10 Neck
11 Supraglenoid tubercle
12 Costal surface
13 Base of coracoid process

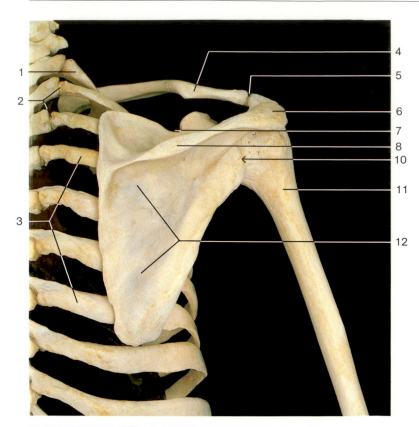

1 1st rib
2 Position of costotransverse joints
3 4th–7th ribs
4 Clavicle
5 Position of acromioclavicular joint
6 Acromion
7 Scapular notch
8 Spine of scapula
9 Head of humerus
10 Glenoid cavity
11 Surgical neck of humerus
12 Dorsal surface of scapula
13 Coracoid process
14 Infraglenoid tubercle
15 Greater tubercle of humerus
16 Anatomical neck of humerus

Bones of shoulder joint (dorsal aspect).

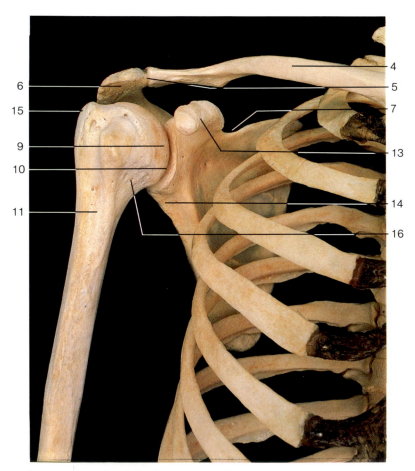

Bones of shoulder joint (ventral aspect).

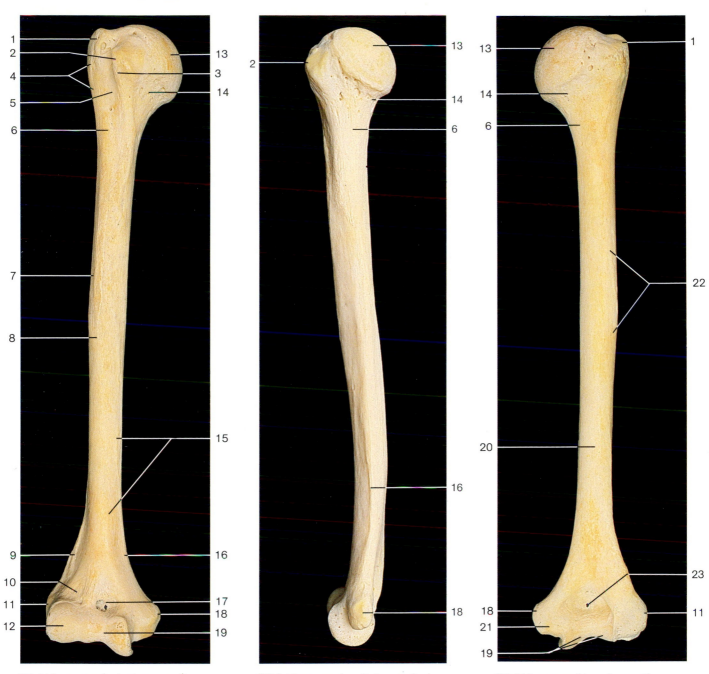

Right humerus (anterior aspect).   **Right humerus** (medial aspect).   **Right humerus** (dorsal aspect).

Humerus

1 Greater tubercle	7 Deltoid tuberosity	13 Head	19 Trochlea
2 Lesser tubercle	8 Anterolateral surface	14 Anatomical neck	20 Posterior surface
3 Crest of lesser tubercle	9 Lateral border	15 Anteromedial surface	21 Groove for ulnar nerve
4 Crest of greater tubercle	10 Radial fossa	16 Medial border	22 Groove for radial nerve
5 Intertubercular sulcus	11 Lateral epicondyle	17 Coronoid fossa	23 Olecranon fossa
6 Surgical neck	12 Capitulum	18 Medial epicondyle	

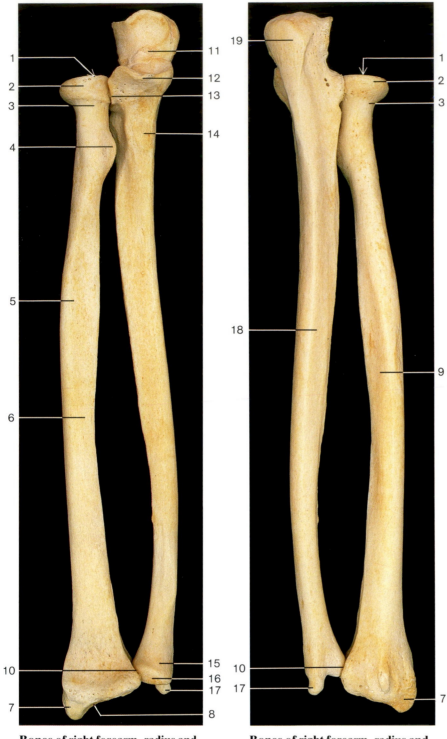

Radius

1 Head
2 Articular circumference
3 Neck
4 Radial tuberosity
5 Shaft
6 Anterior surface
7 Styloid process
8 Articular surface
9 Posterior surface
10 Ulnar notch

Ulna

11 Trochlear notch
12 Coronoid process
13 Radial notch
14 Ulnar tuberosity
15 Head
16 Articular circumference
17 Styloid process
18 Posterior surface
19 Olecranon

Bones of right forearm, radius and ulna (anterior aspect).

Bones of right forearm, radius and ulna (posterior aspect).

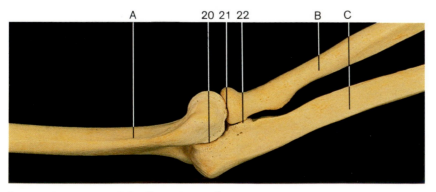

Bones of right elbow joint (lateral aspect).

Articulations at the right elbow

20 Site of humeroulnar joint
21 Site of humeroradial joint
22 Site of proximal radioulnar joint

A Humerus
B Radius
C Ulna

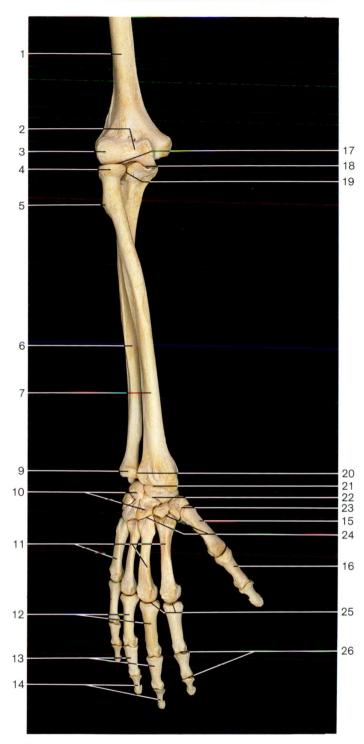

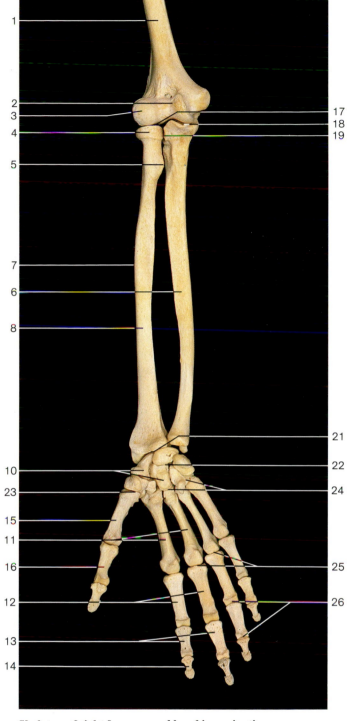

Skeleton of right forearm and hand in pronation.

Skeleton of right forearm and hand in supination.

1	Humerus	11	Metacarpal bones
2	Trochlea of humerus	12	Proximal phalanges
3	Capitulum of humerus	13	Middle phalanges
4	Articular circumference of radius	14	Distal phalanges
5	Radial tuberosity	15	Metacarpal bone of thumb
6	Anterior surface of ulna	16	Proximal phalanx of thumb
7	Posterior surface of radius		
8	Anterior surface of radius		
9	Articular circumference of ulna		
10	Carpal bones		

Sites of joints

17 Humeroradial joint
18 Humeroulnar joint
19 Proximal radioulnar joint
20 Distal radioulnar joint
21 Radiocarpal joint
22 Midcarpal joint
23 Carpometacarpal joint of thumb
24 Carpometacarpal joints
25 Metacarpophalangeal joints
26 Interphalangeal joints of fingers

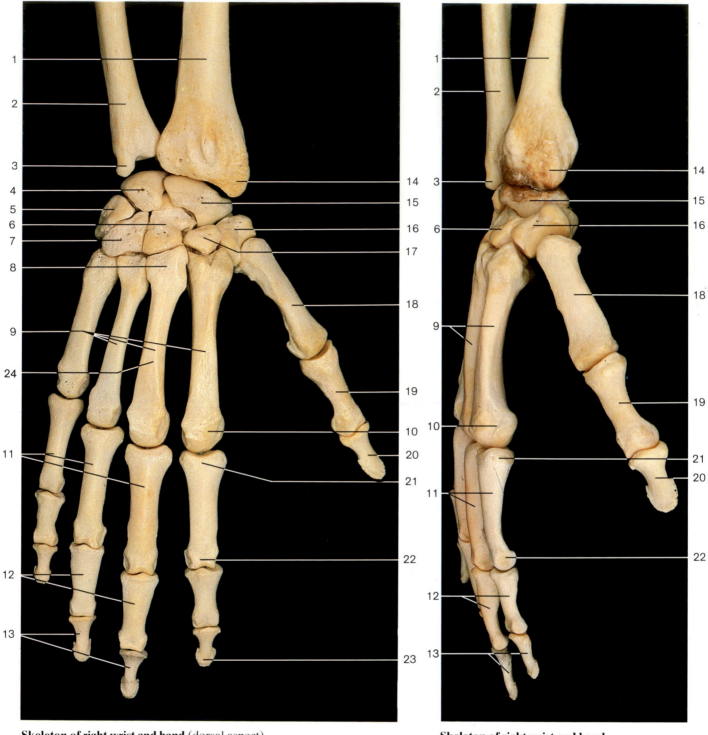

Skeleton of right wrist and hand (dorsal aspect).

Skeleton of right wrist and hand (medial aspect).

1	**Radius**	8	Base of third metacarpal bone	15	Scaphoid bone
2	Ulna	9	Metacarpal bones	16	The trapezium
3	Styloid process of ulna	10	Head of metacarpal bone	17	Trapezoid bone
4	Lunate bone	11	Proximal phalanges of hand	18	Metacarpal bone of thumb
5	Triquetral bone	12	Middle phalanges of hand	19	Proximal phalanx of thumb
6	Capitate bone	13	Distal phalanges of hand	20	Distal phalanx of thumb
7	Hamate bone	14	Styloid process of radius	21	Base of second proximal phalanx

4,5,6,7 } Carpal bones
15,16,17 } Carpal bones

22 Head of second proximal phalanx
23 Tuberosity of distal phalanx
24 Body of third metacarpal bone

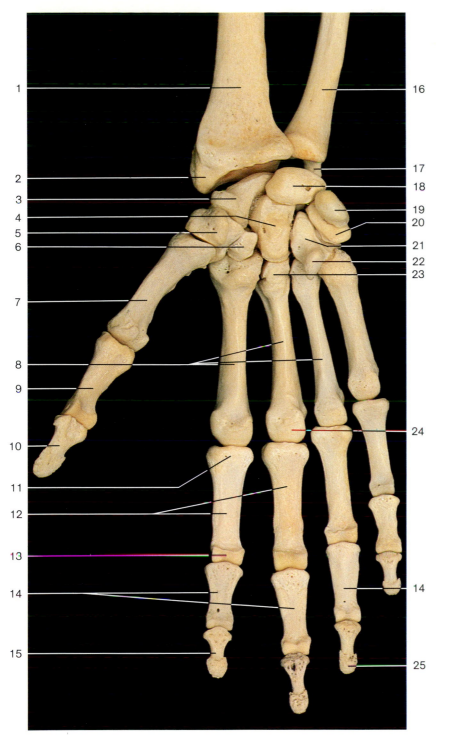

1 Radius
2 Styloid process of radius
3 Scaphoid bone ⎫
4 Capitate bone ⎪
5 Trapezium ⎬ Carpal bones
6 Trapezoid bone ⎭
7 First metacarpal bone
8 Second to fourth metacarpal bones
9 Proximal phalanx of thumb
10 Distal phalanx of thumb
11 Base of second phalanx
12 Proximal phalanges
13 Head of second phalanx
14 Middle phalanges
15 Distal phalanx
16 Ulna
17 Styloid process of ulna
18 Lunate bone ⎫
19 Pisiform bone ⎪
20 Triquetral bone ⎪
21 Hamate bone ⎬ Carpal bones
22 Hamulus or hook ⎪
    of hamate bone ⎭
23 Base of third metacarpal bone
24 Head of metacarpal bone
25 Tuberosity of distal phalanx

Skeleton of right wrist and hand (palmar aspect).

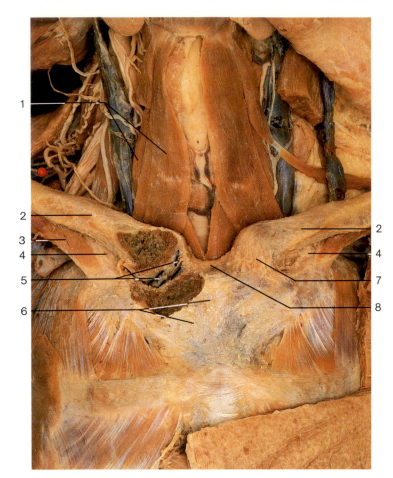

1 Infrahyoid muscles
2 Sternal end of clavicle
3 Subclavius
4 Costoclavicular ligament
5 **Sternoclavicular joint** with articular disc
6 Manubrium of sternum
7 Anterior sternoclavicular ligament
8 Interclavicular ligament
9 Acromial end of clavicle
10 **Acromioclavicular joint**
11 Acromion
12 Tendon of supraspinatus
   (attached to the articular capsule)
13 Coracoacromial ligament
14 Tendon of long head of biceps brachii
15 Tendon of subscapularis
   (attached to the articular capsule)
16 Intertubercular sulcus
17 Articular capsule of shoulder joint
18 Humerus
19 Trapezoid ligament
20 Coracoid process
21 Glenoid labrum
22 **Shoulder joint,** joint cavity
23 Scapula
24 Supraspinatus
25 Cartilage of glenoid cavity
26 Tendon of long head of triceps brachii
27 Head of humerus (articular cartilage)
28 Epiphyseal line

Right sternoclavicular joint (anterior aspect). On the right side the joint has been opened by a coronal section.

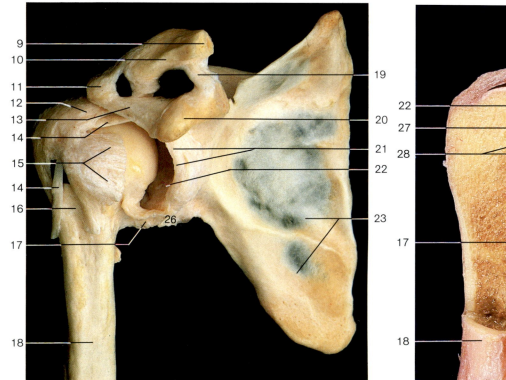

Right shoulder joint. The anterior part of the articular capsule has been removed and the head of the humerus has been slightly rotated outward to show the cavity of the joint.

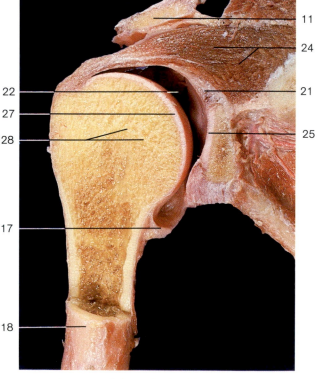

Coronal section of the right shoulder joint (anterior aspect).

1   Humerus
2   Lateral epicondyle of humerus
3   Articular capsule
4   Annular ligament of proximal radioulnar joint
5   Radius
6   Tendon of biceps brachii
7   Medial epicondyle of humerus
8   Ulnar collateral ligament
9   Oblique cord
10 Ulna
11 Interosseous membrane
12 Radial fossa
13 Capitulum of humerus
14 Head of radius
15 Radial collateral ligament
16 Coronoid fossa
17 Trochlea of humerus
18 Coronoid process of ulna
19 Olecranon
20 Radial tuberosity

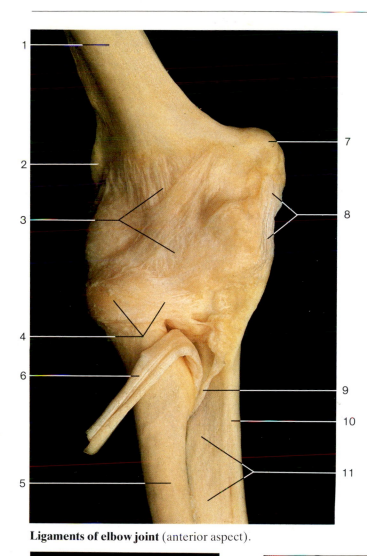

Ligaments of elbow joint (anterior aspect).

Elbow joint with ligaments
(anterior aspect). Articular capsule
has been removed to show the
annular ligament.

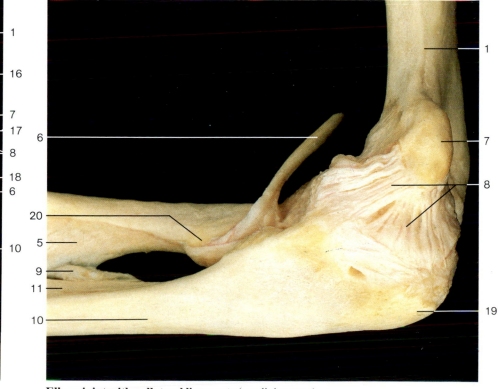

Elbow joint with collateral ligaments (medial aspect).

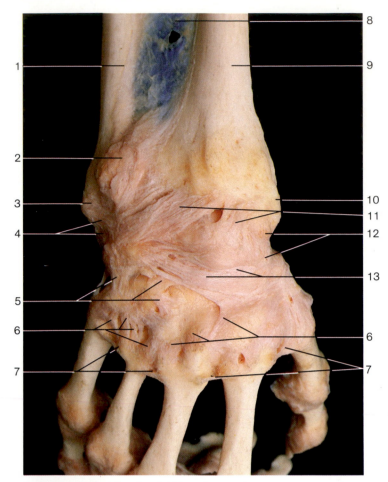

1   Ulna
2   Exostosis (pathological)
3   Head of ulna
4   Ulnar carpal collateral ligament
5   Deep intercarpal ligaments
6   Dorsal carpometacarpal ligaments
7   Dorsal metacarpal ligaments
8   Interosseous membrane
9   Radius
10 Styloid process of radius
11 Dorsal radiocarpal ligament
12 Radial collateral ligament
13 Articular capsule, dorsal intercarpal ligaments
14 Palmar radiocarpal ligament
15 Tendon of flexor carpi radialis (divided)
16 Radiating carpal ligament
17 Palmar carpometacarpal ligaments
18 1st metacarpal bone
19 Palmar ulnocarpal ligament
20 Tendon of flexor carpi ulnaris (divided)
21 Pisohamate ligament
22 Pisometacarpal ligament
23 Palmar metacarpal ligaments
24 5th metacarpal bone

Ligaments of hand and wrist (dorsal aspect).

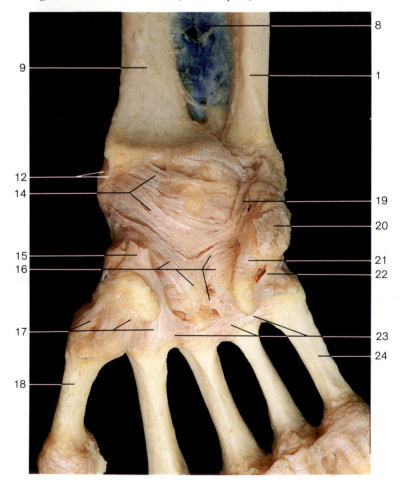

Ligaments of hand and wrist (palmar aspect).

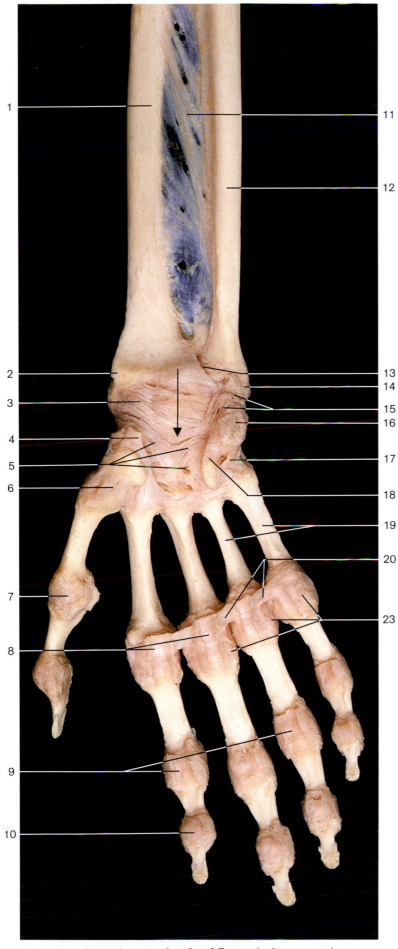

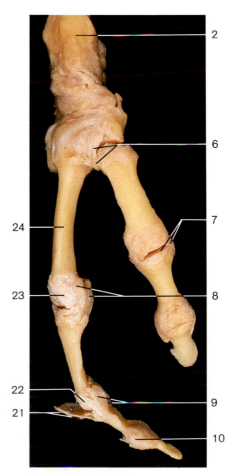

1 Radius
2 Styloid process of radius
3 Palmar radiocarpal ligament
4 Tendon of flexor carpi radialis (cut)
5 Radiating carpal ligament
6 Articular capsule of **carpometacarpal joint of thumb**
7 Articular capsule of **metacarpophalangeal joint of thumb**
8 Palmar ligaments and articular capsule of metacarpophalangeal joints
9 Palmar ligaments and articular capsule of interphalangeal joints
10 Articular capsule
11 Interosseous membrane
12 Ulna
13 **Distal radioulnar joint**
14 Styloid process of ulna
15 Palmar ulnocarpal ligament
16 Pisiform bone with tendon of flexor carpi ulnaris
17 Pisometacarpal ligament
18 Pisohamate ligament
19 Metacarpal bone
20 Deep transverse metacarpal ligament
21 Tendons of extensor muscles and articular capsule
22 Collateral ligament of **interphalangeal joint**
23 Collateral ligaments of **metacarpophalangeal joints**
24 Second metacarpal bone

Ligaments of right forearm, hand and fingers (palmar aspect).
The arrow indicates the location of the carpal tunnel.

Ligaments of fingers
(lateral aspect).

353

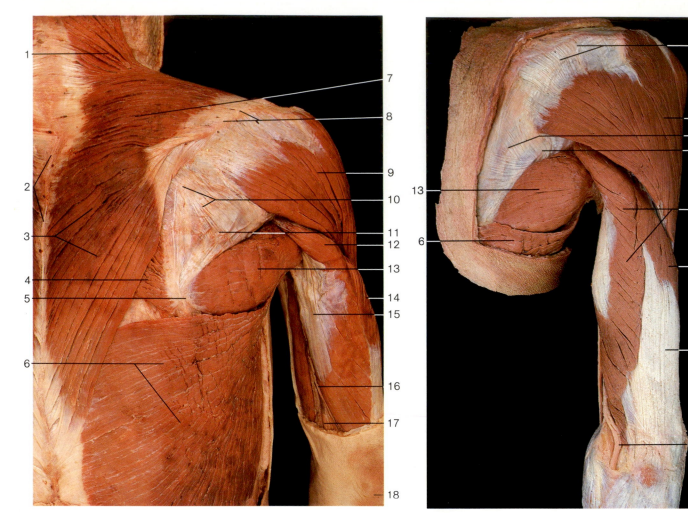

Muscles of shoulder and arm, superficial layer (dorsal aspect).

Dorsal muscles of the right arm, superficial layer (dorsal aspect).

1   Descending fibers of trapezius
2   Spinous processes of thoracic vertebrae
3   Ascending fibers of trapezius
4   Rhomboideus major
5   Inferior angle of scapula
6   Latissimus dorsi
7   Transverse fibers of trapezius
8   Spine of scapula
9   Posterior fibers of deltoid muscle
10 Infraspinatus and infraspinous fascia
11 Teres minor and fascia
12 Long head of triceps brachii
13 Teres major
14 Lateral head of triceps brachii
15 Tendon of triceps brachii
16 Medial intermuscular septum
17 Ulnar nerve
18 Olecranon
19 Acromion

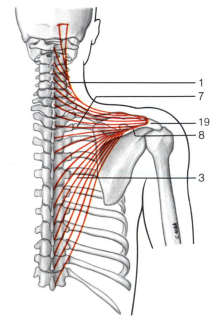

Origin and insertion of trapezius. (Schematic drawing) (W.).

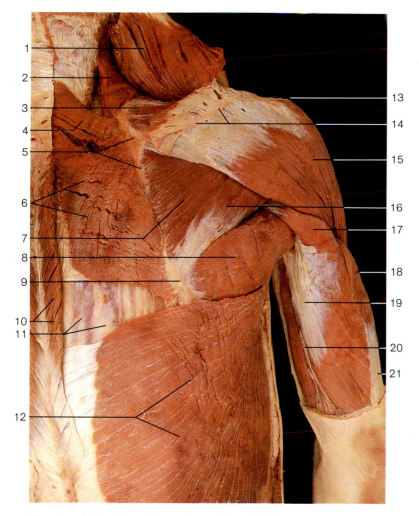

1 Trapezius (reflected)
2 Levator scapulae
3 Supraspinatus
4 Rhomboideus minor
5 Medial border of scapula
6 Rhomboideus major
7 Infraspinatus
8 Teres major
9 Inferior angle of scapula
10 Cut edge of trapezius
11 Intrinsic muscles of back with fascia
12 Latissimus dorsi
13 Acromion
14 Spine of scapula
15 Deltoid muscle
16 Teres minor
17 Long head of triceps brachii
18 Lateral head of triceps brachii
19 Medial head of triceps brachii
20 Medial intermuscular septum
21 Tendon of triceps brachii

Muscles of shoulder and arm, deeper layer (right side, dorsal aspect). The trapezius has been cut near its origin at the vertebral column and reflected upward.

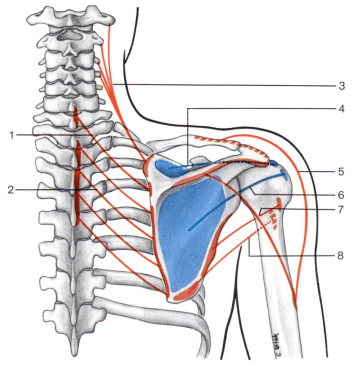

Shoulder muscles, schematic diagram illustrating the course of the main muscles of the dorsal side (W.).

1 Rhomboideus minor (red)
2 Rhomboideus major (red)
3 Levator scapulae (red)
4 Supraspinatus (blue)
5 Deltoid muscle (red)
6 Infraspinatus (blue)
7 Teres minor (red)
8 Teres major (red)

Pectoral Muscles

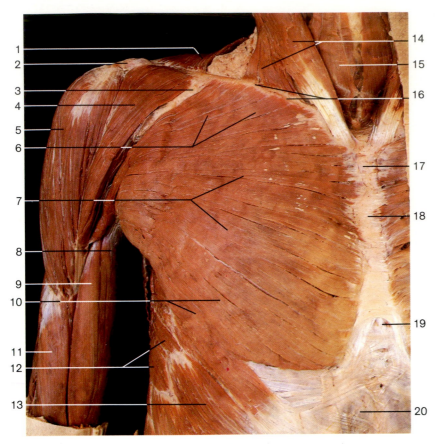

1 Trapezius
2 Acromion
3 Deltopectoral triangle
4 Clavicular part of deltoid muscle
5 Acromial part of deltoid muscle
6 Clavicular part of pectoralis major
7 Sternocostal part of pectoralis major
8 Short head of biceps brachii
9 Long head of biceps brachii
10 Abdominal part of pectoralis major
11 Brachialis
12 Serratus anterior
13 External oblique muscle
14 Sternocleidomastoid muscle
15 Infrahyoid muscles
16 Clavicle
17 Manubrium sterni
18 Body of sternum
19 Xiphoid process
20 Anterior layer of sheath of rectus
   abdominis

Muscles of shoulder and arm, superficial layer (ventral aspect).

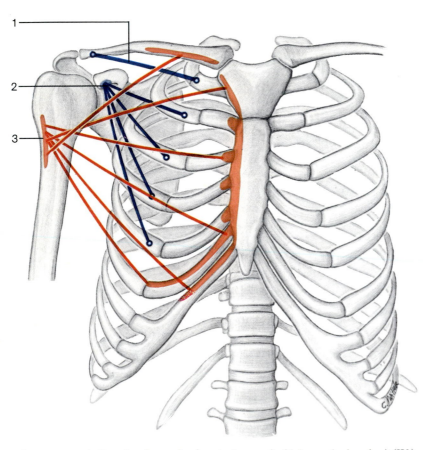

Arrangement of pectoral muscles (ventral aspect). (Schematic drawing) (W.).

1 Subclavius (blue)
2 Pectoralis minor (blue)
3 Pectoralis major (red)

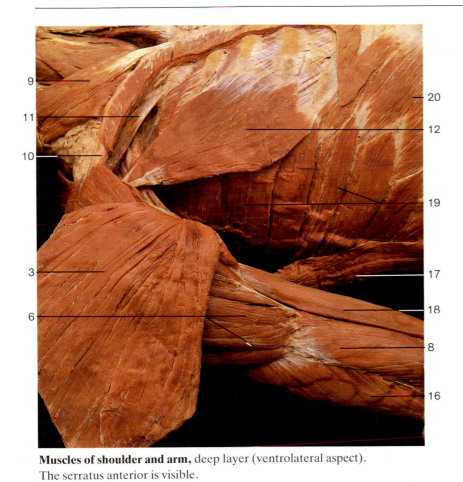

Muscles of shoulder and arm, deep layer (ventrolateral aspect).
The serratus anterior is visible.

Muscles of shoulder and arm, deep layer (ventral aspect).

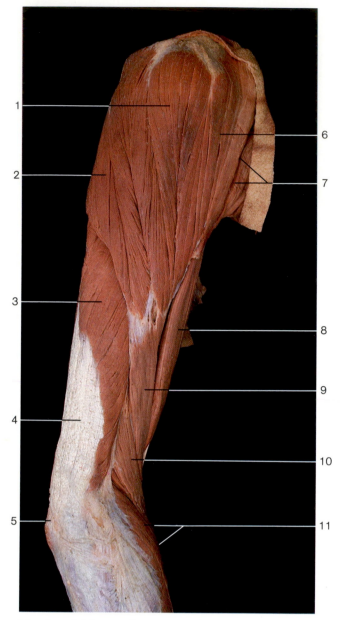

Muscles of right arm (lateral aspect).

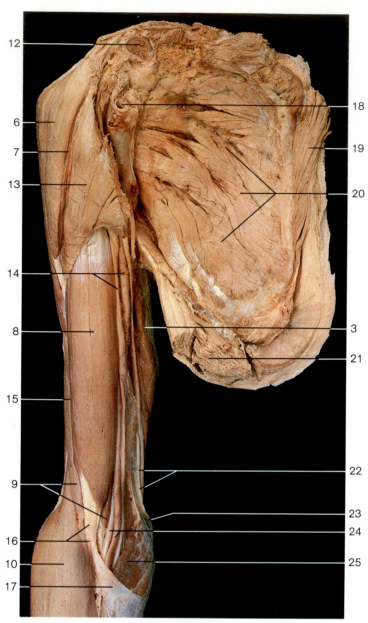

Muscles of right arm (ventral aspect). The arm with the scapula and attached muscles has been removed from the trunk.

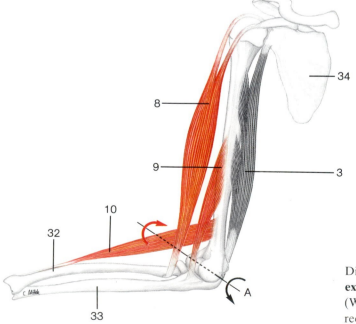

Diagram illustrating the position of the **flexor and extensor muscles of the arm** and their effect on the elbow joint (W.). A = axis; arrows = direction of movements; red = flexion; black = extension.

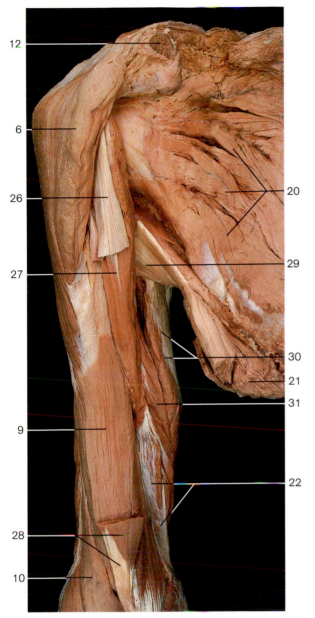

Flexor muscles of right arm (ventral aspect).
Part of the biceps brachii has been removed.

Position and course of flexors of arm. (Schematic drawing) (W.).

1 Subscapularis (red)	3 Biceps brachii (red)
2 Coracobrachialis (blue)	4 Brachialis (blue)

1	Central fibers of deltoid muscle	18	Axillary artery
2	Posterior fibers of deltoid muscle	19	Rhomboideus major
3	Triceps brachii	20	Subscapularis
4	Tendon of triceps brachii	21	Latissimus dorsi (divided)
5	Olecranon	22	Medial intermuscular septum
6	Anterior fibers of deltoid muscle	23	Medial epicondyle of humerus
7	Deltopectoral groove	24	Brachial artery and median nerve
8	Biceps brachii	25	Pronator teres
9	Brachialis	26	Tendon of long head of biceps brachii
10	Brachioradialis	27	Coracobrachialis
11	Extensor carpi radialis longus	28	Distal part of biceps brachii
12	Clavicle (divided)	29	Teres major
13	Pectoralis major	30	Long head of triceps brachii
14	Medial bicipital groove with vessels and nerves	31	Medial head of triceps brachii
15	Lateral bicipital groove	32	Radius
16	Tendon of biceps brachii	33	Ulna
17	Bicipital aponeurosis	34	Scapula

Forearm Muscles

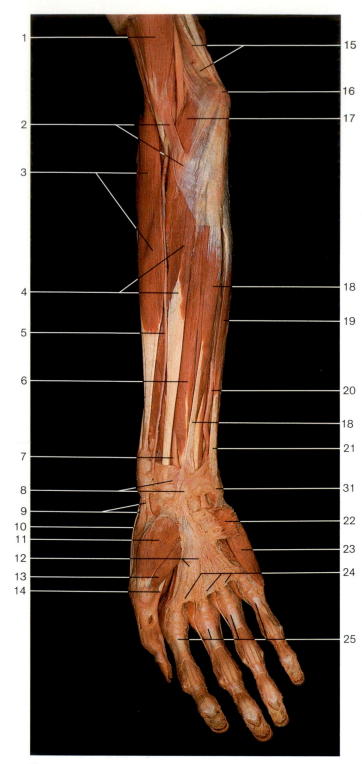

Forearm muscles, superficial layer (ventral aspect).

Forearm muscles, superficial layer (ventral aspect). The palmaris longus and flexor carpi ulnaris have been removed.

1 Biceps brachii
2 Bicipital aponeurosis
3 Brachioradialis
4 Flexor carpi radialis
5 Radial artery
6 Flexor digitorum superficialis
7 Median nerve
8 Flexor retinaculum
9 Tendon of abductor pollicis longus
10 Tendon of extensor pollicis brevis
11 Abductor pollicis brevis

12 Palmar aponeurosis
13 Superficial head of flexor pollicis brevis
14 Tendon of flexor pollicis longus
15 Medial intermuscular septum
16 Medial epicondyle of humerus
17 Humeral head of pronator teres
18 Palmaris longus
19 Flexor carpi ulnaris
20 Ulnar artery
21 Tendon of flexor carpi ulnaris
22 Palmaris brevis

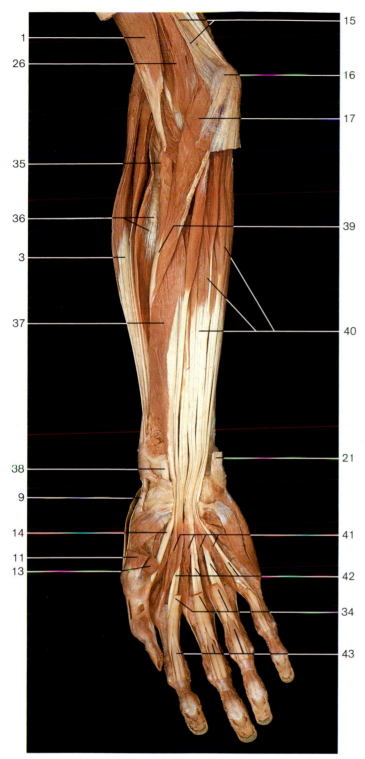

Forearm muscles, middle layer (ventral aspect). The palmaris longus, flexor carpi radialis and ulnaris have been partly removed. The flexor retinaculum has been divided.

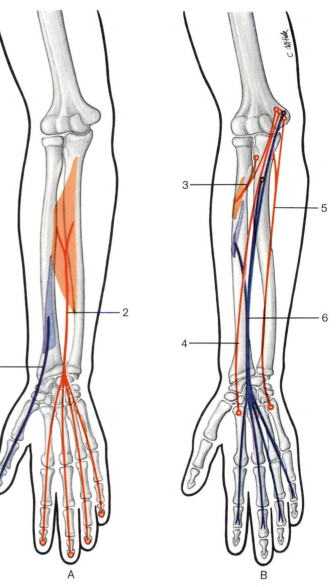

Position of flexors of fingers and hand. (Schematic drawing) (W.).

A Deep layer
B Superficial layer

△
1 Flexor pollicis longus (blue)
2 Flexor digitorum profundus (red)
3 Pronator teres (red)
4 Flexor carpi radialis (red)
5 Flexor carpi ulnaris (red)
6 Flexor digitorum superficialis (blue)

23 Abductor digiti minimi
24 Transverse fasciculi of palmar aponeurosis
25 Digital fibrous sheaths of tendons of flexor digitorum
26 Brachialis
27 Flexor pollicis longus
28 Carpal tunnel (probe)
29 Triceps brachii
30 Flexor digitorum superficialis
31 Pisiform bone
32 Opponens digiti minimi
33 Flexor digiti minimi brevis

34 Tendons of flexor digitorum superficialis
35 Supinator
36 Radius and extensor carpi radialis brevis
37 Flexor pollicis longus
38 Tendon of flexor carpi radialis
39 Pronator teres (insertion on radius)
40 Flexor digitorum profundus
41 Lumbrical muscles
42 Tendons of flexor digitorum profundus
43 Tendons of flexor digitorum profundus having passed through the divided tendons of the flexor digitorum superficialis

361

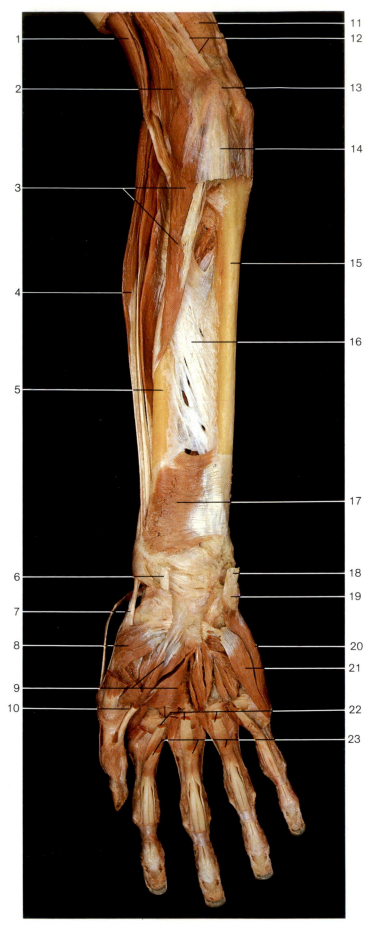

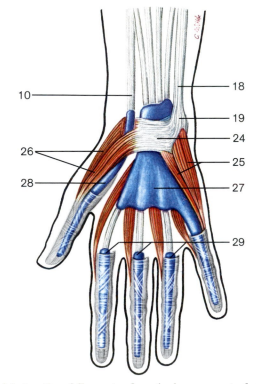

1	Biceps brachii
2	Brachialis
3	Pronator teres
4	Brachioradialis
5	Radius
6	Tendon of flexor carpi radialis
7	Tendon of abductor pollicis longus
8	Opponens pollicis
9	Adductor pollicis
10	Tendon of flexor pollicis longus
11	Triceps brachii
12	Medial intermuscular septum
13	Medial epicondyle of humerus
14	Common flexor mass (divided)
15	Ulna
16	Interosseous membrane
17	Pronator quadratus
18	Tendon of flexor carpi ulnaris
19	Pisiform bone
20	Abductor digiti minimi
21	Flexor digiti minimi brevis
22	Tendons of flexor digitorum profundus
23	Tendons of flexor digitorum superficialis
24	Flexor retinaculum
25	Hypothenar muscles
26	Thenar muscles
27	Common synovial sheath of flexor muscles
28	Synovial sheath of flexor pollicis longus
29	Synovial sheaths of flexor tendons

Muscles of the forearm, deep layer (ventral aspect). All flexors have been removed to display the pronator quadratus and pronator teres muscles together with the interosseous membrane.

Synovial sheaths of flexor tendons (palmar aspect of right hand). (Semischematic drawing) (W.).

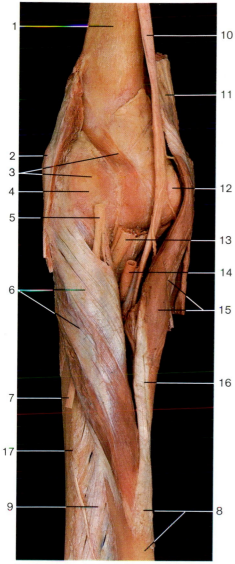

Right supinator and elbow joint
(ventral aspect).

1 Humerus
2 Lateral epicondyle of humerus
3 Articular capsule
4 Position of capitulum of humerus
5 Deep branch of radial nerve
6 Supinator
7 Entrance of deep branch of radial nerve to extensor muscles
8 Radius
9 Interosseous membrane
10 Median nerve
11 Triceps brachii
12 Trochlea of humerus
13 Tendon of biceps brachii
14 Brachial artery
15 Pronator teres
16 Insertion of pronator teres on radius
17 Ulna
18 Pronator quadratus
19 Tendon of flexor carpi radialis
20 Thenar muscles
21 Synovial sheath of tendon of flexor pollicis longus
22 Fibrous sheath of flexor tendons
23 Synovial sheath of flexor tendons
24 Flexor digitorum superficialis
25 Tendon of flexor carpi ulnaris
26 Common synovial sheath of flexor muscles
27 Position of pisiform bone
28 Flexor retinaculum
29 Hypothenar muscles

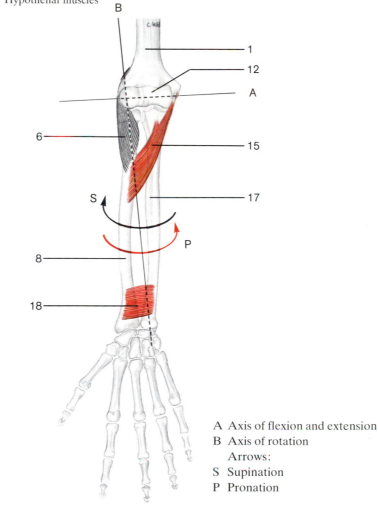

A Axis of flexion and extension
B Axis of rotation
  Arrows:
S Supination
P Pronation

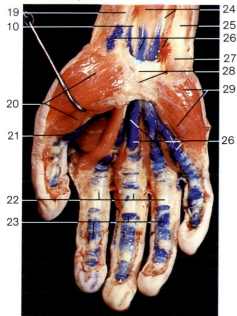

Synovial sheaths of flexor muscles
(palmar aspect of right hand).
Blue PVA-solution has been injected
into the sheaths.

Diagram illustrating the two **axes of the elbow joint** (W.).

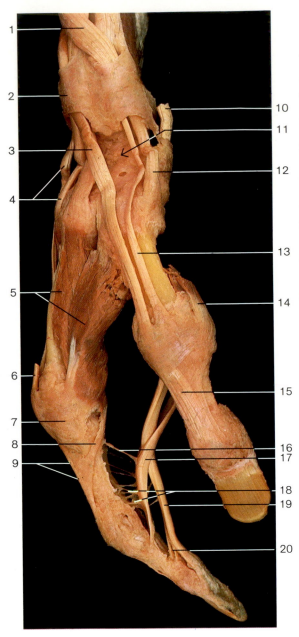

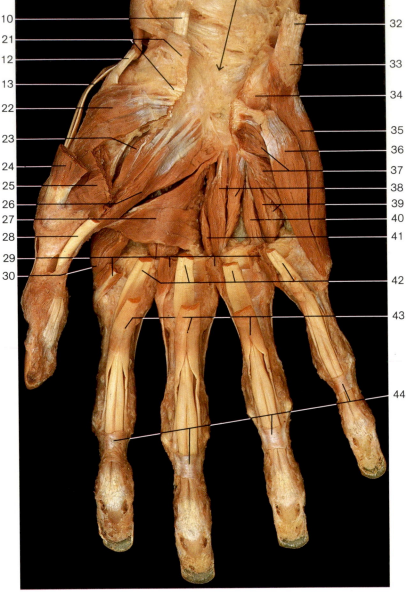

Muscles of thumb and index finger (medial aspect). The tendons of the extensor muscles of the thumb and the insertion of the flexor tendons of the index finger are displayed.

Muscles of hand (palmar aspect). The tendons of the flexor muscles and parts of the thumb muscles have been removed. The carpal tunnel has been opened.

1 Tendons of extensor pollicis brevis and abductor pollicis longus
2 Extensor retinaculum
3 Tendon of extensor pollicis longus
4 Tendons of extensor carpi radialis longus and brevis
5 First dorsal interosseous muscle
6 Tendon of extensor digitorum for index finger
7 Location of metacarpophalangeal joint
8 Tendon of lumbrical muscle
9 Dorsal digital expansion of index finger
10 Tendon of flexor carpi radialis (cut)
11 Anatomical snuffbox
12 Tendon of abductor pollicis longus
13 Tendon of extensor pollicis brevis
14 Tendon of abductor pollicis brevis

15 Dorsal digital expansion of extensor of thumb
16 Vinculum longum
17 Tendons of flexor digitorum superficialis dividing to allow passage of deep tendons
18 Vincula of flexor tendons
19 Tendon of flexor digitorum profundus
20 Vinculum breve
21 Radial carpal eminence (cut edge of flexor retinaculum)
22 Opponens pollicis
23 Deep head of flexor pollicis brevis
24 Abductor pollicis brevis (cut)
25 Superficial head of flexor pollicis brevis (cut)
26 Oblique head of adductor pollicis
27 Transverse head of adductor pollicis
28 Tendon of flexor pollicis longus (cut)

29 Lumbrical muscles (cut)
30 First dorsal interosseous muscle
31 Position of carpal tunnel
32 Tendon of flexor carpi ulnaris
33 Location of pisiform bone
34 Hook of hamate bone
35 Abductor digiti minimi
36 Flexor digiti minimi brevis
37 Opponens digiti minimi
38 2nd palmar interosseous muscle
39 3rd palmar interosseous muscle
40 4th dorsal interosseous muscle
41 3rd dorsal interosseous muscle
42 Tendons of flexor digitorum profundus (cut)
43 Tendons of flexor digitorum superficialis (cut)
44 Fibrous flexor sheaths

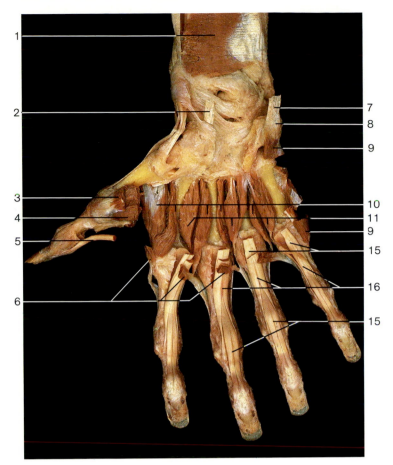

1 Pronator quadratus
2 Tendon of flexor carpi radialis
3 Abductor pollicis brevis (divided)
4 Adductor pollicis (divided)
5 Tendon of flexor pollicis longus
6 Lumbrical muscles (cut)
7 Tendon of flexor carpi ulnaris
8 Pisiform bone
9 Abductor digiti minimi (divided)
10 Dorsal interosseous muscles
11 Palmar interosseous muscles
12 Radius
13 Ulna
14 Flexor retinaculum
15 Tendons of flexor digitorum profundus
16 Tendons of flexor digitorum superficialis

Muscles of right hand, deep layer (palmar aspect). The thenar and hypothenar muscles have been removed to display the interosseous muscles.

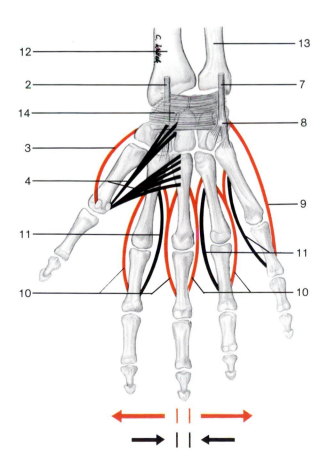

Actions of interosseous muscles in abduction and adduction of fingers. (Schematic drawing) (W.).

Red = **abduction** (dorsal interosseous muscles, abductor digiti minimi and abductor pollicis brevis).
Black = **adduction** (palmar interosseous muscles, adductor pollicis).

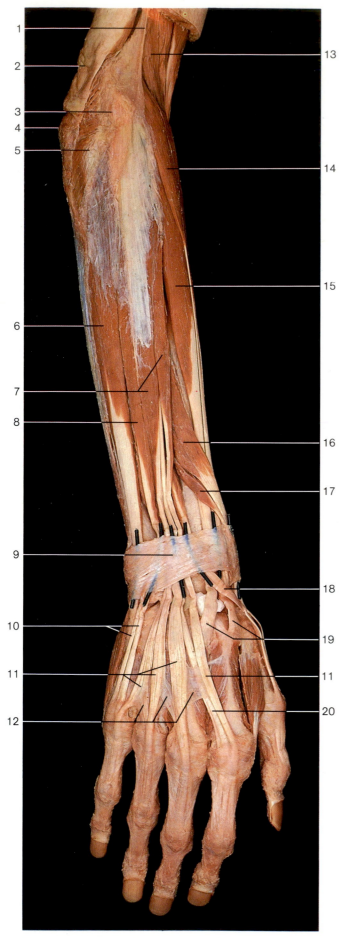

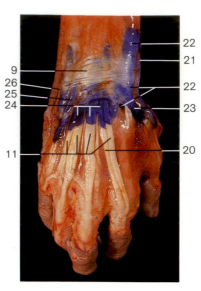

Synovial sheaths of extensor tendons. The sheaths have been injected with blue gelatin.

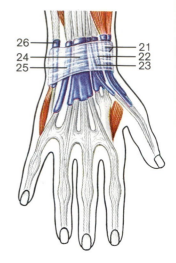

Synovial sheaths of extensor tendons on the back of right wrist (indicated in blue). Notice the six tunnels for the passage of the extensor tendons beneath the extensor retinaculum. (Semischematic drawing) (W.).

1 Lateral intermuscular septum
2 Tendon of triceps brachii
3 Lateral epicondyle of humerus
4 Olecranon
5 Anconeus
6 Extensor carpi ulnaris
7 Extensor digitorum
8 Extensor digit minimi
9 Extensor retinaculum
10 Tendons of extensor digiti minimi
11 Tendons of extensor digitorum
12 Intertendinous connexions
13 Brachioradialis
14 Extensor carpi radialis longus
15 Extensor carpi radialis brevis
16 Abductor pollicis longus
17 Extensor pollicis brevis
18 Tendon of extensor pollicis longus
19 Tendons of both extensor carpi radialis longus and extensor carpi radialis brevis
20 Tendon of extensor indicis
21 1st tunnel: Abductor pollicis longus
          Extensor pollicis brevis
22 2nd tunnel: Extensor carpi radialis longus and brevis
23 3rd tunnel: Extensor pollicis longus
24 4th tunnel: Extensor digitorum
          Extensor indicis
          Synovial sheath of extensor muscles
25 5th tunnel: Extensor digiti minimi
26 6th tunnel: Extensor carpi ulnaris

Extensor muscles of forearm and hand, superficial layer (dorsal aspect). Tunnels for extensor tendons indicated by probes.

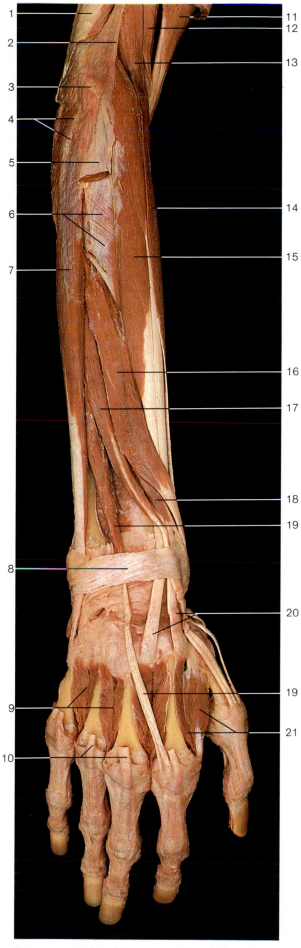

1 Triceps brachii
2 Lateral intermuscular septum
3 Lateral epicondyle of humerus
4 Anconeus
5 Extensor digitorum and extensor digiti minimi (cut)
6 Supinator
7 Extensor carpi ulnaris
8 Extensor retinaculum
9 3rd and 4th dorsal interosseous muscles
10 Tendons of extensor digitorum (cut)
11 Biceps brachii
12 Brachialis
13 Brachioradialis
14 Extensor carpi radialis longus
15 Extensor carpi radialis brevis
16 Abductor pollicis longus
17 Extensor pollicis longus
18 Extensor pollicis brevis
19 Extensor indicis
20 Tendons of the extensor carpi radialis longus and extensor carpi radialis brevis
21 1st dorsal interosseous muscle

Extensor muscles of forearm and hand, deep layer (dorsal aspect).

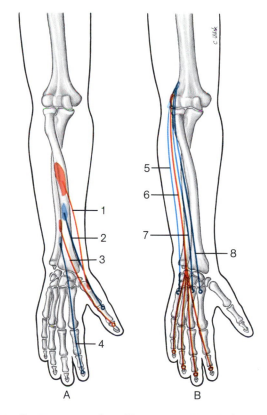

Position of extensor muscles of forearm and hand. (Semischematic drawing) (W.).

A Extensors of thumb
B Extensors of fingers and hand

1 Abductor pollicis longus (red) 5 Extensor carpi ulnaris (blue)
2 Extensor pollicis brevis (blue) 6 Extensor digitorum (red)
3 Extensor pollicis longus (red) 7 Extensor carpi radialis brevis (blue)
4 Extensor indicis (blue) 8 Extensor carpi radialis longus (blue)

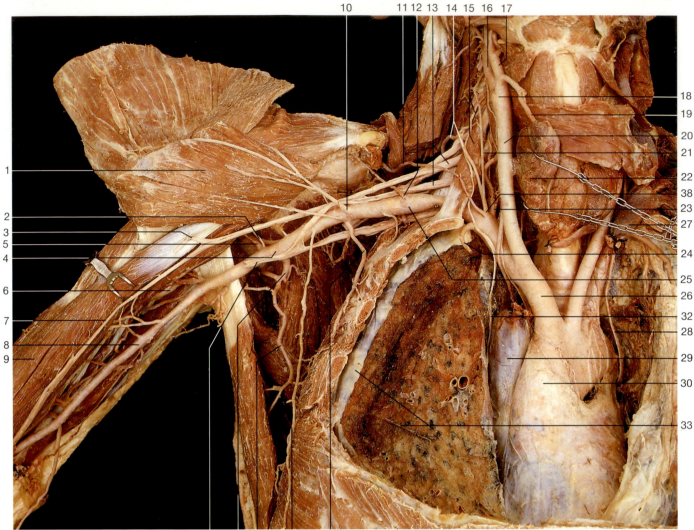

Main branches of right subclavian and axillary arteries (anterior aspect). Pectoralis muscles have been reflected, clavicle and anterior wall of thorax removed and right lung divided. Left lung with pleura and thyroid gland have been reflected laterally to display aortic arch and common carotid artery with their branches.

1 Pectoralis minor (reflected)	22 Thyroid gland	43 Radial collateral artery
2 Anterior circumflex humeral artery	23 Inferior thyroid artery	44 Radial recurrent artery
3 Musculocutaneous nerve (divided)	24 Internal thoracic artery	45 **Radial artery**
4 **Axillary artery**	25 Right subclavian artery	46 Anterior and posterior interosseous arteries
5 Posterior circumflex humeral artery	26 Brachiocephalic trunk	47 Princeps pollicis artery
6 **Profunda brachii artery**	27 Left brachiocephalic vein (divided)	48 **Deep palmar arch**
7 Median nerve (var.)	28 Left vagus nerve	49 Common palmar digital arteries
8 **Brachial artery**	29 Superior vena cava (divided)	50 Ulnar recurrent artery
9 Biceps brachii	30 **Ascending aorta**	51 Recurrent interosseous artery
10 Thoracoacromial artery	31 Median nerve (divided)	52 Common interosseous artery
11 Suprascapular artery	32 Phrenic nerve	53 **Ulnar artery**
12 Descending scapular artery	33 Right lung (divided), pulmonary pleura	54 **Superficial palmar arch**
13 Brachial plexus	34 Thoracodorsal artery	55 Median nerve and brachial artery
14 Transverse cervical artery	35 Subscapular artery	56 Biceps brachii
15 Scalenus anterior muscle, phrenic nerve	36 Lateral mammary branches (var.)	57 Ulnar nerve
16 Right internal carotid artery	37 Lateral thoracic artery	58 Flexor pollicis longus
17 Right external carotid artery	38 **Thyrocervical trunk**	59 Palmar digital arteries
18 Carotid sinus	39 Superior thoracic artery	60 Anterior interosseous artery
19 Superior thyroid artery	40 Superior ulnar collateral artery	61 Flexor carpi ulnaris
20 Right common carotid artery	41 Inferior ulnar collateral artery	62 Superficial palmar branch of radial artery
21 Ascending cervical artery	42 Middle collateral artery	

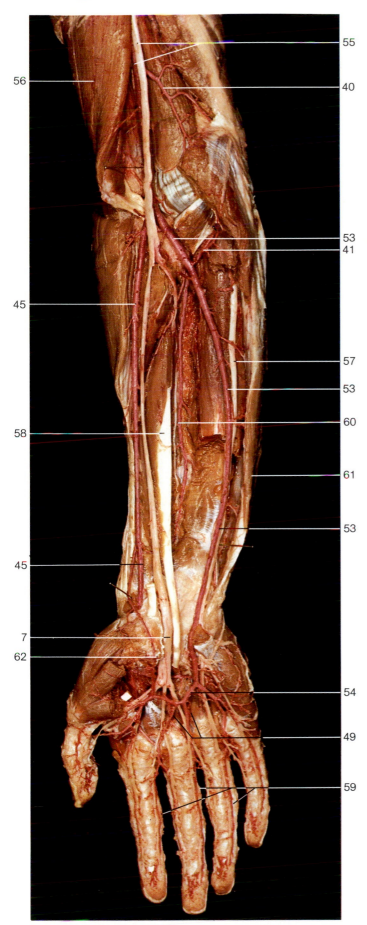

Dissection of the arteries of forearm and hand. The superficial flexors have been removed, the carpal tunnel opened and the flexor retinaculum cut. The arteries have been filled with colored resin.

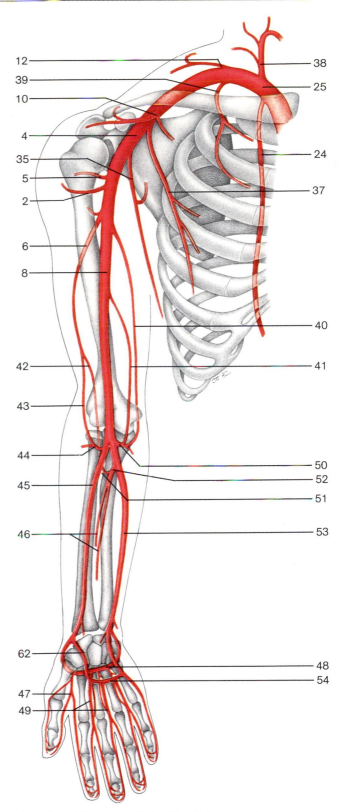

Arteries of the upper limb. (Semischematic drawing) (O.).

369

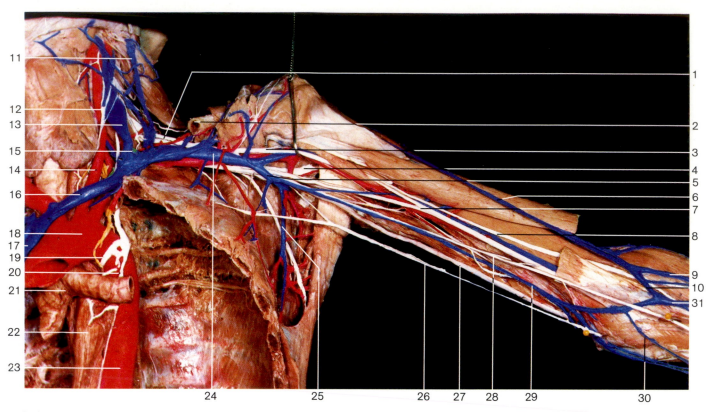

Veins and nerves of the axilla and left arm (ventral aspect). Part of the clavicle and the anterior wall of the thorax have been removed. The shoulder is slightly reflected. The vessels have been injected with colored resin.

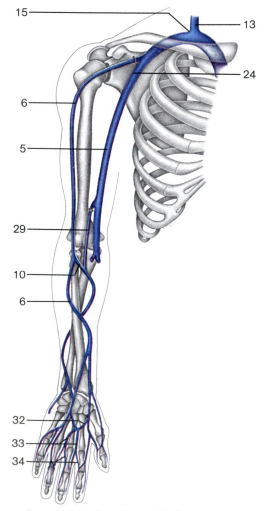

Superficial veins of upper limb.
(Semischematic drawing) (O.).

1   Brachial plexus
2   Clavicle (cut)
3   Lateral cord of brachial plexus
4   Axillary nerve
5   **Brachial vein**
6   **Cephalic vein**
7   Median nerve
8   Musculocutaneous nerve
9   Accessory cephalic vein
10 Median cubital vein
11 External jugular vein
12 Ansa cervicalis
13 **Internal jugular vein**
14 Common carotid artery
15 Venous angle [on the left side entrance of thoracic duct (green)]
16 **Brachiocephalic vein**
17 **Superior vena cava**
18 Aortic arch
19 Recurrent laryngeal nerve
20 Vagus nerve
21 Bifurcation of trachea
22 Esophagus
23 Descending (thoracic) aorta
24 **Axillary vein**
25 **Thoracoepigastric vein**
26 Medial cutaneous nerve of arm
27 Ulnar nerve
28 Medial cutaneous nerve of forearm
29 **Basilic vein**
30 Median basilic vein
31 Median vein of forearm
32 Dorsal venous network of hand
33 Dorsal metacarpal veins
34 Palmar digital veins

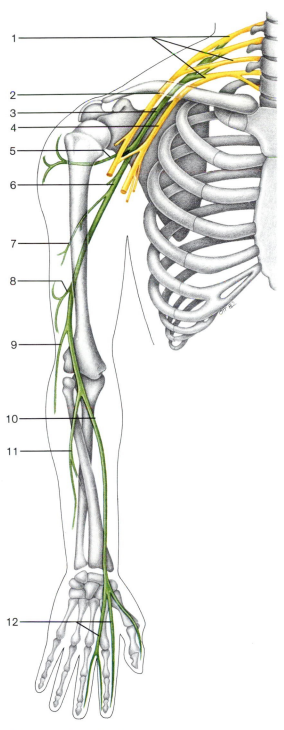

Main branches of radial nerve. (Schematic drawing) (O.).

Main branches of musculocutaneous, median and ulnar nerves. (Schematic drawing) (O.).

1 Brachial plexus	13 Roots of median nerve
2 Lateral cord of brachial plexus	14 Musculocutaneous nerve
3 Posterior cord of brachial plexus	15 **Median nerve**
4 Medial cord of brachial plexus	16 **Ulnar nerve**
5 **Axillary nerve**	17 Medial cutaneous nerves of arm and forearm
6 **Radial nerve**	18 Lateral cutaneous nerve of forearm
7 Posterior cutaneous nerve of arm	19 Anterior interosseous nerve
8 Lower lateral cutaneous nerve of arm	20 Palmar branch of median nerve
9 Posterior cutaneous nerve of forearm	21 Dorsal branch of ulnar nerve
10 Superficial branch of radial nerve	22 Deep branch of ulnar nerve
11 Deep branch of radial nerve	23 Common palmar digital nerves of median nerve
12 Dorsal digital nerves	24 Superficial branch of ulnar nerve

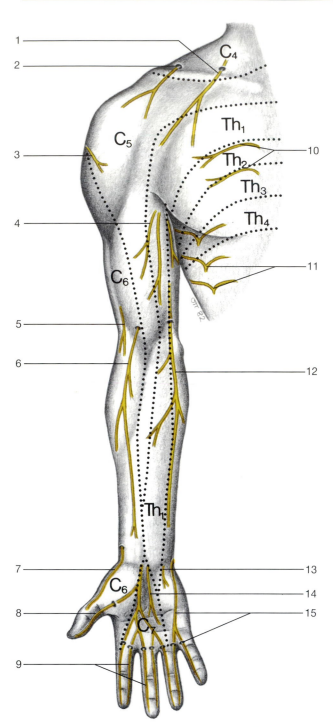

Cutaneous nerves of right upper limb (ventral aspect). (Semischematic drawing) (O.).

Cutaneous nerves of the upper limb (dorsal aspect). (Semischematic drawing) (O.).

1 Medial supraclavicular nerve
2 Intermediate supraclavicular nerve
3 Upper lateral cutaneous nerve of arm
4 Terminal branches of intercostobrachial nerves
5 Lower lateral cutaneous nerve of arm
6 Lateral cutaneous nerve of forearm
7 Terminal branch of superficial branch of radial nerve
8 Palmar digital nerve of thumb (branch of median nerve)
9 Palmar digital nerves of median nerve
10 Anterior cutaneous branches of intercostal nerves
11 Lateral cutaneous branches of intercostal nerves
12 Medial cutaneous nerve of forearm

13 Palmar cutaneous branch of ulnar nerve
14 Palmar branch of median nerve
15 Palmar digital branches of ulnar nerve
16 Cutaneous branches of dorsal rami of spinal nerves
17 Dorsal branch of ulnar nerve
18 Dorsal digital nerves
19 Posterior supraclavicular nerve
20 Posterior cutaneous nerve of arm ⎫
21 Posterior cutaneous nerve of forearm ⎬ from radial nerve
22 Superficial branch ⎭
23 Dorsal digital branches

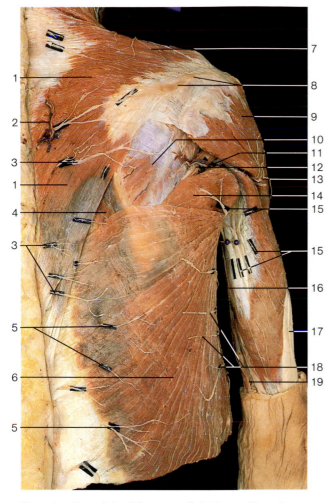

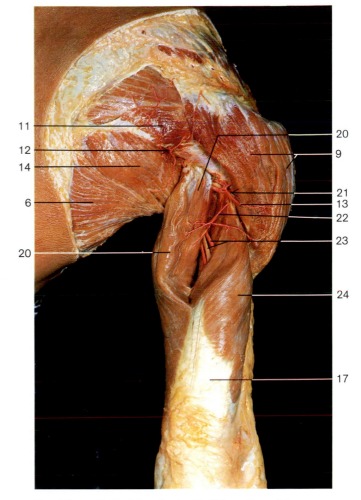

Dorsal region of shoulder, superficial layer. Note the segmental arrangement of the cutaneous nerves of the back.

Shoulder and arm (dorsal aspect). Dissection of the quadrangular and triangular spaces of the axillary region.

1 Trapezius
2 Dorsal branches of posterior intercostal artery and vein (medial cutaneous branches)
3 Medial branches of dorsal rami of spinal nerves
4 Rhomboideus major
5 Lateral branches of dorsal rami of spinal nerves
6 Latissimus dorsi
7 Posterior supraclavicular nerves
8 Spine of scapula
9 Deltoid muscle
10 Infraspinatus
11 Teres minor
12 **Triangular space** with circumflex scapular artery and vein
13 Upper lateral cutaneous nerve of arm with artery
14 Teres major
15 Terminal branches of intercostobrachial nerve
16 Medial cutaneous nerve of arm
17 Tendon of triceps brachii
18 Lateral cutaneous branches of intercostal nerves
19 Medial cutaneous nerve of forearm
20 Long head of triceps brachii
21 **Quadrangular space** with axillary nerve and posterior humeral circumflex artery
22 Anastomosis between profunda brachii artery and posterior humeral circumflex artery
23 Course of radial nerve and profunda brachii artery
24 Lateral head of triceps brachii
25 Course of descending scapular artery and dorsal scapular nerve
26 Course of suprascapular nerve, artery and vein

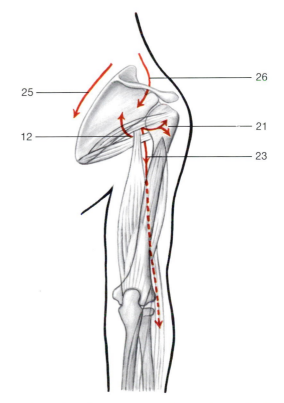

Course of vessels and nerves to shoulder and upper limb. (Schematic drawing.)

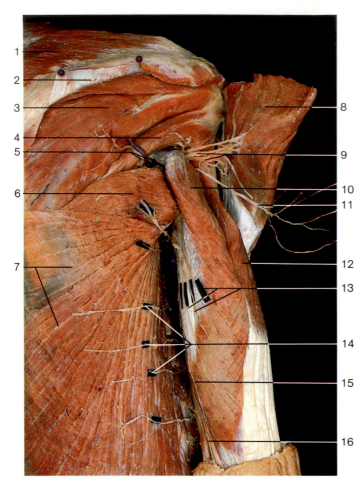

Scapular region, arm and shoulder, deep layer (dorsal aspect). Part of deltoid muscle has been cut and reflected to display the quadrangular and triangular spaces of the axillary region.

Scapular region and posterior brachial region; arm and shoulder, deep layer (dorsal aspect). The lateral head of the triceps brachii has been cut to display the radial nerve and accompanying vessels.

1   Trapezius
2   Spine of scapula
3   Infraspinatus
4   Teres minor
5   **Triangular space** containing circumflex scapular artery and vein
6   Teres major
7   Latissimus dorsi
8   Deltoid muscle (cut and reflected)
9   **Quadrangular space** containing axillary nerve and posterior circumflex humeral artery and vein
10 Long head of triceps brachii
11 Cutaneous branch of axillary nerve
12 Lateral head of triceps brachii
13 Terminal branches of intercostobrachial nerve
14 Lateral cutaneous branches of intercostal nerves
15 Medial cutaneous nerve of arm
16 Medial cutaneous nerve of forearm
17 Upper lateral cutaneous nerve of arm
18 Anastomosis between profunda brachii artery and posterior humeral circumflex artery
19 Humerus
20 **Profunda brachii artery**
21 **Radial nerve**
22 Radial collateral artery
23 Medial collateral artery
24 Lower lateral cutaneous nerve of arm
25 Posterior cutaneous nerve of forearm
26 Tendon of triceps brachii

374

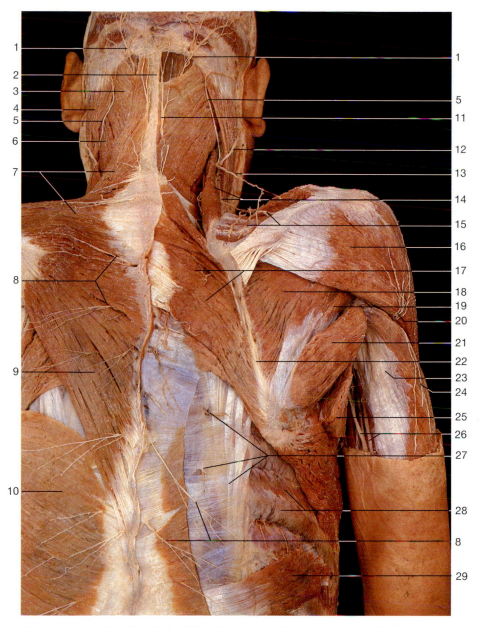

Dorsal regions of neck and shoulder (dorsal aspect). Left side: superficial layer; right side: trapezius and latissimus dorsi removed. Dissection of dorsal branches of spinal nerves.

1	Greater occipital nerve	16	Deltoid muscle
2	Ligamentum nuchae	17	Rhomboideus major
3	Splenius capitis	18	Infraspinatus muscle
4	Sternocleidomastoid	19	Teres minor
5	Lesser occipital nerve	20	Upper lateral cutaneous nerve of arm (branch of axillary nerve)
6	Splenius cervicis	21	Teres major
7	Descending and transverse fibers of trapezius	22	Medial margin of scapula
8	Medial cutaneous branches of dorsal rami of spinal nerves	23	Long head of triceps muscle
9	Ascending fibers of trapezius	24	Posterior cutaneous nerve of arm (branch of radial nerve)
10	Latissimus dorsi	25	Latissimus dorsi (divided)
11	Cutaneous branch of third occipital nerve	26	Ulnar nerve, brachial artery
12	Great auricular nerve	27	Lateral cutaneous branches of dorsal rami of spinal nerves, iliocostalis thoracis
13	Accessory nerve (n. XI)	28	External intercostal muscle, seventh rib
14	Posterior supraclavicular nerve, levator scapulae	29	Serratus posterior inferior
15	Branches of suprascapular artery		

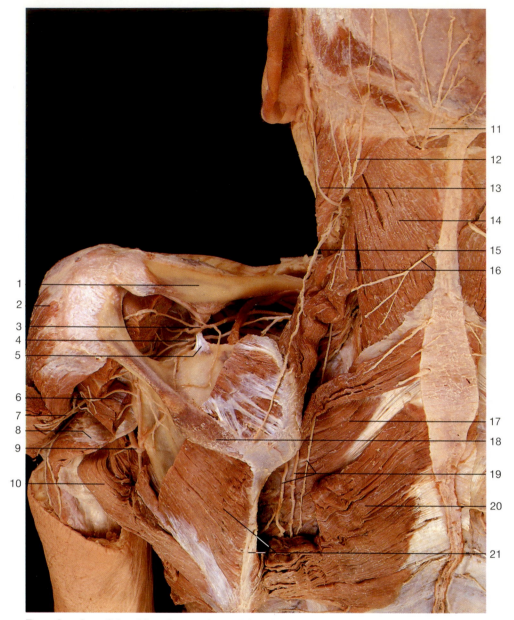

1 Clavicle
2 Deltoid muscle
3 **Suprascapular artery**
4 Suprascapular nerve
5 Superior transverse scapular ligament
6 Teres minor
7 Axillary nerve, posterior circumflex humeral artery
8 Long head of triceps
9 **Circumflex scapular artery**
10 Teres major
11 Greater occipital nerve
12 Lesser occipital nerve
13 Great auricular nerve
14 Splenius capitis
15 Accessory nerve (n. XI)
16 Third occipital nerve, levator scapulae
17 Serratus posterior superior
18 Spine of scapula
19 Descending scapular artery, dorsal scapular nerve
20 Rhomboideus major
21 Infraspinatus, medial margin of scapula
22 Radial nerve, profunda brachii artery
23 Thoracodorsal artery
24 Thyrocervical trunk
25 Brachial plexus

Dorsal region of shoulder; deepest layer. Rhomboid and scapular muscles fenestrated; posterior part of deltoid muscle reflected.

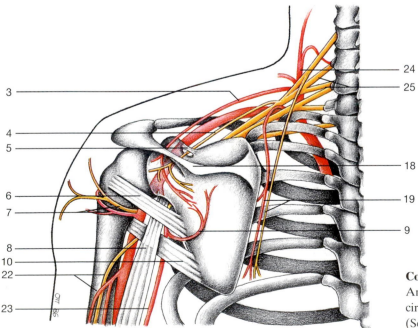

Collateral circulation of shoulder.
Anastomosis of suprascapular and circumflex scapular arteries. (Semischematic drawing) (O.).

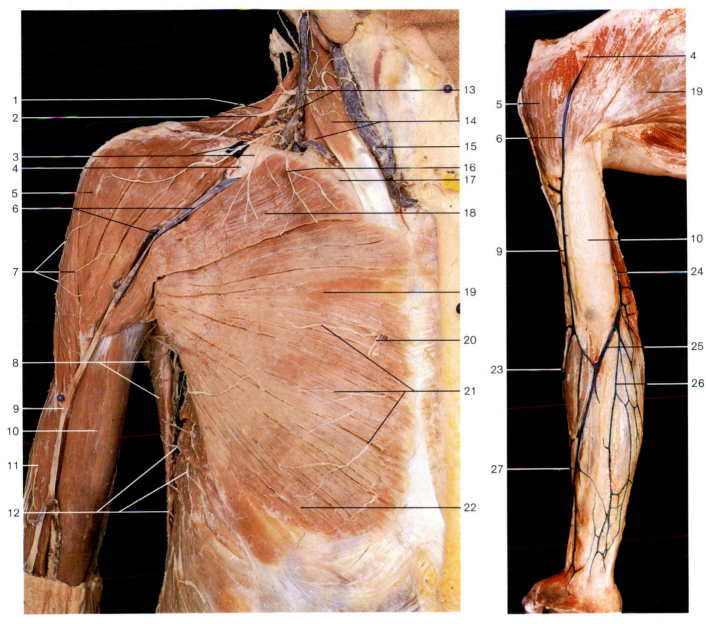

Right shoulder and thoracic wall, superficial layer (anterior aspect). Dissection of the cutaneous nerves and veins.

Superficial veins of right arm have been injected with blue gelatin.

1   Trapezius
2   Posterior supraclavicular nerve
3   Middle supraclavicular nerve
4   Deltopectoral triangle
5   Deltoid muscle
6   Cephalic vein within the deltopectoral groove
7   Upper lateral cutaneous nerve of arm
    (branch of axillary nerve)
8   Latissimus dorsi
9   Cephalic vein within the lateral bicipital groove
10 Biceps brachii
11 Triceps brachii
12 Lateral cutaneous branches of intercostal nerves
13 Transverse cervical nerve and external jugular vein

14 Sternocleidomastoid muscle
15 Anterior jugular vein
16 Anterior supraclavicular nerve
17 Clavicle
18 Clavicular part of pectoralis major
19 Sternocostal part of pectoralis major
20 Perforating branch of internal thoracic artery
21 Anterior cutaneous branches of intercostal nerves
22 Abdominal part of pectoralis major
23 Accessory cephalic vein
24 Basilic vein
25 Median cubital vein
26 Median vein of forearm
27 Cephalic vein in the forearm

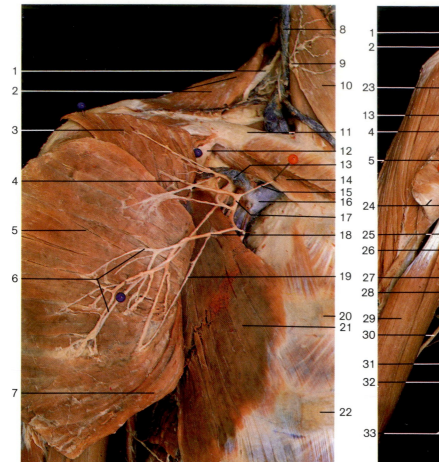

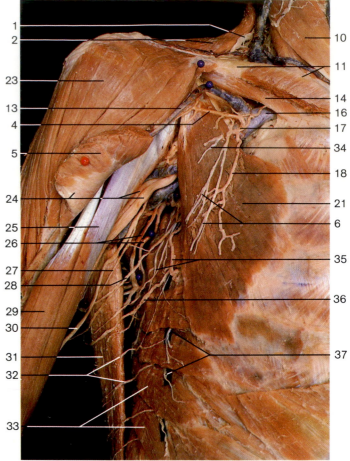

Right deltopectoral triangle, infraclavicular region (anterior aspect). The pectoralis major has been cut and reflected.

Thoracic wall and shoulder, deep layer. **Right axillary region** (anterior aspect). The pectoralis major has been cut and partly removed.

1   Accessory nerve
2   Trapezius
3   Pectoralis major (clavicular part)
4   Acromial branch of thoracoacromial artery
5   Pectoralis major
6   Lateral pectoral nerve
7   Abdominal part of pectoralis major
8   External jugular vein
9   Cutaneous branches of cervical plexus
10   Sternocleidomastoid
11   Clavicle
12   Clavipectoral fascia
13   Cephalic vein
14   Subclavius
15   Clavicular branch of thoracoacromial artery
16   Subclavian vein
17   Thoracoacromial artery
18   Pectoral branch of thoracoacromial artery
19   Medial pectoral nerve
20   2nd rib

21   Pectoralis minor
22   3rd rib
23   Deltoid muscle
24   Brachial artery and median nerve
25   Short head of biceps brachii
26   Thoracodorsal artery and nerve
27   Medial cutaneous nerve of arm
28   Intercostobrachial nerve (T$_2$)
29   Long head of biceps brachii
30   Medial cutaneous nerve of forearm
31   Latissimus dorsi
32   Lateral cutaneous branches of intercostal nerves (posterior branches)
33   Serratus anterior
34   Medial pectoral nerve
35   Long thoracic nerve and lateral thoracic artery
36   Intercostobrachial nerve (T$_3$)
37   Lateral cutaneous branches of intercostal nerves (anterior branches)

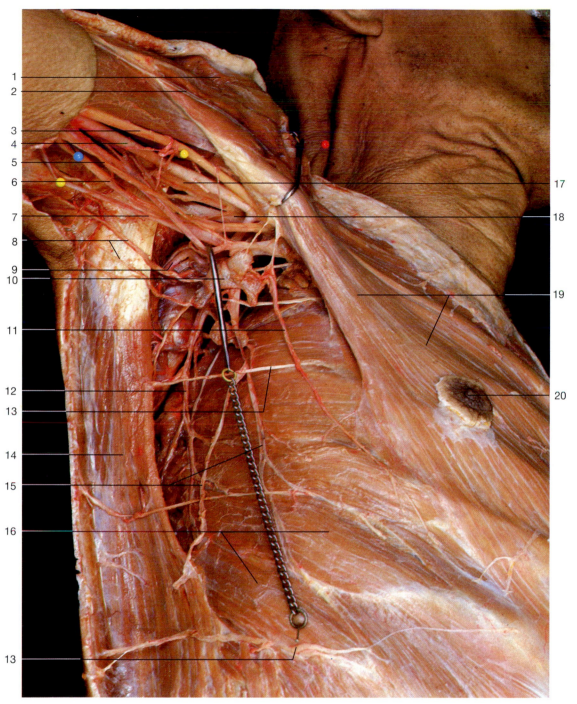

Right axillary region (inferior aspect). **Dissection of superficial axillary nodes and lymphatic vessels.** The pectoralis major has been slightly elevated.

1	Deltoid muscle	12	Thoracodorsal artery
2	Cephalic vein	13	Lateral cutaneous branch of intercostal nerve
3	Median nerve	14	Latissimus dorsi
4	Brachial artery	15	Thoracoepigastric vein
5	Medial cutaneous nerves of arm and forearm	16	Serratus anterior
6	Ulnar nerve	17	Musculocutaneous nerve
7	Basilic Vein	18	Radial nerve
8	Intercostobrachial nerves	19	Pectoralis major
9	Circumflex scapular artery	20	Nipple
10	**Superficial axillary nodes**		
11	Lateral thoracic artery		

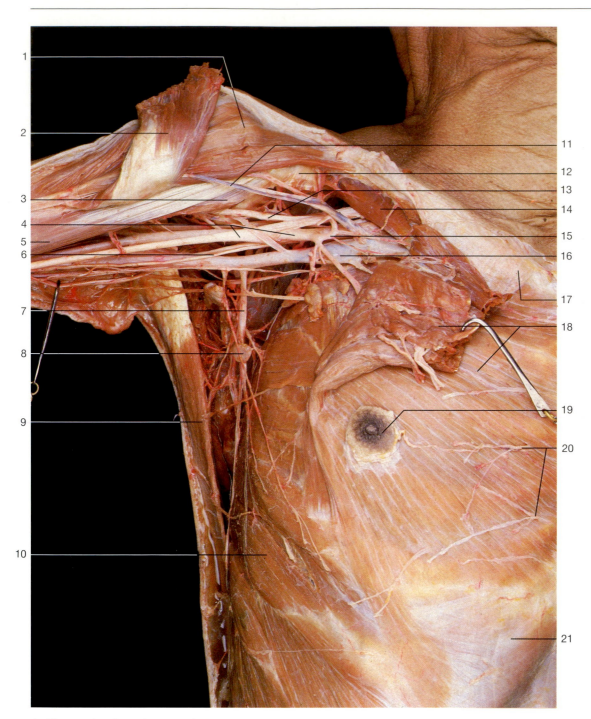

Axillary region (anterior aspect). Dissection of deep axillary nodes. Pectoralis major and minor divided and reflected. Shoulder girdle and arm elevated and reflected.

1 Deltoid muscle
2 Insertion of pectoralis major
3 Coracobrachialis
4 Roots of **median nerve, axillary artery**
5 Short head of biceps brachii
6 **Ulnar nerve**
7 Thoracoepigastric vein
8 Deep axillary node
9 Latissimus dorsi
10 Serratus anterior
11 Cephalic vein
12 Insertion of pectoralis minor, coracoid process

13 **Musculocutaneous nerve**
14 Subclavius muscle
15 Thoracoacromial artery
16 **Axillary vein**
17 Clavicle
18 Pectoralis major and minor (reflected)
19 Nipple
20 Anterior cutaneous branches of intercostal nerves
21 Anterior layer of rectus sheaths

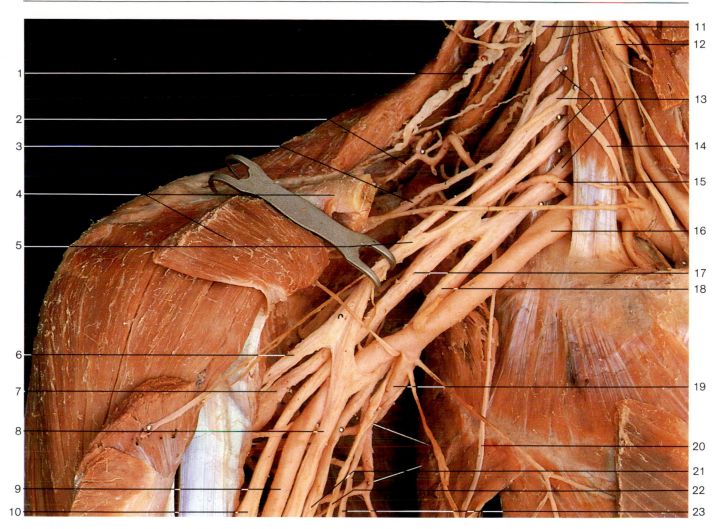

Brachial plexus (anterior aspect). Clavicle and pectoralis muscles have been partly removed.

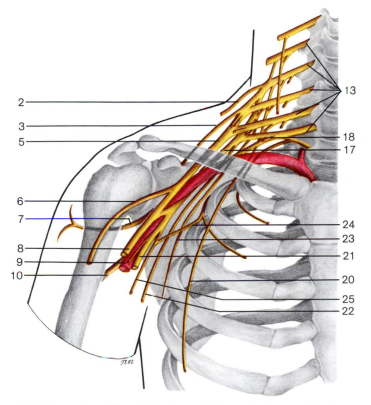

Main branches of brachial plexus. (Schematic drawing) (Tr.).

1 Accessory nerve
2 Dorsal scapular nerve
3 Suprascapular nerve
4 Clavicle and pectoralis minor
5 **Lateral cord** of brachial plexus
6 Musculocutaneous nerve
7 Axillary nerve
8 Median nerve
9 Brachial artery
10 Radial nerve and profunda brachii artery
11 Cervical plexus
12 Common carotid artery
13 Roots of brachial plexus (C_5–T_1)
14 Phrenic nerve
15 Descending scapular artery
16 Subclavian artery
17 **Posterior cord** of brachial plexus
18 **Medial cord** of brachial plexus
19 Subscapular artery
20 Long thoracic nerve
21 Ulnar nerve
22 Medial cutaneous nerve of forearm
23 Thoracodorsal nerve
24 Intercostobrachial nerve
25 Medial cutaneous nerve of arm

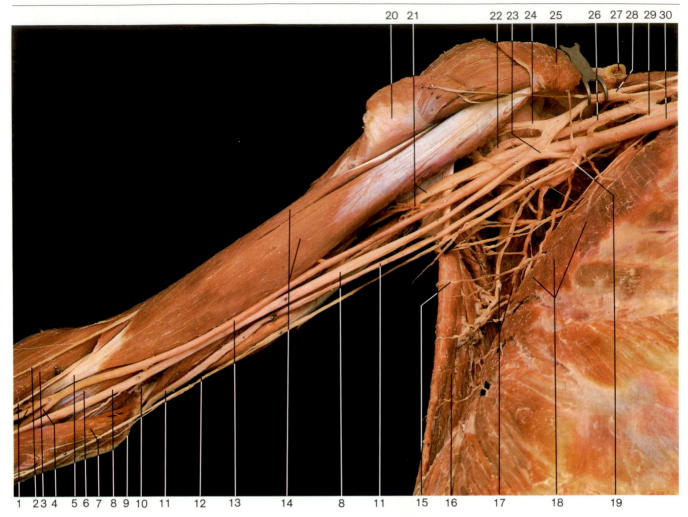

Right arm. Dissection of vessels and nerves (medial aspect). Shoulder girdle has been reflected slightly.

1 Radial artery and superficial branch of radial nerve
2 Lateral cutaneous nerve of forearm
3 Brachioradialis
4 Ulnar artery
5 Tendon of biceps brachii
6 Brachialis
7 Pronator teres
8 Median nerve
9 Medial epicondyle of humerus
10 Inferior ulnar collateral artery
11 Ulnar nerve
12 Medial cutaneous nerve of forearm
13 Brachial artery
14 Biceps brachii
15 Intercostobrachial nerve (T$_3$)
16 Latissimus dorsi
17 Thoracodorsal nerve and artery
18 Serratus anterior
19 Subscapular artery
20 Pectoralis major (reflected) and lateral pectoral nerve
21 Radial nerve and profunda brachii artery
22 Axillary nerve
23 Roots of the median nerve with axillary artery
24 Musculocutaneous nerve
25 Pectoralis minor (reflected) and medial pectoral nerve
26 Posterior cord of brachial plexus
27 Clavicle (cut)
28 Lateral cord of brachial plexus
29 Medial cord of brachial plexus
30 Subclavian artery

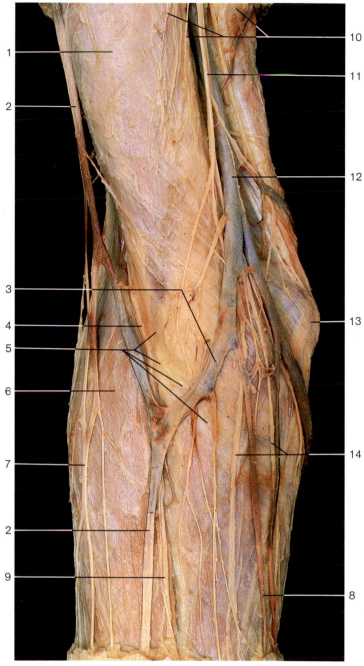

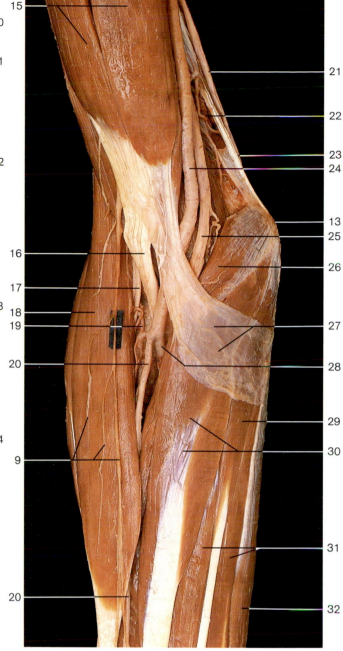

Cubital region (anterior aspect), dissection of cutaneous nerves and veins.

Cubital region, superficial layer (anterior aspect). The fasciae of the muscles have been removed.

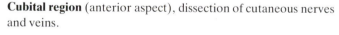

1 Biceps brachii with fascia
2 Cephalic vein
3 Median cubital vein
4 Musculocutaneous nerve
5 Tendon and aponeurosis of biceps brachii
   (covered by the antebrachial fascia)
6 Brachioradialis with fascia
7 Accessory cephalic vein
8 Median vein of forearm
9 Cutaneous branches of musculocutaneous nerve
10 Terminal branches of medial cutaneous nerve of arm
11 Medial antebrachial cutaneous nerve
12 Basilic vein
13 Medial epicondyle of humerus
14 Terminal branches of medial cutaneous nerve
   of forearm
15 Biceps brachii

16 Tendon of biceps brachii
17 Radial nerve
18 Brachioradialis
19 Radial recurrent artery
20 Radial artery
21 Ulnar nerve
22 Inferior ulnar collateral artery
23 Medial intermuscular septum
24 Brachial artery
25 Median nerve
26 Pronator teres
27 Bicipital aponeurosis
28 Ulnar artery
29 Palmaris longus
30 Flexor carpi radialis
31 Flexor digitorum superficialis
32 Flexor carpi ulnaris

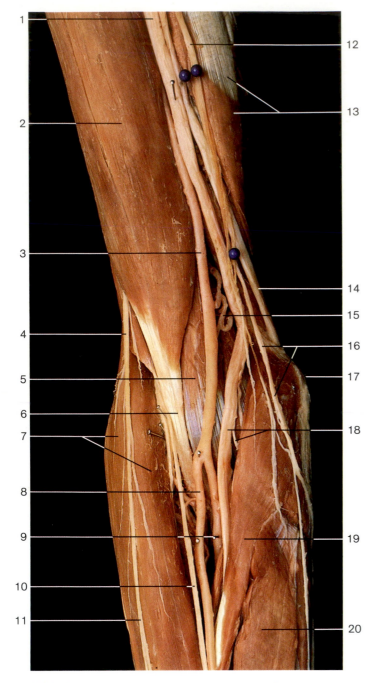

Cubital region, middle layer (anterior aspect). The bicipital aponeurosis has been removed.

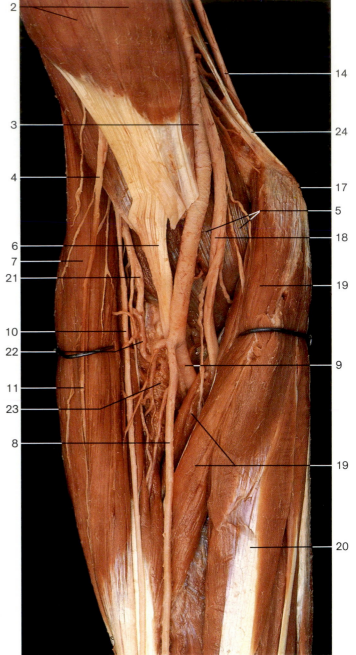

Cubital region, middle layer (anterior aspect). The pronator teres and brachioradialis have been slightly reflected.

1 Median nerve	15 Inferior ulnar collateral artery
2 Biceps brachii	16 Terminal branches of medial cutaneous nerve of forearm
3 Brachial artery	17 Medial epicondyle of humerus
4 Musculocutaneous nerve	18 Median nerve with branches to pronator teres
5 Brachialis	19 Pronator teres
6 Tendon of biceps brachii	20 Flexor carpi radialis
7 Brachioradialis	21 Deep branch of radial nerve
8 Radial artery	22 Radial recurrent artery
9 Ulnar artery	23 Supinator
10 Superficial branch of radial nerve	24 Medial intermuscular septum of arm
11 Lateral cutaneous nerve of forearm	
12 Medial cutaneous nerve of forearm	
13 Triceps brachii	
14 Ulnar nerve	

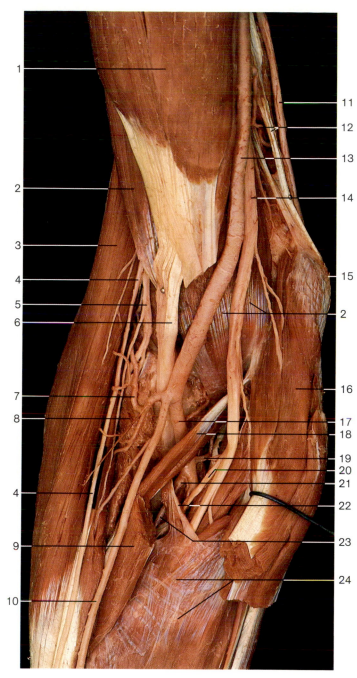

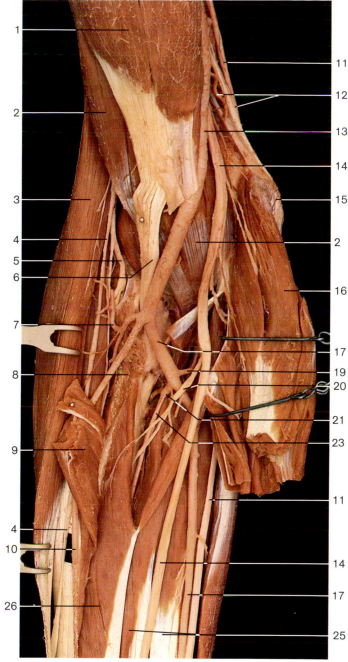

Cubital region, deep layer (anterior aspect). The pronator teres and flexor carpi ulnaris have been cut and reflected.

Cubital region, deepest layer (anterior aspect). The flexor digitorum superficialis and the ulnar head of the pronator teres have been cut and reflected.

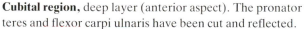

1	Biceps brachii	14	Median nerve
2	Brachialis	15	Medial epicondyle of humerus
3	Brachioradialis	16	Humeral head of pronator teres
4	Superficial branch of radial nerve	17	Ulnar artery
5	Deep branch of radial nerve	18	Ulnar head of pronator teres
6	Tendon of biceps brachii	19	Ulnar recurrent artery
7	Radial recurrent artery	20	Anterior interosseous nerve
8	Supinator	21	Common interosseous artery
9	Insertion of pronator teres	22	Tendinous arch of flexor digitorum superficialis
10	Radial artery	23	Anterior interosseous artery
11	Ulnar nerve	24	Flexor digitorum superficialis
12	Medial intermuscular septum of arm and inferior ulnar collateral artery	25	Flexor digitorum profundus
13	Brachial artery	26	Flexor pollicis longus

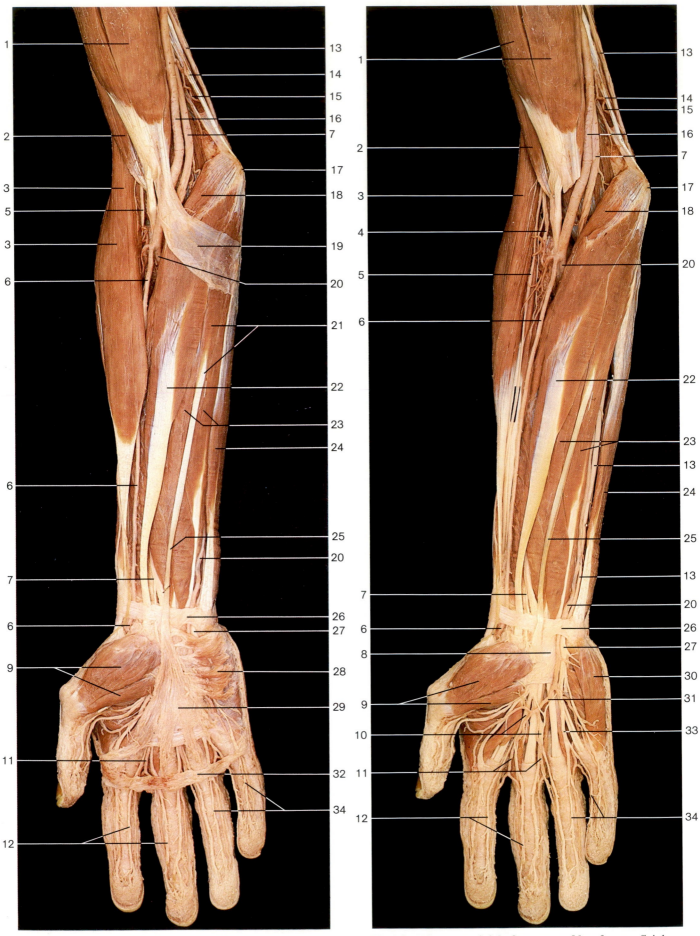

Vessels and nerves of right forearm and hand, superficial layer (palmar aspect).

Vessels and nerves of right forearm and hand, superficial layer (palmar aspect). The palmar aponeurosis of the hand and the bicipital aponeurosis have been removed.

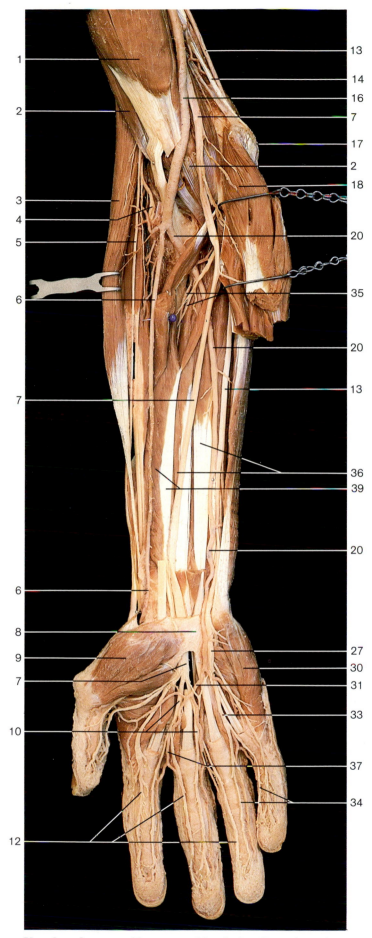

1. Biceps brachii
2. Brachialis
3. Brachioradialis
4. Deep branch of radial nerve
5. Superficial branch of radial nerve
6. Radial artery
7. Median nerve
8. Flexor retinaculum
9. Thenar muscles
10. Common palmar digital branches of median nerve
11. Common palmar digital arteries
12. Proper palmar digital nerves (median nerve)
13. Ulnar nerve
14. Medial intermuscular septum of arm
15. Inferior ulnar collateral artery
16. Brachial artery
17. Medial epicondyle of humerus
18. Pronator teres
19. Bicipital aponeurosis
20. Ulnar artery
21. Palmaris longus
22. Flexor carpi radialis
23. Flexor digitorum superficialis
24. Flexor carpi ulnaris
25. Tendon of palmaris longus
26. Remnant of antebrachial fascia
27. Superficial branch of ulnar nerve
28. Palmaris brevis
29. Palmar aponeurosis
30. Hypothenar muscles
31. **Superficial palmar arch**
32. Superficial transverse metacarpal ligament
33. Common palmar digital branch of ulnar nerve
34. Proper palmar digital branches of ulnar nerve
35. Anterior interosseous artery and nerve
36. Flexor digitorum profundus
37. Common palmar digital arteries
38. Palmar branch of median nerve
39. Flexor pollicis longus
40. Palmar branch of ulnar nerve

Vessels and nerves of forearm and hand, deep layer (anterior aspect). The superficial layer of the flexor muscles has been removed.

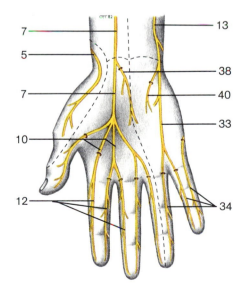

Cutaneous innervation of hand, palmar surface.
(Schematic drawing) (O.).
Cutaneous innervation of palmar surface:
3½ digits by median nerve,
1½ digits by ulnar nerve.

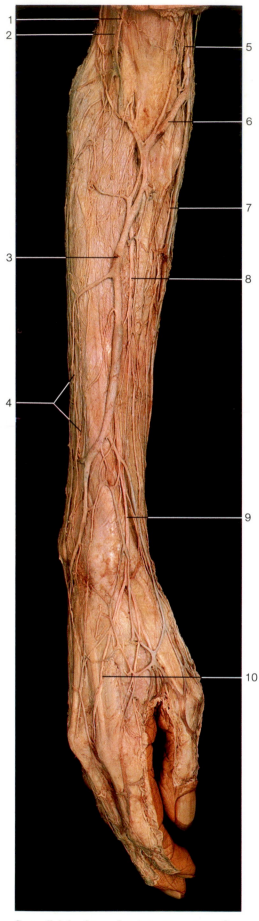

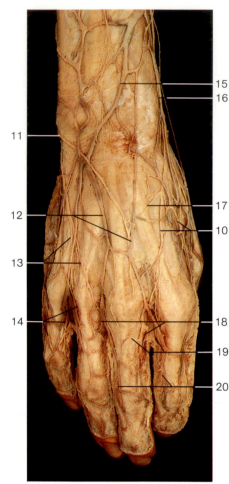

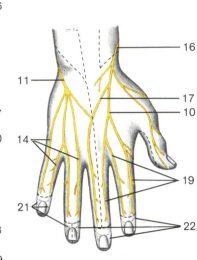

Dorsum of hand, superficial layer. Venous network and cutaneous nerves are shown.

Cutaneous innervation of hand (dorsal aspect). (Semischematic drawing). (O.). Innervation pattern of dorsal surface: 2½ digits by radial nerve, 2½ digits by ulnar nerve. Notice that the terminal branches to the dorsal surfaces of the distal phalanges are derived from the palmar digital nerves.

Superficial veins and cutaneous nerves of forearm and hand (anteromedial aspect).

1 Musculocutaneous nerve
2 Cephalic vein in the lateral bicipital groove
3 Cephalic vein in the forearm
4 Posterior cutaneous nerves of forearm
5 Basilic vein
6 Median cubital vein
7 Medial cutaneous nerve of forearm
8 Lateral cutaneous nerve of forearm
9 Superficial branch of radial nerve
10 Dorsal digital branches of radial nerve
11 Dorsal branch of ulnar nerve
12 Venous network on the dorsum of the hand
13 Common dorsal digital branches of ulnar nerve
14 Proper dorsal digital branches of ulnar nerve
15 Cephalic vein (roots at the wrist)
16 Superficial branch of radial nerve
17 Communicating branch with ulnar nerve
18 Intercapital veins
19 Dorsal digital nerves (radial nerve)
20 Dorsal digital veins
21 Palmar digital nerves (ulnar nerve)
22 Proper palmar digital nerves (median nerve)

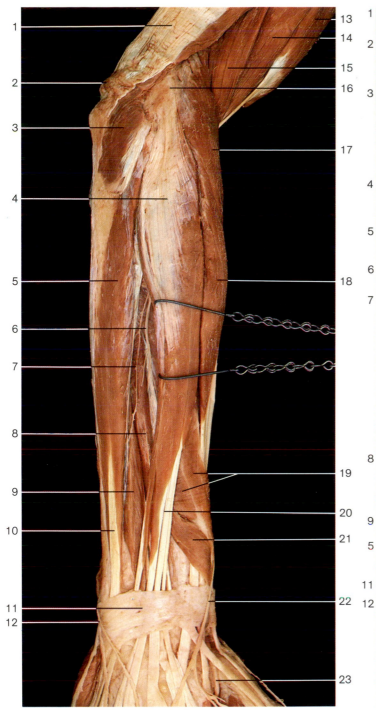

Vessels and nerves of right forearm, superficial layer (dorsal aspect).

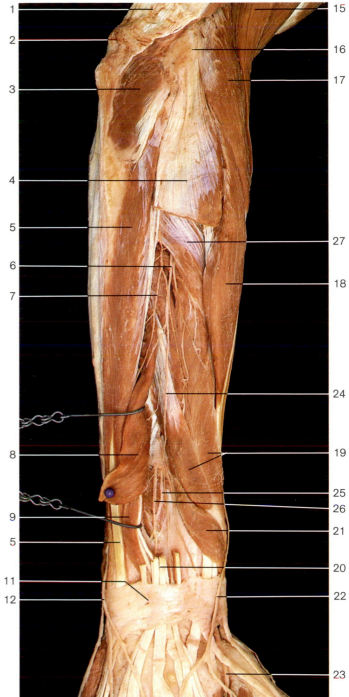

Vessels and nerves of right forearm, deep layer (dorsal aspect).

1 Tendon of triceps brachii	10 Tendon of extensor carpi ulnaris	19 Abductor pollicis longus
2 Olecranon	11 Extensor retinaculum	20 Tendons of extensor digitorum
3 Anconeus	12 Dorsal branch of ulnar nerve	21 Extensor pollicis brevis
4 Extensor digitorum	13 Biceps brachii	22 Superficial branch of radial nerve
5 Extensor carpi ulnaris	14 Brachialis	23 Radial artery
6 Deep branch of radial nerve	15 Brachioradialis	24 Posterior interosseous nerve
7 Posterior interosseous artery	16 Lateral epicondyle of humerus	25 Anterior interosseous nerve
8 Extensor pollicis longus	17 Extensor carpi radialis longus	26 Anterior interosseous artery
9 Extensor indicis	18 Extensor carpi radialis brevis	27 Supinator

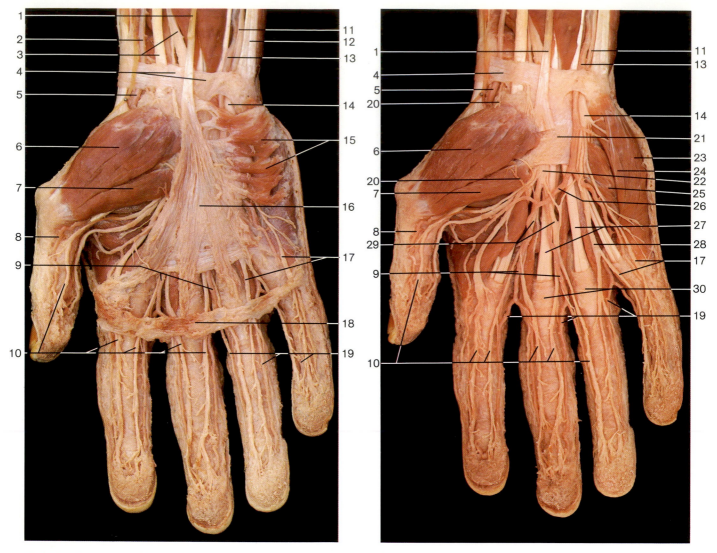

Right hand, superficial layer, dissection of vessels and nerves (palmar aspect).

Right hand, superficial layer, dissection of vessels and nerves (palmar aspect). The palmar aponeurosis has been removed to display the superficial palmar arch.

1 Tendon of palmaris longus
2 **Radial artery**
3 Tendon of flexor carpi radialis and median nerve
4 Distal part of antebrachial fascia
5 Radial artery turning into the anatomical snuffbox
6 Abductor pollicis brevis
7 Superficial head of flexor pollicis brevis
8 Palmar digital artery of thumb
9 Common palmar digital arteries
10 Proper palmar digital nerves (median nerve)
11 **Ulnar nerve**
12 Tendon of flexor carpi ulnaris
13 **Ulnar artery**
14 Superficial branch of ulnar nerve
15 Palmaris brevis
16 Aponeurosis of palmaris longus

17 Palmar digital nerves (ulnar nerve)
18 Superficial transverse metacarpal ligament
19 Proper palmar digital arteries
20 Superficial palmar branch of radial artery (contributing to the superficial palmar arch)
21 Flexor retinaculum
22 **Median nerve**
23 Abductor digiti minimi
24 Flexor digiti minimi brevis
25 Opponens digiti minimi
26 **Superficial palmar arch**
27 Tendons of flexor digitorum superficialis
28 Common palmar digital branch of ulnar nerve
29 Common palmar digital branch of median nerve
30 Fibrous sheath of flexor tendons

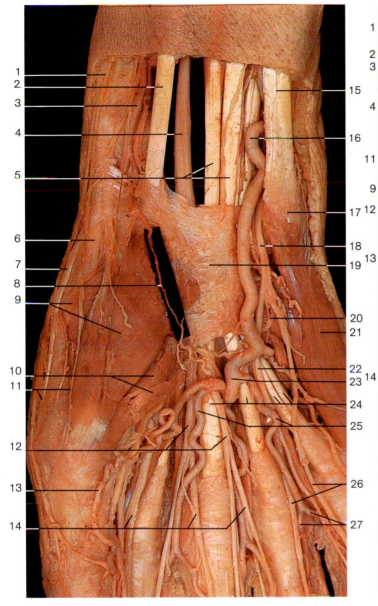

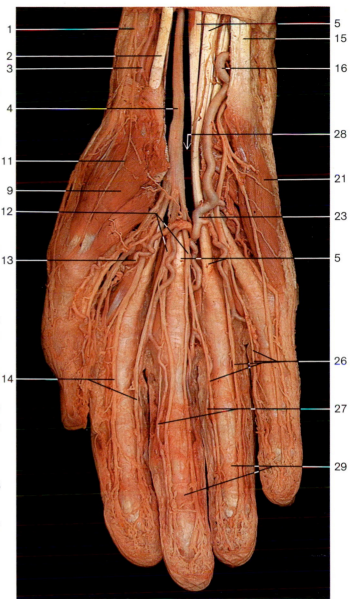

Right hand, superficial layer (palmar aspect). Dissection of the superficial palmar arch.

Right hand, middle layer (palmar aspect). The flexor retinaculum has been removed.

1   Superficial branch of radial nerve
2   Tendon of flexor carpi radialis
3   Radial artery
4   Median nerve
5   Tendon of flexor digitorum superficialis
6   Tendon of abductor pollicis longus
7   Tendon of extensor pollicis brevis
8   Superficial palmar branch of radial artery
9   Abductor pollicis brevis
10 Superficial head of flexor pollicis brevis
11 Terminal branches of superficial branch of radial nerve
12 Common palmar digital nerves (median nerve)
13 Palmar digital artery of thumb
14 Proper palmar digital nerves (median nerve)
15 Tendon of flexor carpi ulnaris
16 Ulnar artery

17 Position of pisiform bone
18 Superficial branch of ulnar nerve
19 Flexor retinaculum
20 Deep branch of ulnar nerve
21 Abductor digiti minimi
22 Common palmar digital nerves (ulnar nerve)
23 Superficial palmar arch
24 Tendons of flexor digitorum muscles
25 Common palmar digital arteries
26 Palmar digital nerves (ulnar nerve)
27 Proper palmar digital arteries
28 Carpal tunnel
29 Fibrous sheaths for the tendons of the flexors of fingers

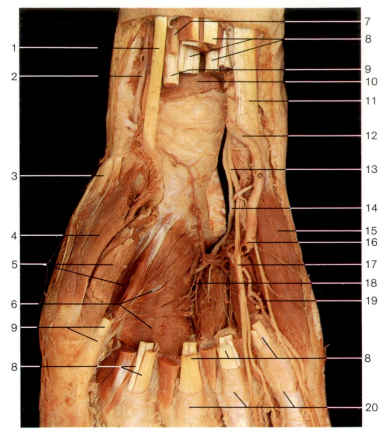

Right hand, deep layer (palmar aspect). The carpal tunnel has been opened, the tendons of the flexor muscles have been removed and the superficial palmar arch has been cut.

1 Tendon of flexor carpi radialis
2 Radial artery
3 Tendon of abductor pollicis longus
4 Abductor pollicis brevis
5 Superficial and deep heads of flexor pollicis brevis
6 Oblique and transverse heads of adductor pollicis
7 Median nerve
8 Tendons of flexores digitorum longus et brevis
9 Tendon of flexor pollicis longus
10 Pronator quadratus
11 Tendon of flexor carpi ulnaris
12 Ulnar artery
13 Superficial branch of ulnar nerve
14 Deep branch of ulnar nerve
15 Abductor digiti minimi
16 **Superficial palmar arch** (cut end)
17 Common palmar digital nerves (ulnar nerve)
18 Palmar metacarpal arteries of deep palmar arch
19 Palmar digital artery of the 5th finger
20 Fibrous sheaths of flexores digitorum
21 Palmar interosseous muscles
22 Opponens pollicis (cut)
23 **Deep palmar arch**
24 1st dorsal interosseous muscle
25 1st lumbrical muscle

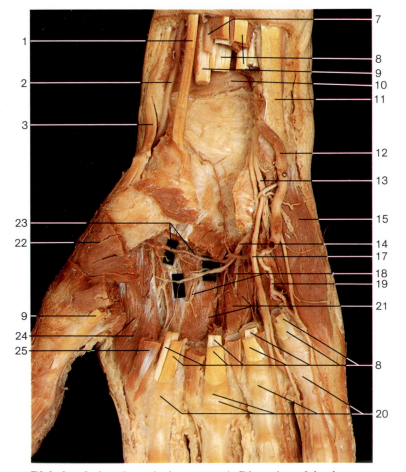

Right hand, deep layer (palmar aspect). Dissection of the deep palmar arch.

Chapter IX

Lower Limb

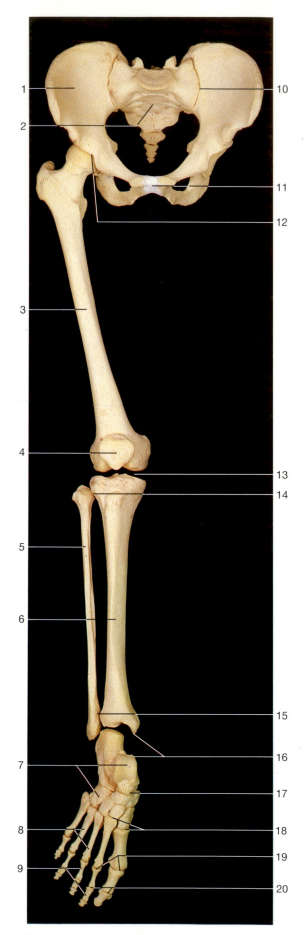

A	Pelvic girdle	9	Phalanges
B	Thigh	10	Sacroiliac joint
C	Leg	11	Pubic symphysis
D	Foot	12	Hip joint
1	Right hip bone	13	Knee joint
2	Sacrum	14	Proximal tibiofibular joint
3	Femur	15	Distal tibiofibular joint
4	Patella	16	Talocrural joint
5	Fibula	17	Talocalcaneonavicular joint
6	Tibia	18	Tarsometatarsal joints
7	Tarsal bones	19	Metatarsophalangeal joints
8	Metatarsal bones	20	Interphalangeal joints

The pelvic girdle is firmly connected to the vertebral column at the sacroiliac joint. Therefore the body can be kept upright more easily even if only one limb is used for support (as in walking). The mobility of the lower limb is more limited than that of the upper limb.

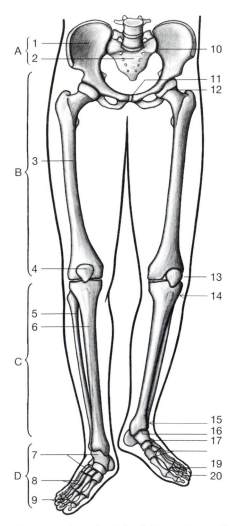

Skeleton of pelvic girdle and lower limb (anterior aspect). The talocrural joint has been dislocated.

Organization of pelvic girdle and lower limb.

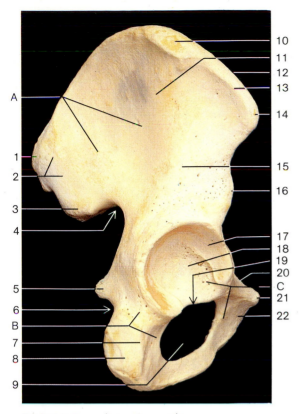

Right hip bone (lateral aspect).

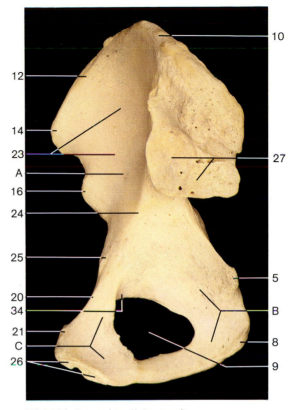

Right hip bone (medial aspect).

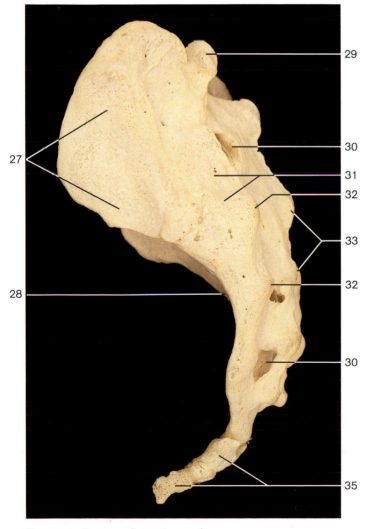

Sacrum and coccyx (lateral aspect).

A   Ilium
B   Ischium
C   Pubis

1   Posterior superior iliac spine
2   Posterior gluteal line
3   Posterior inferior iliac spine
4   Greater sciatic notch
5   Spine of ischium
6   Lesser sciatic notch
7   Body of ischium
8   Ischial tuberosity
9   Obturator foramen
10 Iliac crest
11 Anterior gluteal line
12 Internal lip of iliac crest
13 External lip of iliac crest
14 Anterior superior iliac spine
15 Inferior gluteal line
16 Anterior inferior iliac spine
17 Lunate surface of acetabulum
18 Acetabular fossa
19 Acetabular notch
20 Pecten pubis
21 Pubic tubercle
22 Body of pubis
23 Iliac fossa
24 Arcuate line
25 Iliopubic eminence
26 Articular surface of pubis
27 Auricular surface of sacrum
28 Pelvic surface of sacrum
29 Superior articular process of sacrum
30 Dorsal sacral foramina
31 Sacral tuberosity
32 Lateral sacral crest
33 Median sacral crest
34 Obturator groove
35 Coccyx

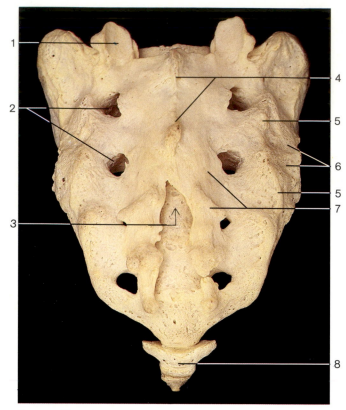

Sacrum (dorsal aspect).

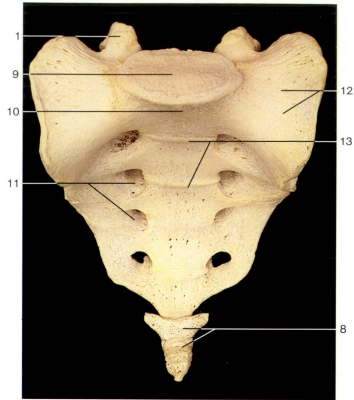

Sacrum (ventral aspect).

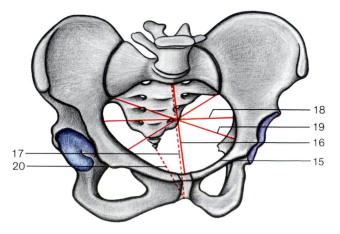

Sacrum (superior aspect).

1 Superior articular process of sacrum
2 Dorsal sacral foramina
3 Sacral hiatus
4 Median sacral crest
5 Lateral sacral crest
6 Sacral tuberosity
7 Intermediate sacral crest
8 Coccyx
9 Base of sacrum
10 Promontory
11 Anterior sacral foramina
12 Lateral part of sacrum
13 Transverse line of sacrum
14 Sacral canal
15 Linea terminalis
16 True conjugate
17 Diagonal conjugate
18 Transverse diameter
19 Oblique diameter
20 Inferior pelvic aperture or outlet

Diameters of pelvis (oblique superior aspect). (Schematic drawing) (W.).

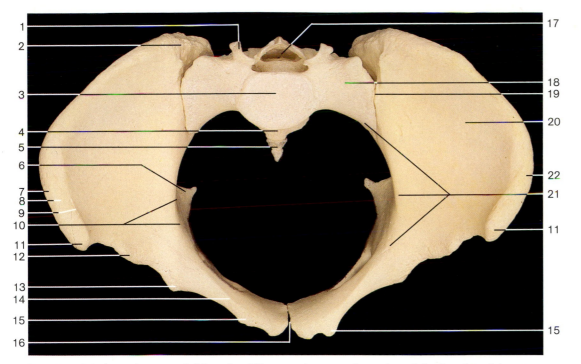

Female pelvis (superior aspect). Note the differences between the male and the female pelvis, predominantly in the form and dimensions of the sacrum, the superior and inferior apertures and the alae of the ilium.

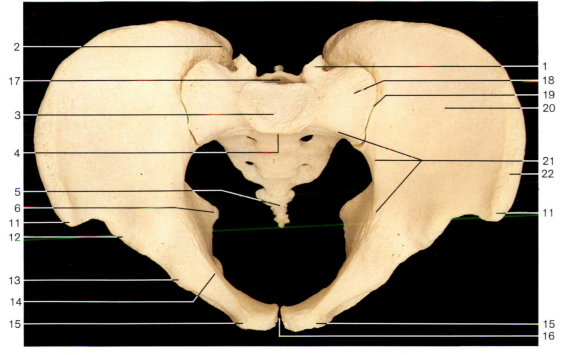

Male pelvis (superior aspect). Compare with the female pelvis (depicted above).

1	Superior articular process of sacrum	12	Anterior inferior iliac spine
2	Posterior superior iliac spine	13	Iliopubic eminence
3	Base of sacrum	14	Pecten pubis
4	Promontory	15	Pubic tubercle
5	Coccyx	16	Pubic symphysis
6	Spine of ischium	17	Sacral canal
7	External lip ⎫	18	Sacrum
8	Intermediate line ⎬ of iliac crest	19	Position of sacroiliac joint
9	Internal lip ⎭	20	Iliac fossa
10	Arcuate line	21	Linea terminalis
11	Anterior superior iliac spine	22	Iliac crest

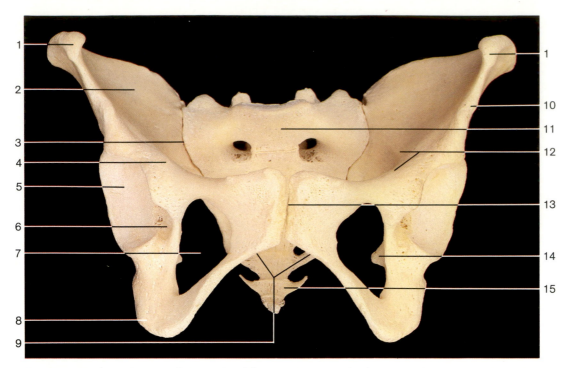

Female pelvis (anterior aspect). Note the differences between the form and dimensions of the male and the female pelvis. The female pubic arch is wider than the male. The obturator foramen in the female pelvis is triangular, while that in the male pelvis is ovoid.

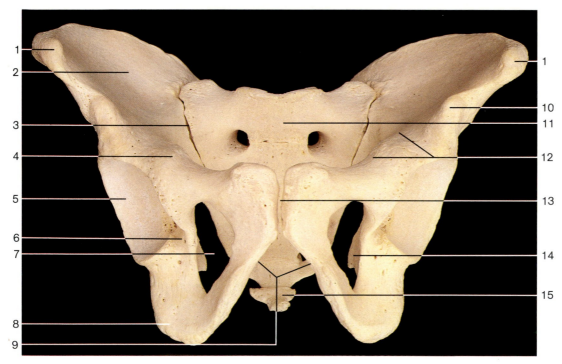

Male pelvis (anterior aspect). Compare with foregoing figure.

1 Anterior superior iliac spine	
2 Iliac fossa	9 Pubic arch
3 Position of sacroiliac joint	10 Anterior inferior iliac spine
4 Iliopubic eminence	11 Sacrum
5 Lunate surface of acetabulum	12 Linea terminalis (at margin of superior aperture)
6 Acetabular notch	13 Pubic symphysis
7 Obturator foramen	14 Spine of ischium
8 Ischial tuberosity	15 Coccyx

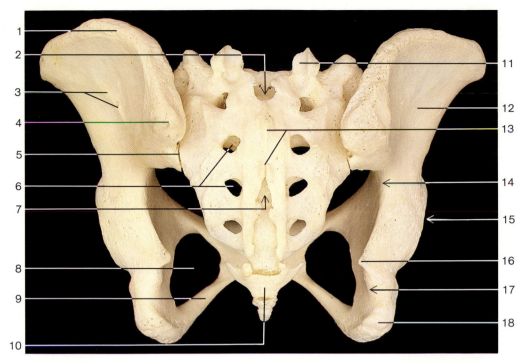

Female pelvis (dorsal inferior aspect). Note the differences between the female and male pelvis, especially with respect to the inferior aperture, the shape of the sacrum, the two sciatic notches and the pubic arch.

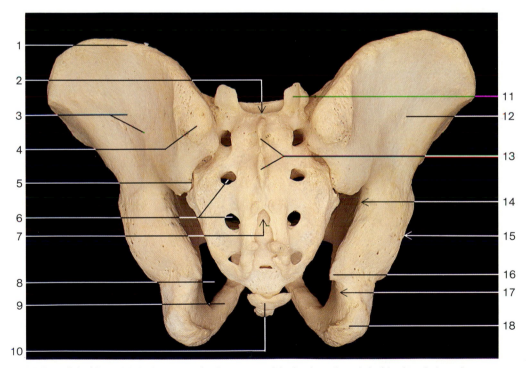

Male pelvis (dorsal inferior aspect). Compare with the female pelvis (depicted above).

1 Iliac crest	10 Coccyx
2 Sacral canal	11 Superior articular process of sacrum
3 Posterior gluteal line	12 Gluteal surface of ilium
4 Posterior superior iliac spine	13 Median sacral crest
5 Position of sacroiliac joint	14 Greater sciatic notch
6 Dorsal sacral foramina	15 Position of acetabulum
7 Sacral hiatus	16 Spine of ischium
8 Obturator foramen	17 Lesser sciatic notch
9 Ramus of ischium	18 Ischial tuberosity

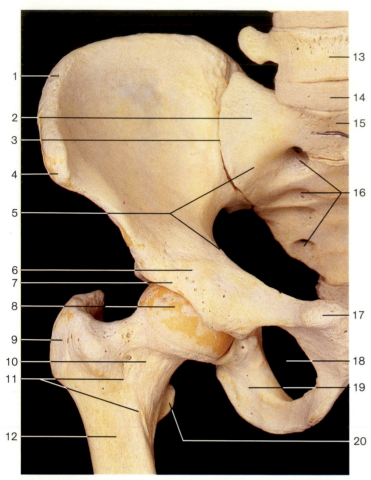

1   Iliac crest
2   Lateral part of sacrum
3   Position of sacroiliac joint
4   Anterior superior iliac spine
5   Linea terminalis
6   Iliopubic eminence
7   Bony margin of acetabulum
8   Head of femur
9   Greater trochanter
10 Neck of femur
11 Intertrochanteric line
12 Shaft of femur
13 5th lumbar vertebra
14 Imitation intervertebral disc between 5th lumbar
    vertebra and sacrum
15 Promontory
16 Anterior sacral foramina
17 Pubic tubercle
18 Obturator foramen
19 Ramus of ischium
20 Lesser trochanter
21 Dorsal sacral foramina
22 Greater sciatic notch
23 Spine of ischium
24 Pubic symphysis
25 Pubis
26 Ischial tuberosity
27 Intertrochanteric crest

Bones of right hip joint (ventral aspect).

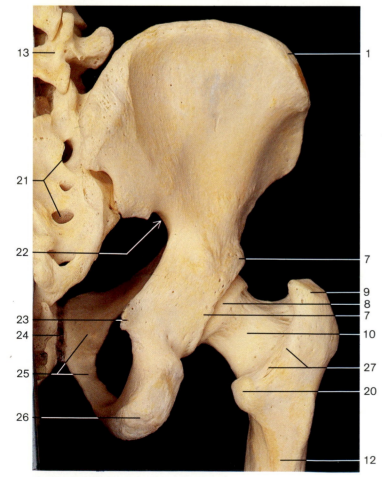

Bones of right hip joint (dorsal aspect).

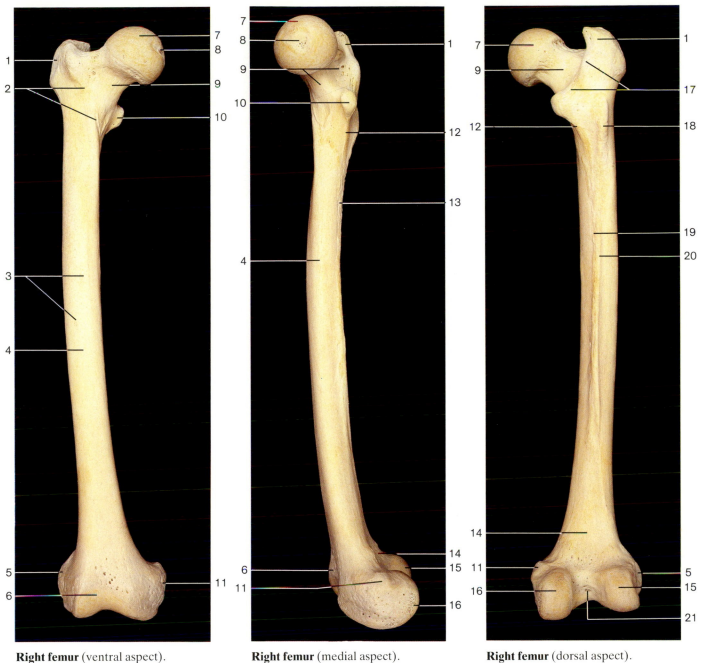

Right femur (ventral aspect). **Right femur** (medial aspect). **Right femur** (dorsal aspect).

1	Greater trochanter	8	Fovea of head	15	Lateral condyle
2	Intertrochanteric line	9	Neck	16	Medial condyle
3	Nutrient foramina	10	Lesser trochanter	17	Intertrochanteric crest
4	Shaft of femur (diaphysis)	11	Medial epicondyle	18	Third trochanter
5	Lateral epicondyle	12	Pectineal line	19	Medial lip of linea aspera
6	Patellar surface	13	Linea aspera	20	Lateral lip of linea aspera
7	Head	14	Popliteal surface	21	Intercondylar fossa

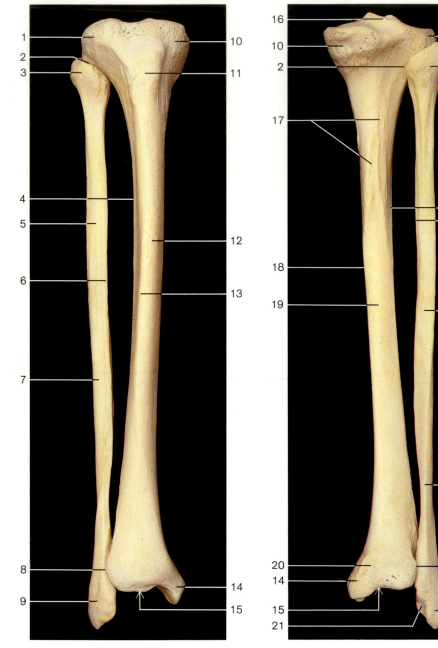

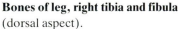

1	Lateral condyle of tibia
2	Position of tibiofibular joint
3	Head of fibula
4	Interosseous border of tibia
5	Shaft of fibula
6	Interosseous border of fibula
7	Lateral surface of fibula
8	Position of tibiofibular joint
9	Lateral malleolus
10	Medial condyle of tibia
11	Tuberosity of tibia
12	Shaft of tibia (diaphysis)
13	Anterior margin of tibia
14	Medial malleolus
15	Inferior articular surface of tibia
16	Intercondylar eminence
17	Soleal line
18	Medial border of tibia
19	Posterior surface of tibia
20	Malleolar sulcus of tibia
21	Malleolar articular surface of fibula
22	Apex of head of fibula
23	Posterior surface of fibula
24	Posterior border of fibula
25	Medial intercondylar tubercle
26	Posterior intercondylar area
27	Anterior intercondylar area
28	Lateral intercondylar tubercle

Bones of leg, right tibia and fibula (ventral aspect).

Bones of leg, right tibia and fibula (dorsal aspect).

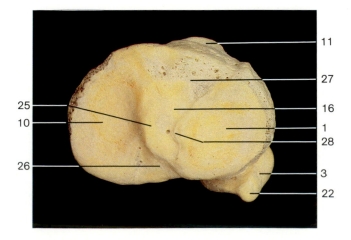

Upper end of right tibia with fibula (from above), anterior margin of tibia above. Superior articular surface of tibia.

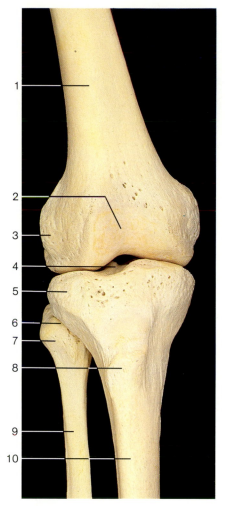

Bones of right knee joint
(anterior aspect).

Bones of right knee joint
(dorsal aspect).

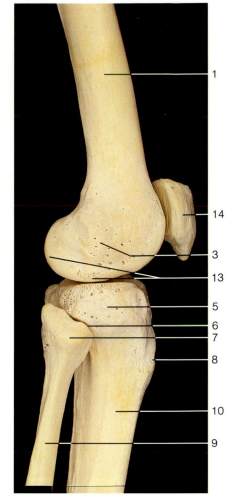

Bones of right knee joint
(lateral aspect).

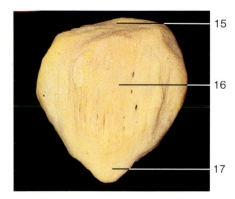

Right patella (anterior aspect).

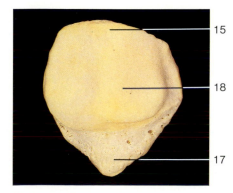

Right patella (posterior aspect).

1 **Femur**
2 Patellar surface of femur
3 Lateral epicondyle of femur
4 Intercondylar eminence of tibia
5 Lateral condyle of tibia
6 Position of tibiofibular joint
7 Head of fibula
8 Tuberosity of **tibia**
9 **Fibula**
10 Shaft of tibia
11 Popliteal surface of femur
12 Intercondylar fossa of femur
13 Lateral condyle of femur
14 **Patella**
15 Base of patella
16 Anterior surface of patella
17 Apex of patella
18 Articular surface of patella

Bones of the Foot

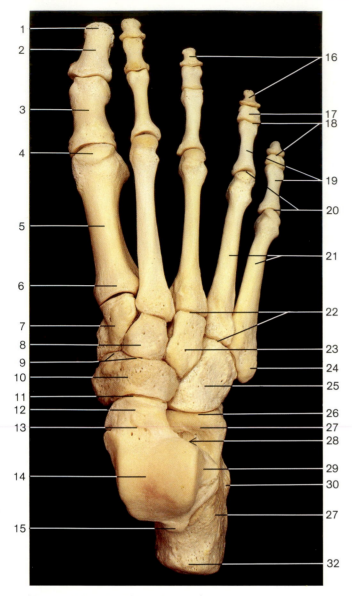

Bones of right foot (dorsal aspect).

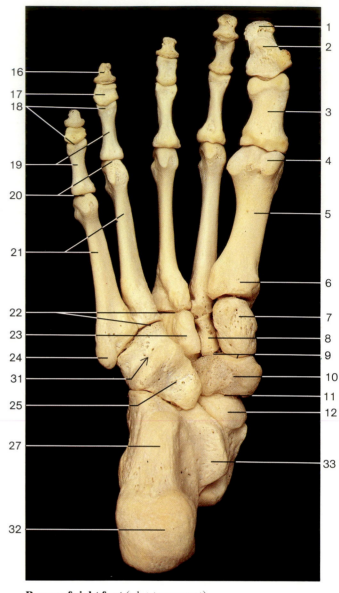

Bones of right foot (plantar aspect).

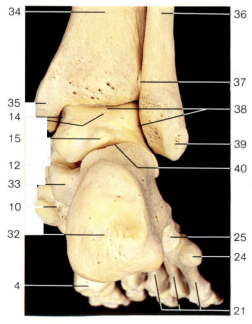

Bones of right foot together with tibia and fibula (posterior aspect).

1   Tuberosity of distal phalanx of great toe
2   Distal phalanx of great toe
3   Proximal phalanx of great toe
4   Head of first metatarsal bone
5   First metatarsal bone
6   Base of first metatarsal bone
7   Medial cuneiform bone
8   Intermediate cuneiform bone
9   Position of **cuneonavicular joint**
10 Navicular bone

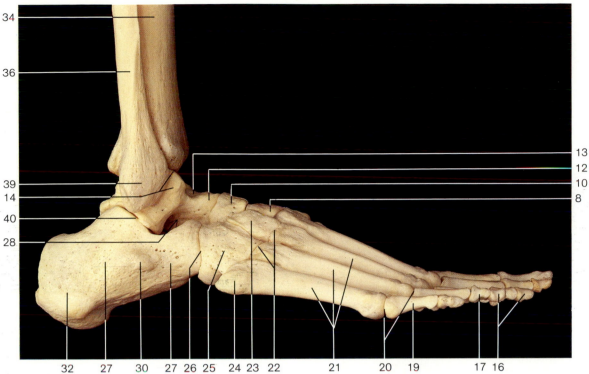

Bones of right foot, tibia and fibula (lateral aspect).

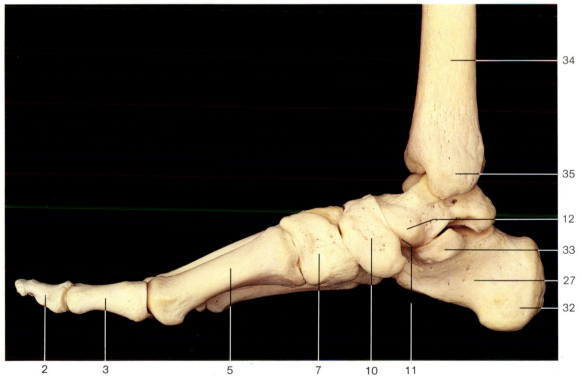

Bones of right foot, tibia and fibula (medial aspect).

11	Position of **talocalcaneonavicular joint**	21	Metatarsal bones	31	Groove for tendon of peroneus longus
12	Head of talus	22	Position of **tarsometatarsal joints**	32	Calcaneal tuberosity
13	Neck of talus	23	Lateral cuneiform bone	33	Sustentaculum tali
14	Trochlea of talus	24	Tuberosity of 5th metatarsal bone	34	Tibia
15	Posterior talar process	25	Cuboid bone	35	Medial malleolus
16	Distal phalanges	26	Position of **calcaneocuboid joint**	36	Fibula
17	Middle phalanges	27	Calcaneus	37	Position of tibiofibular syndesmosis
18	Position of **interphalangeal joints**	28	Tarsal sinus	38	Position of **talocrural joint**
19	Proximal phalanges	29	Lateral malleolar surface of talus	39	Lateral malleolus
20	Position of **metatarsophalangeal joints**	30	Peroneal trochlea of calcaneus	40	Position of **subtalar joint**

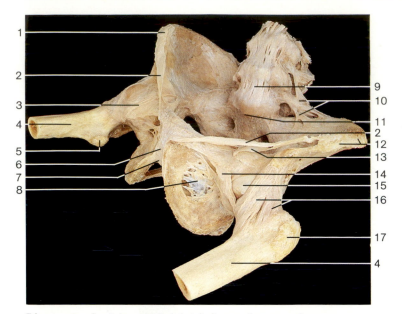

Ligaments of pelvis and hip joint (left anterior aspect).

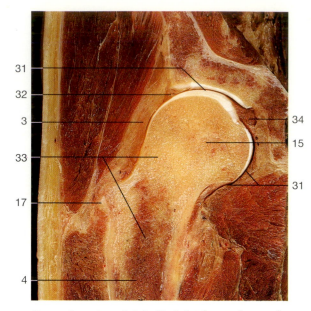

Coronal section of right hip joint (ventral aspect).

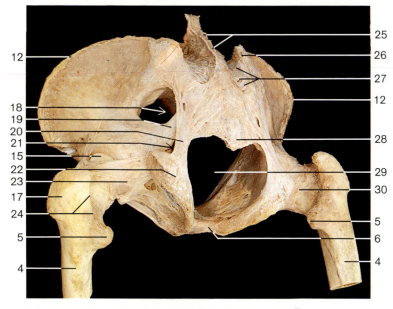

Ligaments of pelvis and hip joint (left posterior aspect).

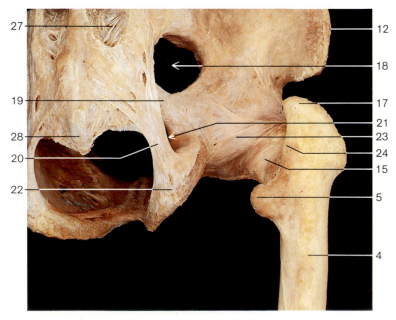

Ligaments of hip joint (dorsal aspect).

1   Anterior superior iliac spine
2   Inguinal ligament
3   Articular capsule of hip joint
4   Femur
5   Lesser trochanter
6   Pubic symphysis
7   Arcuate pubic ligament
8   Obturator membrane
9   5th lumbar vertebra
10 Iliolumbar ligament
11 Promontory
12 Iliac crest
13 Iliopectineal arch
14 Pubofemoral ligament
15 Head of femur
16 Iliofemoral ligament
17 Greater trochanter
18 Greater sciatic foramen
19 Sacrospinous ligament
20 Sacrotuberous ligament
21 Lesser sciatic foramen
22 Ischial tuberosity
23 Ischiofemoral ligament
24 Intertrochanteric crest
25 Spinous processes of lumbar vertebrae
     with supraspinous ligament
26 Posterior superior iliac spine
27 Dorsal sacroiliac ligaments
28 Coccyx with superficial dorsal sacrococcygeal
     ligament
29 Inferior pelvic aperture or outlet
30 Zona orbicularis
31 Articular cavity of hip joint
32 Acetabular lip
33 Spongy bone
34 Ligament of head of femur

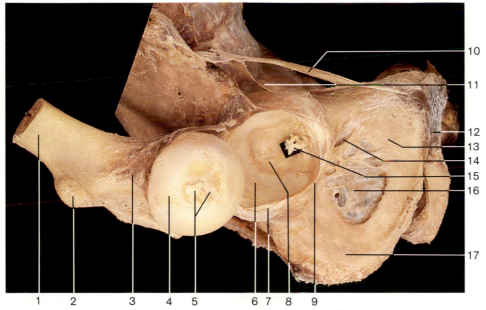

Right hip joint (opened, lateral anterior aspect). The ligament of the head of the femur has been divided and the femur has been posteriorly reflected.

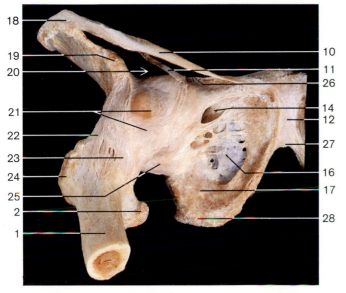

Ligaments of right hip joint (anterior inferior aspect).

1 Femur
2 Lesser trochanter
3 Neck of femur
4 Head of femur
5 Fovea of head with remnants of ligament of head
6 Lunate surface of acetabulum
7 Acetabular lip
8 Acetabular fossa
9 Transverse acetabular ligament
10 Inguinal ligament
11 Iliopectineal arch
12 Pubic symphysis
13 Pubic bone
14 Obturator canal
15 Ligament of head of femur
16 Obturator membrane
17 Ischium
18 Anterior superior iliac spine
19 Anterior inferior iliac spine
20 **Muscular space**
21 Sulcus for iliopsoas
22 Iliofemoral ligament (horizontal band)
23 Iliofemoral ligament (vertical band)
24 Greater trochanter
25 Ischiofemoral ligament
26 **Vascular space**
27 Arcuate pubic ligament
28 Ischial tuberosity
29 Intertrochanteric line

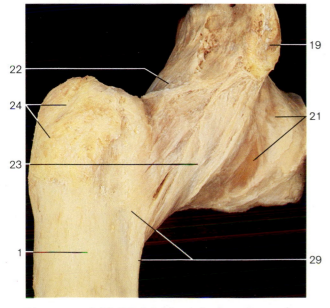

Ligaments of right hip joint (anterior lateral aspect).

Ligaments of the Knee Joint

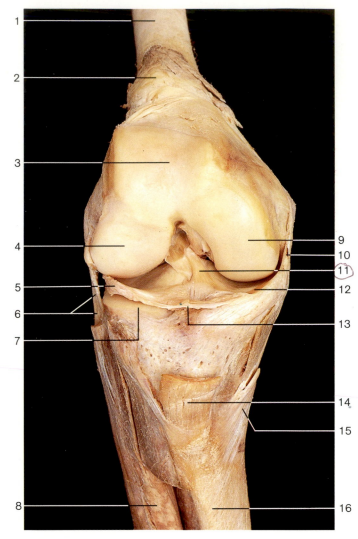

Right knee joint (opened) **with ligaments** (anterior aspect). The patella and articular capsule have been removed and the femur slightly flexed.

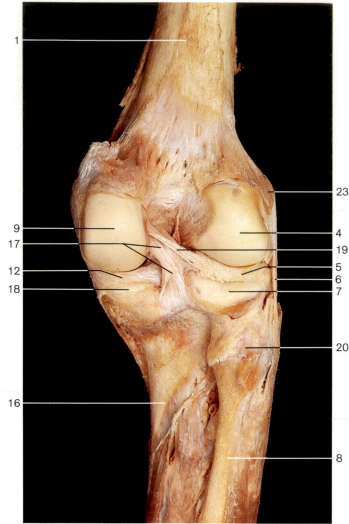

Right joint with ligaments (posterior aspect). The joint is extended and the articular capsule has been removed.

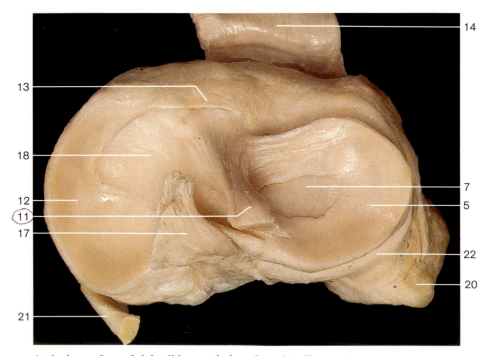

Articular surface of right tibia, menisci, and cruciate ligaments (superior aspect). Anterior margin of tibia above.

1 Femur
2 Articular capsule with suprapatellar bursa
3 Patellar surface
4 Lateral condyle of femur
5 Lateral meniscus of knee joint
6 Fibular collateral ligament
7 Lateral condyle of tibia (superior articular surface)
8 Fibula
9 Medial condyle of femur
10 Tibial collateral ligament
11 Anterior cruciate ligament
12 Medial meniscus of knee joint
13 Transverse ligament of knee
14 Patellar ligament
15 Common tendon of sartorius, semitendinosus and gracilis
16 Tibia
17 Posterior cruciate ligament
18 Medial condyle of tibia (superior articular surface)
19 Posterior meniscofemoral ligament
20 Head of fibula
21 Tendon of semimembranosus muscle
22 Posterior attachment of articular capsule of knee joint
23 Lateral epicondyle of femur

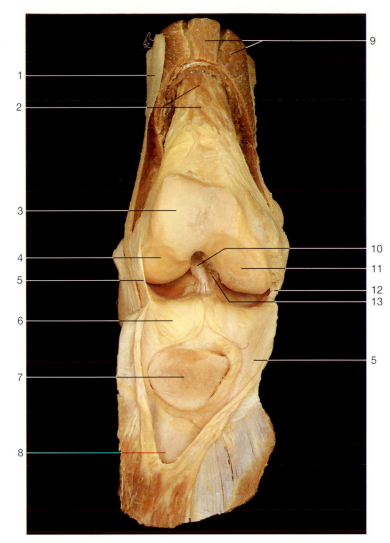

1 Iliotibial tract
2 Articularis genus
3 Patellar surface
4 Lateral condyle of femur
5 Articular capsule
6 Infrapatellar fat pad
7 **Patella,** articular surface
8 **Suprapatellar bursa**
9 Quadriceps muscle of thigh (divided)
10 **Anterior cruciate ligament**
11 Medial condyle of femur
12 Tibial collateral ligament
13 **Posterior cruciate ligament**
14 Medial epicondyle of femur
15 Intercondylar fossa of femur
16 Fibular collateral ligament
17 **Medial meniscus** of knee joint
18 Medial intercondylar tubercle
19 Femur
20 Lateral epicondyle of femur
21 **Lateral meniscus** of knee joint
22 Epiphyseal line of tibia
23 Tibia

Right knee joint, opened (anterior aspect). Patellar ligament with patella reflected.

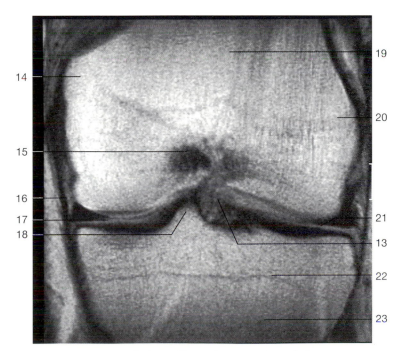

Right knee joint. MR-Scan. Frontal section through the central part of the joint (posterior aspect).

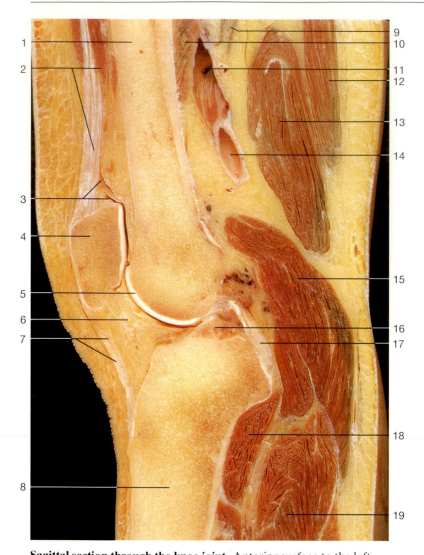

1	**Femur**
2	Quadriceps femoris
3	Suprapatellar bursa, articular cavity
4	**Patella**
5	Patellar surface (articular cartilage)
6	Infrapatellar fat pad
7	Patellar ligament
8	**Tibia**
9	Tibial nerve
10	Adductor magnus
11	Popliteal vein
12	Semitendinosus
13	Semimembranosus
14	**Popliteal artery**
15	Gastrocnemius
16	Anterior cruciate ligament
17	Posterior cruciate ligament
18	Popliteus
19	Soleus muscle
20	Deep flexor muscles of leg
21	Tendo calcaneus
22	Epiphyseal line of tibia
23	Calcaneus
24	**Talocrural joint**
25	Talus

Sagittal section through the knee joint. Anterior surface to the left.

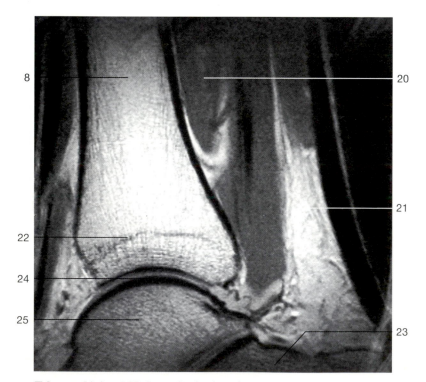

Talocrural joint. MR-Scan. Sagittal section; anterior part to the left.

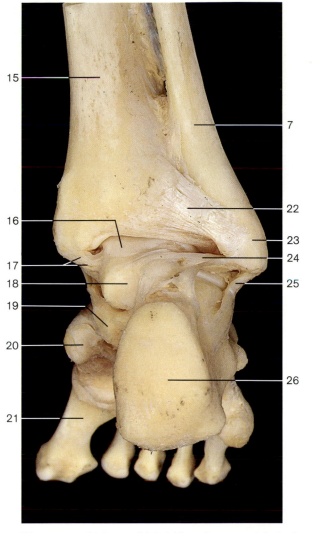

Ligaments of talocrural joint (dorsal aspect, right leg).

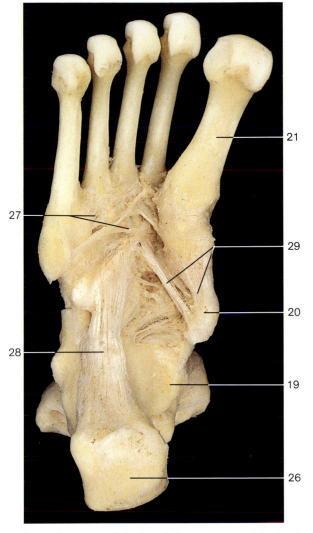

Deep ligaments of the foot (plantar aspect, right foot).
The toes have been removed.

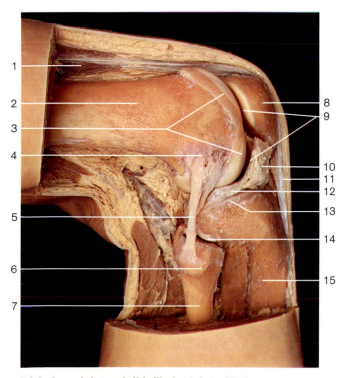

Right knee joint and tibiofibular joint with ligaments.
Note the position of the lateral meniscus.

1 Quadriceps femoris
2 Femur
3 Patellar surface
4 Lateral epicondyle of femur
5 Fibular collateral ligament
6 Head of fibula
7 Fibula
8 Patella
9 Articular cavity of knee joint
10 Infrapatellar fat pad
11 Patellar ligament
12 Lateral meniscus of knee joint
13 Lateral condyle of tibia (superior articular facet)
14 Tibiofibular joint
15 Tibia
16 Trochlea of talus, superior surface
17 Deltoid ligament of ankle (posterior tibiotalar part)
18 Talus
19 Sustentaculum tali
20 Navicular bone
21 1st metatarsal bone
22 Posterior tibiofibular ligament
23 Lateral malleolus
24 Posterior talofibular ligament
25 Calcaneofibular ligament
26 Calcaneal tuberosity
27 Plantar tarsometatarsal ligaments
28 Long plantar ligament
29 Plantar cuneonavicular ligaments

413

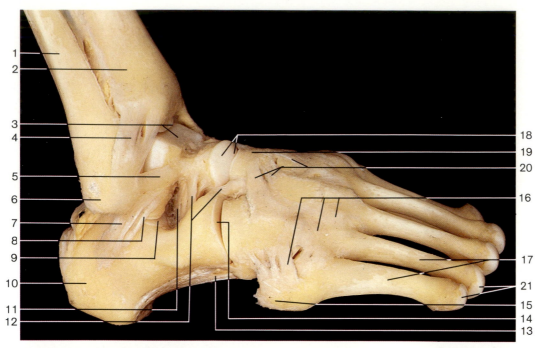

Ligaments of right foot (lateral aspect).

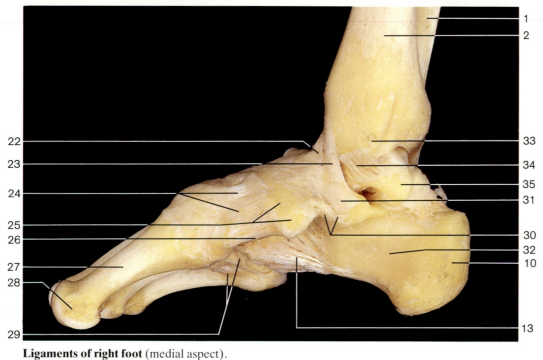

Ligaments of right foot (medial aspect).

1 Fibula
2 Tibia
3 Trochlea of talus
4 Anterior tibiofibular ligament **(talocrural joint)**
5 Anterior talofibular ligament
6 Lateral malleolus
7 Calcaneofibular ligament
8 Lateral talocalcaneal ligament
9 **Subtalar joint**
10 Tuber calcanei
11 Interosseous talocalcaneal ligament
12 Bifurcate ligament
13 Long plantar ligament
14 **Calcaneocuboid joint**
15 Tuberosity of 5th metatarsal bone
16 Dorsal tarsometatarsal ligaments
17 Metatarsal bones

18 Head of talus **(talocalcaneonavicular joint)**
19 Navicular bone
20 Dorsal cuneonavicular ligaments
21 Heads of metatarsal bones
22 Medial or deltoid ligament of ankle, tibionavicular part
23 Medial or deltoid ligament of ankle, tibiocalcaneal part
24 Dorsal cuneonavicular ligaments
25 Navicular bone
26 Plantar cuneonavicular ligament
27 1st metatarsal bone
28 Head of 1st metatarsal bone
29 Plantar tarsometatarsal ligaments
30 Plantar calcaneonavicular ligament
31 Sustentaculum tali
32 Calcaneus
33 Medial malleolus
34 Medial or deltoid ligament of ankle, posterior part
35 Talus

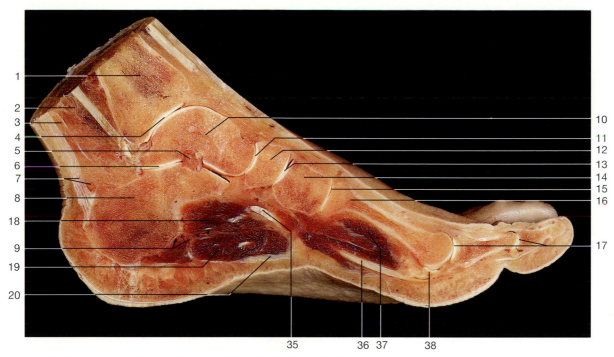

Longitudinal section through the foot at the level of first phalanx.

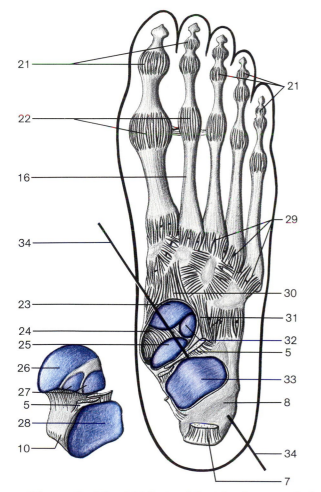

Ligaments of the right foot and the talocalcaneonavicular joint (dorsal aspect). The talus has been rotated to show the corresponding articular surfaces of the three interconnected bones. (Schematic drawing) (W.).

1   Tibia
2   Deep flexors
3   Superficial flexors
4   **Talocrural joint**
5   Interosseous talocalcaneal ligament
6   **Subtalar joint**
7   Tendo calcaneus or Achilles tendon and bursa
8   Calcaneus
9   Vessels and nerves of foot
10 Talus
11 **Talocalcaneonavicular joint**
12 Navicular bone
13 **Cuneonavicular joint**
14 Intermediate cuneiform bone
15 **Tarsometatarsal joints**
16 Metatarsal bones
17 **Metacarpophalangeal** and **interphalangeal joints**
18 Quadratus plantae with flexor tendons
19 Flexor digitorum brevis
20 Plantar aponeurosis
21 Articular capsules of interphalangeal joints
22 Articular capsules of metatarsophalangeal joints
23 Articular surface of navicular bone
24 Plantar calcaneonavicular ligament
25 Middle talar articular surface of calcaneus
26 Navicular articular surface of talus
27 Anterior and middle calcaneal surfaces of talus
28 Posterior calcaneal surface of talus
29 Dorsal tarsometatarsal ligaments
30 Talonavicular ligament
31 Bifurcate ligament
32 Anterior talar articular surface of calcaneus
33 Posterior talar articular surface of calcaneus
34 Axis for inversion and eversion
35 Tendon of tibialis posterior
36 Tendon of flexor hallucis longus
37 Flexor hallucis brevis
38 Sesamoid bone

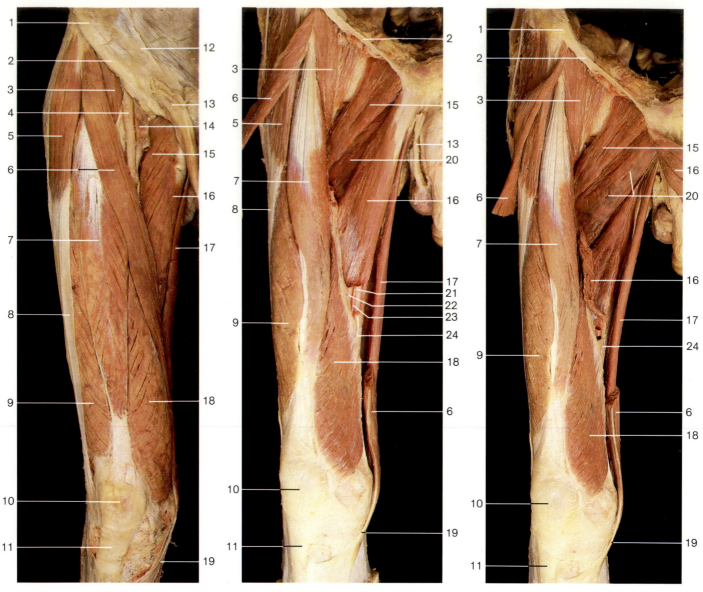

Extensor and adductor muscles of thigh (right thigh, ventral aspect).

Quadriceps femoris and superficial layer of adductor muscles (right thigh, ventral aspect). The sartorius has been divided.

Quadriceps and middle layer of adductor muscles (right thigh, ventral aspect). The sartorius and adductor longus have been divided.

1	Anterior superior iliac spine	13	Spermatic cord
2	Inguinal ligament	14	Femoral vein
3	Iliopsoas	15	**Pectineus**
4	Femoral artery	16	**Adductor longus**
5	Tensor fasciae latae	17	Gracilis
6	Sartorius	18	Vastus medialis
7	Rectus femoris	19	Common tendon of sartorius, gracilis and semitendinosus
8	Iliotibial tract	20	**Adductor brevis**
9	Vastus lateralis	21	Femoral artery
10	Patella	22	Femoral vein
11	Patellar ligament	23	Saphenous nerve
12	Aponeurosis of external oblique muscle of abdomen	24	Vastoadductory lamina of fascia beneath sartorius

21 Femoral artery
22 Femoral vein } entering the adductor canal
23 Saphenous nerve

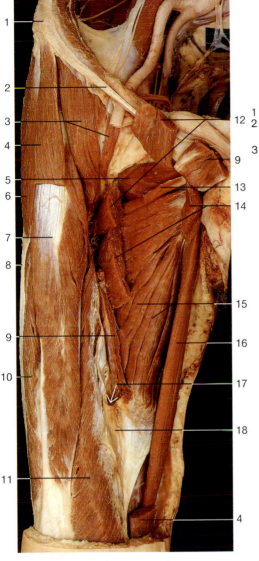

Deep layer of adductor muscles.
Adductor magnus (ventral aspect).
Pectineus, adductor longus and brevis
have been divided.

Course of adductor muscles.
(Schematic drawing) (W.).

1 Pectineus (blue)
2 Adductor minimus (red)
3 Adductor brevis (blue)
4 Adductor longus (blue)
5 Adductor magnus (red)
6 Gracilis (blue)

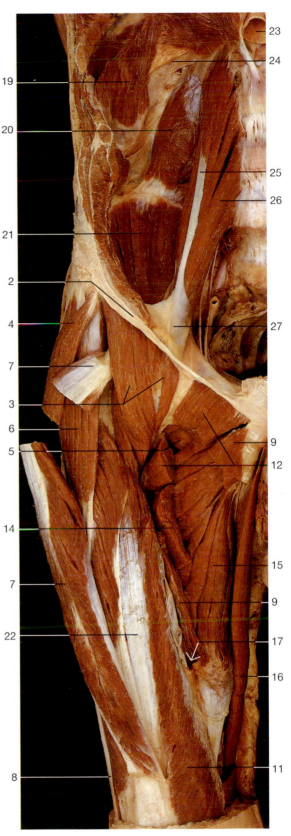

Iliopsoas and adductor muscles; deepest layer
(ventral aspect). Pectineus, adductor longus and
brevis, rectus femoris have been divided.

1 Anterior superior iliac spine	15 **Adductor magnus**
2 Inguinal ligament	16 Gracilis
3 **Iliopsoas muscle**	17 Adductor hiatus
4 Sartorius	18 Vastoadductor membrane
5 Obturator externus	19 Diaphragm
6 Tensor fasciae latae	20 Quadratus lumborum
7 Rectus femoris	21 **Iliacus muscle**
8 Iliotibial tract	22 Vastus intermedius
9 Adductor longus (divided)	23 Aorta in aortic hiatus
10 Vastus lateralis	24 Twelfth rib
11 Vastus medialis	25 **Psoas minor**
12 Pectineus (divided)	26 **Psoas major**
13 Adductor minimus	27 Iliopectineal arch
14 Adductor brevis (divided)	

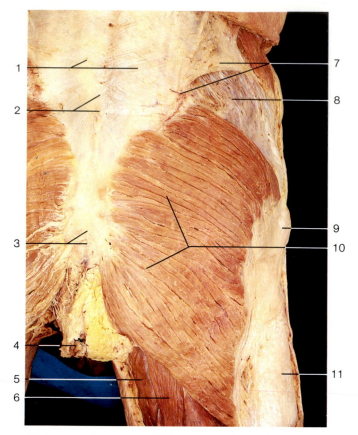

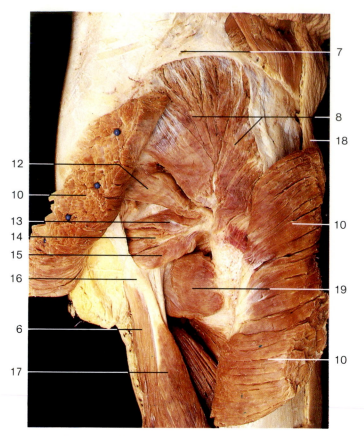

Gluteal muscles, superficial layer (dorsal aspect).

Gluteal muscles, deeper layer (dorsal aspect).

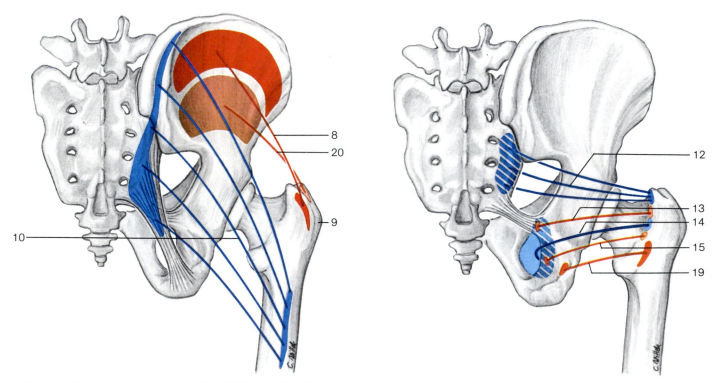

Course of gluteal muscles of superficial (left) and **deep layers** (right). (Schematic drawing) (W.).

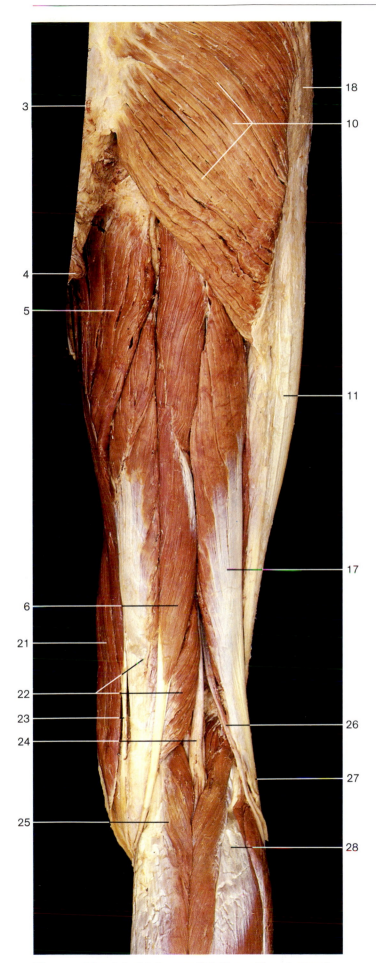

1 Thoracolumbar fascia
2 Spinous processes of lumbar vertebrae
3 Coccyx
4 Anus
5 Adductor magnus
6 Semitendinosus
7 Iliac crest
8 **Gluteus medius**
9 Greater trochanter
10 **Gluteus maximus**
11 Iliotibial tract
12 Piriformis
13 Superior gemellus
14 Obturator internus
15 Inferior gemellus
16 Ischial tuberosity
17 Long head of biceps femoris
18 Tensor fasciae latae
19 Quadratus femoris
20 **Gluteus minimus**
21 Sartorius
22 Semimembranosus
23 Tendon of gracilis
24 Tibial nerve
25 Medial head of gastrocnemius
26 Common peroneal nerve
27 Tendon of biceps femoris
28 Lateral head of gastrocnemius
29 Rectus femoris
30 Vastus medialis
31 Vastus intermedius
32 Vastus lateralis
33 Sciatic nerve
34 Gluteus maximus (insertion)
35 Great saphenous vein
36 Femoral artery
37 Femoral vein
38 Adductor longus
39 Femur
40 Gracilis
41 Septum between semitendinosus
   and semimembranosus

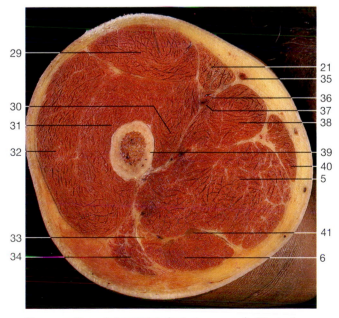

Flexors of the right thigh, superficial layer (dorsal aspect).

Cross section of right thigh (inferior aspect). Ventral side on top.

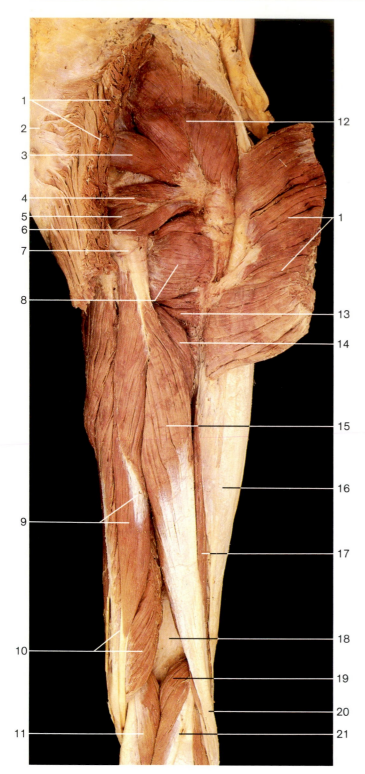

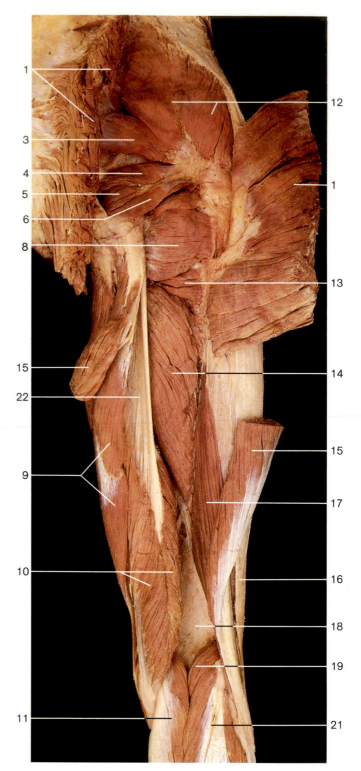

Dorsal muscles of right thigh (posterior aspect).
The gluteus maximus has been divided and reflected.

Dorsal muscles of right thigh (posterior aspect).
The gluteus maximus and the long head of biceps femoris
have been divided and displaced.

1	Gluteus maximus (divided)	9	Semitendinosus muscle with intermediate tendon
2	Position of coccyx	10	Semimembranosus
3	Piriformis	11	Medial head of gastrocnemius
4	Superior gemellus	12	Gluteus medius
5	Obturator internus	13	Adductor minimus
6	Inferior gemellus	14	Adductor magnus
7	Ischial tuberosity	15	Long head of biceps femoris
8	Quadratus femoris	16	Iliotibial tract

17	Short head of biceps femoris
18	Popliteal surface of femur
19	Plantaris
20	Tendon of biceps femoris
21	Lateral head of gastrocnemius
22	Membranous part of semimembranosus

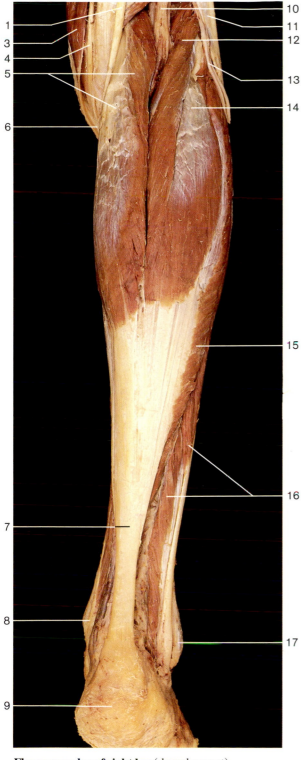

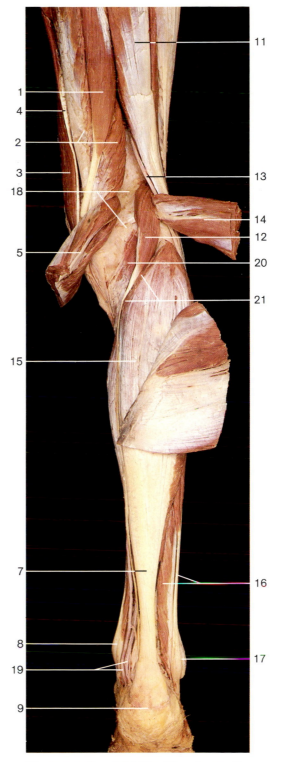

Flexor muscles of right leg (dorsal aspect).

Flexor muscles of right leg (dorsal aspect). Both heads of the gastrocnemius have been divided and reflected.

1	Semitendinosus	8	Medial malleolus
2	Semimembranosus	9	Calcaneal tuberosity
3	Sartorius	10	Tibial nerve
4	Tendon of gracilis	11	Biceps femoris
5	Medial head of gastrocnemius	12	Plantaris
6	Common tendon of gracilis, sartorius and semitendinosus	13	Common peroneal nerve
		14	Lateral head of gastrocnemius
7	Tendo calcaneus (Achilles tendon)	15	Soleus muscle

16	Peroneus longus and brevis
17	Lateral malleolus
18	Popliteal fossa
19	Tibial nerve and posterior tibial artery
20	Popliteus
21	Tendinous arch of soleus

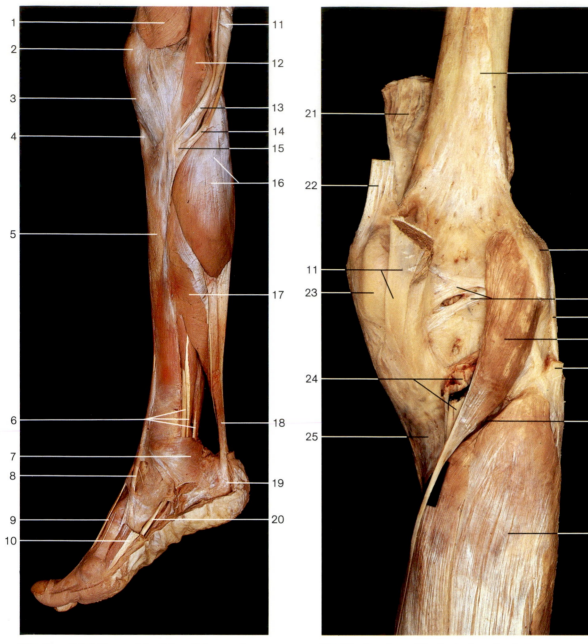

Muscles of right leg and foot (medial aspect).

Popliteal region with plantaris and soleus
(right side, dorsal aspect). Notice the insertion of
the tendon of semimembranosus.

1 Vastus medialis	16 Medial head of gastrocnemius
2 Patella	17 Soleus
3 Patellar ligament	18 Tendo calcaneus (Achilles tendon)
4 Tibial tuberosity	19 Calcaneus
5 Tibia	20 Tendon of flexor hallucis longus
6 Tendons of deep flexor muscles (from anterior to posterior:	21 Quadriceps femoris (divided)
1. tibialis posterior; 2. flexor digitorum longus; 3. flexor hallucis	22 Tendon of adductor magnus (divided)
longus)	23 Medial condyle of femur
7 Flexor retinaculum	24 Popliteal artery and vein, tibial nerve
8 Tendon of tibialis anterior	25 Tibia
9 Tendon of extensor hallucis longus	26 Femur
10 Abductor hallucis	27 Lateral epicondyle of femur
11 Semimembranosus	28 Oblique popliteal ligament
12 Sartorius	29 Lateral collateral ligament
13 Tendon of gracilis	30 Plantaris
14 Tendon of semitendinosus	31 Tendon of biceps femoris (divided)
15 Common tendon of gracilis, semitendinosus and sartorius	32 Tendinous arch of soleus

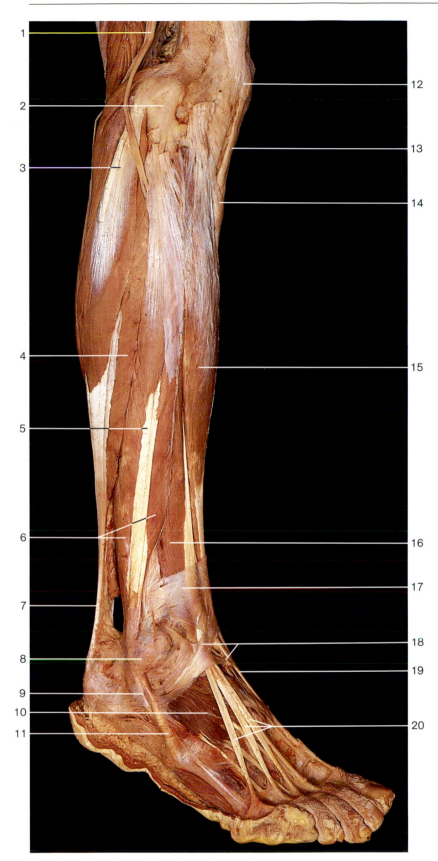

Muscles of right leg and foot (lateral aspect).

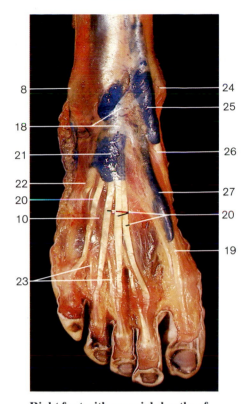

Right foot with synovial sheaths of extensor muscles (dorsal aspect). The synovial sheaths have been injected with blue solution.

1 Common peroneal nerve
2 Head of fibula
3 Lateral head of gastrocnemius
4 Soleus
5 Peroneus longus
6 Peroneus brevis
7 Tendo calcaneus (Achilles tendon)
8 Lateral malleolus
9 Tendon of peroneus longus
10 Extensor digitorum brevis
11 Tendon of peroneus brevis
12 Patella
13 Patellar ligament
14 Tuberosity of tibia
15 Tibialis anterior
16 Extensor digitorum longus
17 Superior extensor retinaculum
18 Inferior extensor retinaculum
19 Tendon of extensor hallucis longus
20 Tendons of extensor digitorum longus
21 Common synovial sheath of extensor digitorum longus
22 Tendon of extensor digitorum longus to the lateral margin of foot (peroneus tertius)
23 Tendons of extensor digitorum brevis
24 Medial malleolus
25 Synovial sheath of tendon of tibialis anterior
26 Tendon of tibialis anterior
27 Synovial sheath of tendon of extensor hallucis longus

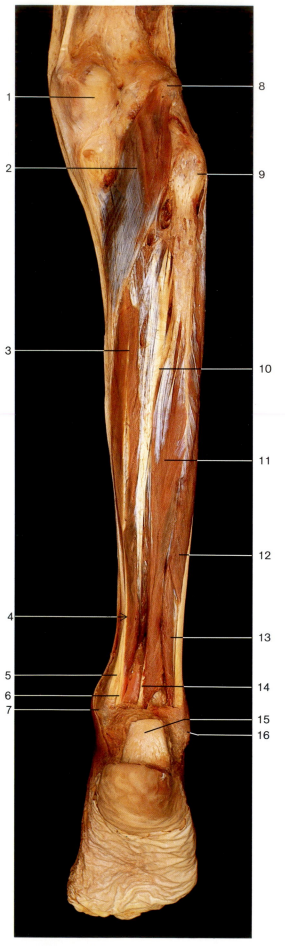

1 Medial condyle of femur
2 Popliteus
3 Flexor digitorum longus
4 Crossing of tendons in leg
5 Tendon of tibialis posterior
6 Tendon of flexor digitorum longus
7 Medial malleolus
8 Lateral condyle of femur
9 Head of fibula
10 Tibialis posterior
11 Flexor hallucis longus
12 Peroneus longus
13 Peroneus brevis
14 Tendon of flexor hallucis longus
15 Tendo calcaneus (divided)
16 Lateral malleolus

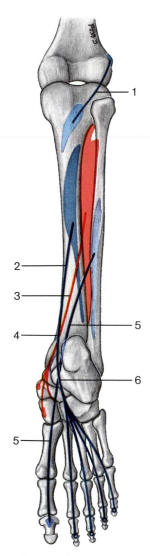

Course of deep flexors of leg. (Schematic drawing) (W.).

1 Popliteus (blue)
2 Flexor digitorum longus (blue)
3 Tibialis posterior (red)
4 Crossing of tendons in leg
5 Flexor hallucis longus (blue)
6 Crossing of tendons in sole

Deep flexors of right leg (dorsal aspect).

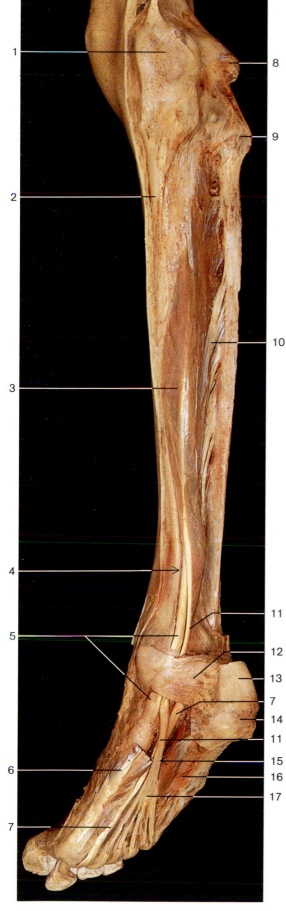

1   Medial condyle of femur
2   Tibia
3   Flexor digitorum longus
4   Crossing of tendons in leg
5   Tendon of tibialis posterior
6   Abductor hallucis
7   Tendon of flexor hallucis longus
8   Lateral condyle of femur
9   Head of fibula
10 Tibialis posterior
11 Tendon of flexor digitorum longus
12 Flexor retinaculum
13 Tendo calcaneus
14 Tuber calcanei
15 Crossing of tendons in sole
16 Quadratus plantae
17 Tendons of flexor digitorum longus
18 Tendon of tibialis anterior
19 Area of insertion of tibialis posterior
20 Lumbrical muscles
21 Flexor hallucis longus

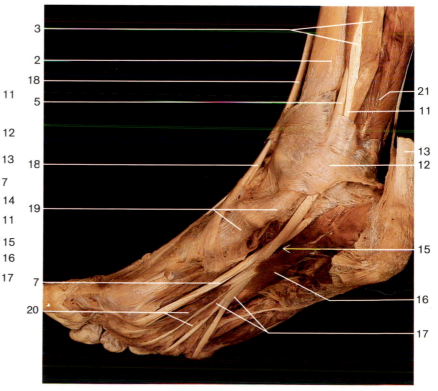

Deep flexors of right leg and foot (posterior oblique medial aspect). Flexor digitorum brevis and flexor hallucis longus have been removed.

Sole of foot; tendons of long flexor muscles (oblique medial and inferior aspect).

425

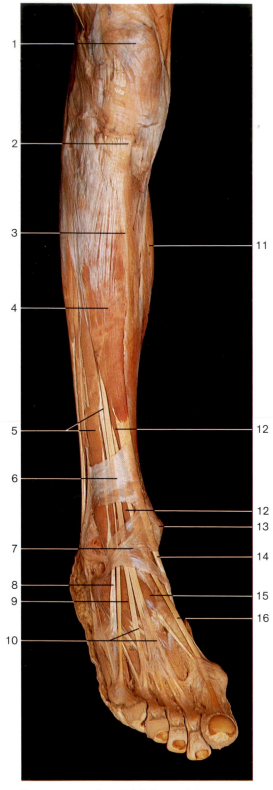

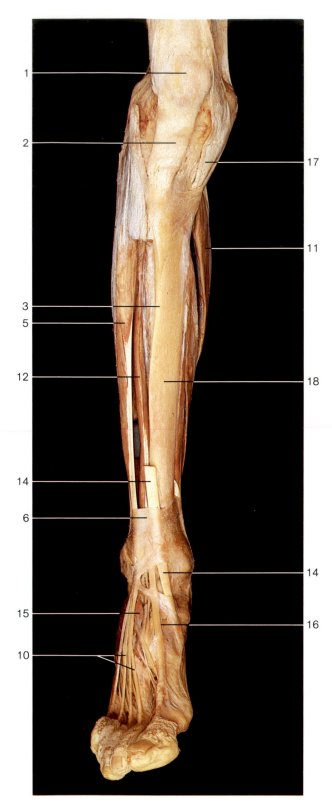

Extensor muscles of right leg and foot
(oblique anterolateral aspect).

Extensors of the right leg and foot
(anterior aspect). Part of the tibialis anterior has been
removed.

1 Patella	8 Tendon of peroneus tertius	15 Extensor hallucis brevis
2 Patellar ligament	9 Extensor digitorum brevis	16 Tendon of extensor hallucis
3 Anterior margin of tibia	10 Tendons of extensor digitorum longus	longus
4 Tibialis anterior	11 Soleus	17 Common tendon of gracilis,
5 Extensor digitorum longus	12 Extensor hallucis longus	semitendinosus and sartorius
6 Superior extensor retinaculum	13 Medial malleolus	18 Tibia
7 Inferior extensor retinaculum	14 Tendon of tibialis anterior	

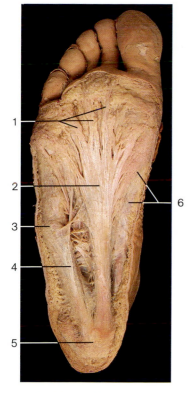

Sole of foot, plantar aponeurosis (from below).

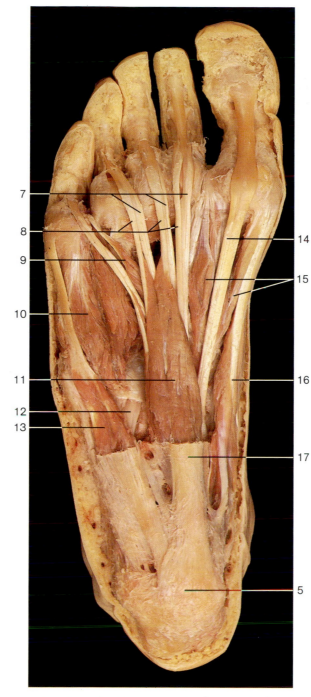

Sole of foot, first layer of muscles (from below).
The plantar aponeurosis and the fasciae of the
superficial muscles have been removed.

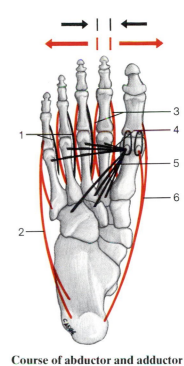

**Course of abductor and adductor
muscles of foot.** (Schematic
drawing) (W.).
Red arrows = abduction.
Black arrows = adduction.

1 Plantar interossei (black)
2 Abductor digiti minimi (red)
3 Dorsal interossei (red)
4 Transverse head of adductor
   hallucis (black)
5 Oblique head of adductor
   hallucis (black)
6 Abductor hallucis (red)

1 Longitudinal bands of plantar aponeurosis
2 Plantar aponeurosis
3 Position of tuberosity of 5th metatarsal bone
4 Muscles of 5th toe with fascia
5 Tuber calcanei
6 Muscles of great toe with fascia
7 Tendons of flexor digitorum longus
8 Tendons of flexor digitorum brevis
9 Lumbrical muscle
10 Flexor digiti minimi brevis
11 Flexor digitorum brevis
12 Tendon of peroneus longus
13 Abductor digiti minimi
14 Tendon of flexor hallucis longus
15 Flexor hallucis brevis
16 Abductor hallucis
17 Plantar aponeurosis (divided)

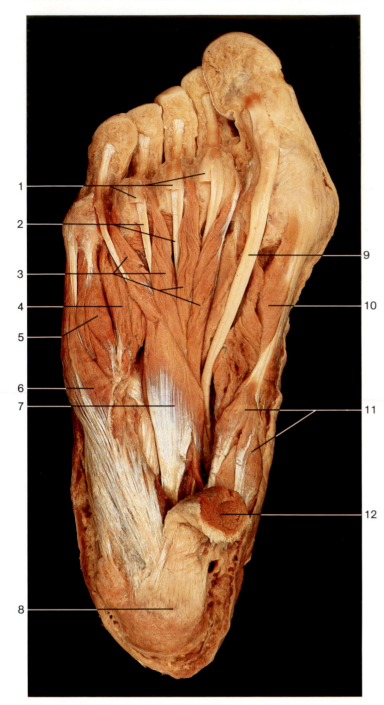

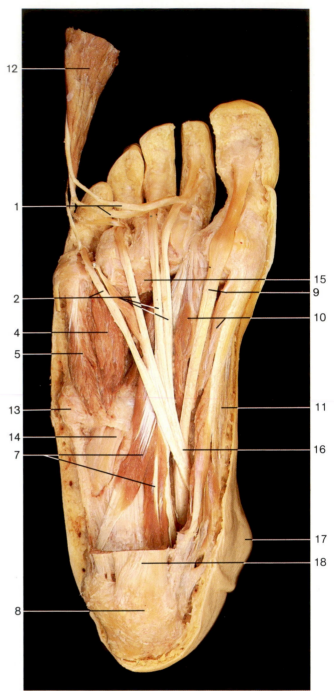

Muscles of sole of foot, second layer (from below).
The flexor digitorum brevis has been divided.

Muscles of sole of foot, second layer (from below).
The tendons of the flexor muscles and the crossing
of tendons are displayed. The flexor digitorum brevis
has been divided and reflected.

1	Tendons of flexor digitorum brevis	7	Quadratus plantae	13	Tuberosity of 5th metatarsal bone
2	Tendons of flexor digitorum longus	8	Tuber calcanei	14	Tendon of peroneus longus
3	Lumbrical muscles	9	Tendon of flexor hallucis longus	15	Transverse head of adductor hallucis
4	Interossei	10	Flexor hallucis brevis	16	Crossing of tendons in sole of foot
5	Flexor digiti minimi brevis	11	Abductor hallucis	17	Medial malleolus
6	Abductor digiti minimi	12	Flexor digitorum brevis (divided)	18	Plantar aponeurosis (divided)

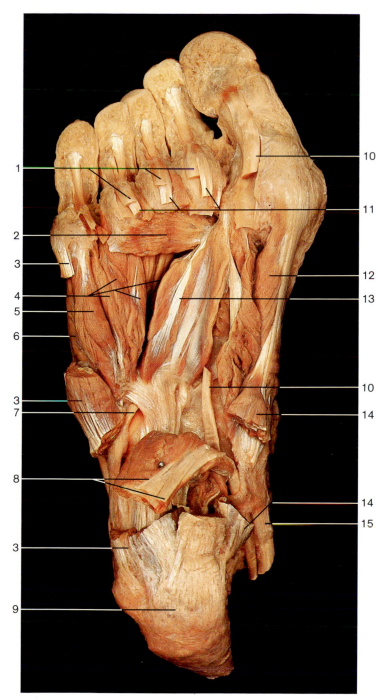

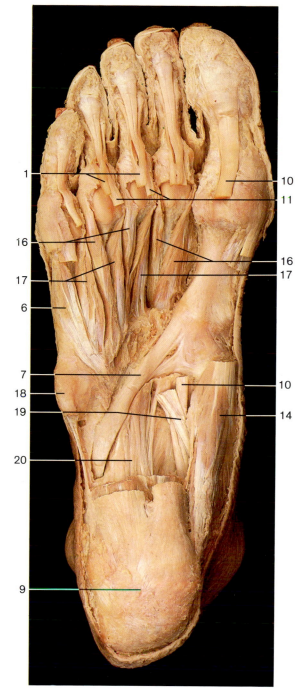

Muscles of sole of foot, third layer (from below). The flexor digitorum brevis has been removed, and the quadratus plantae and the abductor muscles of the little and great toes have been divided.

Muscles of sole of foot, fourth layer (from below). The interosseous muscles and the canal for the tendon of peroneus longus are displayed.

1 Tendons of flexor digitorum brevis	8 Quadratus plantae with tendon of flexor digitorum longus	14 Abductor hallucis (divided)
2 Transverse head of adductor hallucis	9 Calcaneal tuberosity	15 Tendon of tibialis posterior
3 Abductor digiti minimi	10 Tendon of flexor hallucis longus (divided)	16 Dorsal interossei
4 Interosseous muscles	11 Tendon of flexor digitorum longus	17 Plantar interossei
5 Flexor digiti minimi brevis	12 Flexor hallucis brevis	18 Tuberosity of 5th metatarsal bone
6 Opponens digiti minimi	13 Oblique head of adductor hallucis	19 Crossing of plantar tendons
7 Tendon of peroneus longus		20 Long plantar ligament

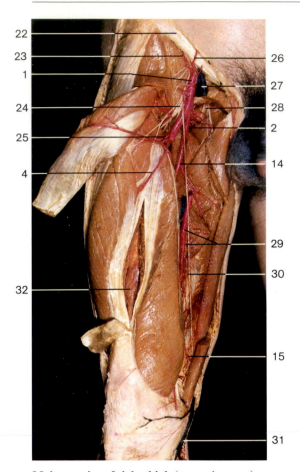

Main arteries of right thigh (ventral aspect).
Femoral artery and vein partly removed.
Red = arteries; blue = veins.

1 **Femoral artery**
2 **Profunda femoris artery**
3 Ascending branch of lateral circumflex femoral artery
4 Descending branch of lateral circumflex femoral artery
5 Lateral superior genicular artery
6 Popliteal artery
7 Lateral inferior genicular artery
8 **Anterior tibial artery**
9 Peroneal artery
10 Lateral plantar artery
11 Arcuate artery with dorsal metatarsal arteries
12 **Plantar arch** with plantar metatarsal arteries
13 Medial circumflex femoral artery
14 Profunda femoris artery with perforating arteries
15 Descending genicular artery
16 Medial superior genicular artery
17 Middle genicular artery
18 Medial inferior genicular artery
19 **Posterior tibial artery**
20 Dorsalis pedis artery
21 Medial plantar artery
22 Inguinal ligament
23 Superficial circumflex iliac artery
24 Femoral nerve
25 Lateral circumflex femoral artery
26 Superficial epigastric artery
27 Femoral vein
28 Obturator nerve
29 Femoral artery and vein
30 Saphenous nerve
31 Great saphenous vein
32 Vastus intermedius

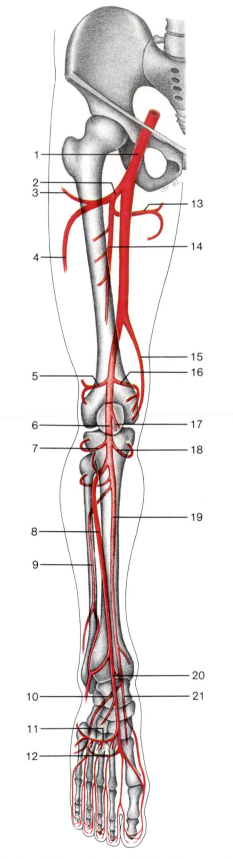

Main arteries of lower extremity (right side, ventral aspect).
(Schematic drawing) (O.).

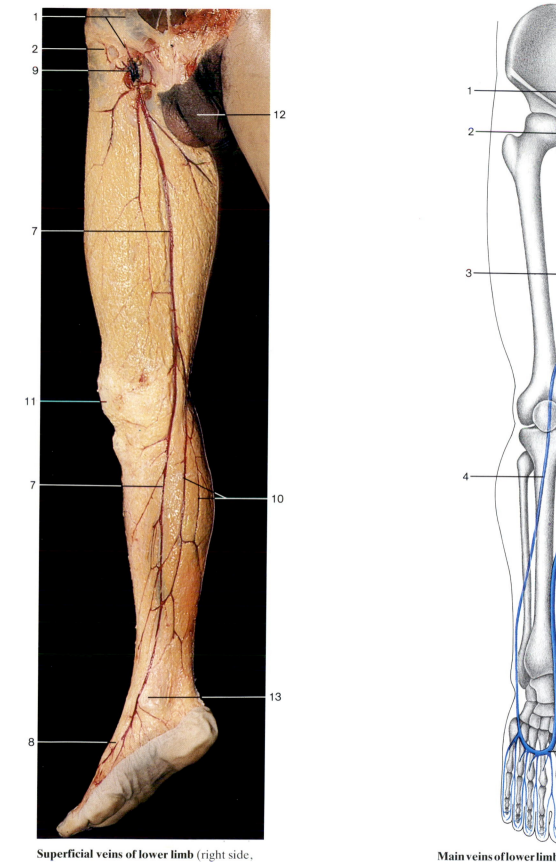

Superficial veins of lower limb (right side, medial anterior aspect). The veins have been injected with red solution.

Main veins of lower limb (right side, anterior aspect). (Schematic drawing) (O.).

1 Superficial epigastric vein
2 Superficial circumflex iliac vein
3 Femoral vein
4 Small saphenous vein
5 External iliac vein

6 External pudendal vein
7 Great saphenous vein
8 Dorsal venous arch
9 Saphenous opening with femoral vein

10 Venous anastomoses of small saphenous vein with great saphenous vein
11 Patella
12 Penis
13 Medial malleolus

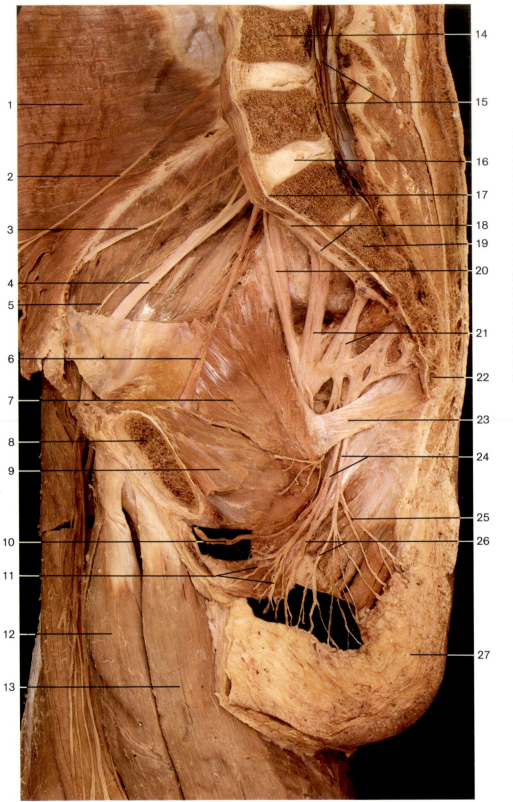

1   Transversus abdominis
2   Iliohypogastric nerve
3   Ilioinguinal nerve
4   **Femoral nerve**
5   Lateral femoral cutaneous nerve
6   Obturator nerve
7   Obturator internus
8   Pubic bone (cut edge)
9   Levator ani (remnant)
10 Dorsal nerve of penis
11 Posterior scrotal nerves
12 Adductor longus
13 Gracilis
14 Body of 4th lumbar vertebra
15 Cauda equina
16 Intervertebral disc
17 Promontory
18 Sympathetic trunk
19 Sacrum
20 **Lumbosacral trunk**
21 **Sciatic plexus**
22 Coccyx
23 Sacrospinous ligament
24 **Pudendal nerve**
25 Inferior rectal nerves
26 Perineal nerves
27 Subcutaneous fat tissue
    of gluteal region

Lumbosacral plexus in situ (right side, medial aspect).
Pelvic organs with peritoneum and part of the levator ani have been removed.

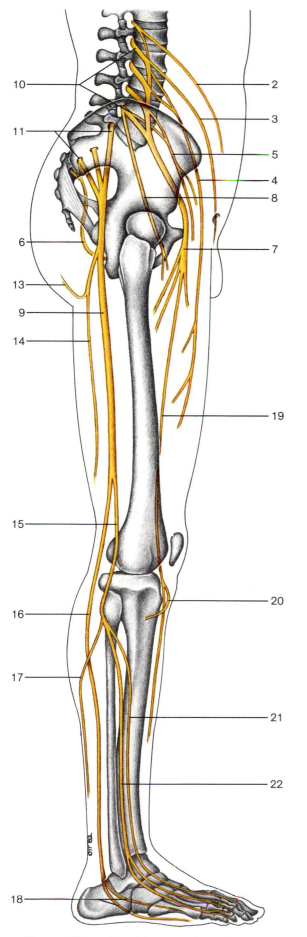

1   Subcostal nerve
2   Iliohypogastric nerve
3   Ilioinguinal nerve
4   Lateral femoral cutaneous nerve
5   Genitofemoral nerve
6   **Pudendal nerve**
7   **Femoral nerve**
8   Obturator nerve
9   **Sciatic nerve**
10   Lumbar plexus (T_{12}-L_3)
11   Sacral plexus (L_4-S_3)   }   lumbosacral plexus
12   "Pudendal" plexus (S_2-S_4)
13   Inferior clunial nerve
14   Posterior femoral cutaneous nerve
15   Common peroneal nerve
16   **Tibial nerve**
17   Lateral sural cutaneous nerve
18   Medial and lateral plantar nerve
19   Saphenous nerve
20   Infrapatellar branch of saphenous nerve
21   **Deep peroneal nerve**
22   **Superficial peroneal nerve**

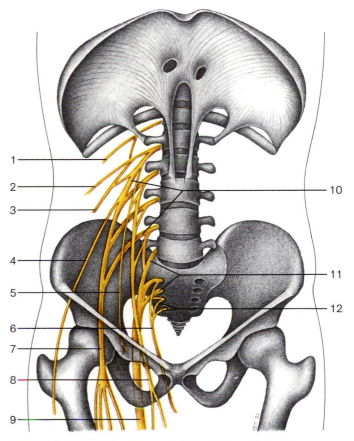

Nerves of lower limb (right side, lateral aspect). (Schematic drawing) (O.).

Main branches of lumbosacral plexus (ventral aspect). (Schematic drawing) (O.).

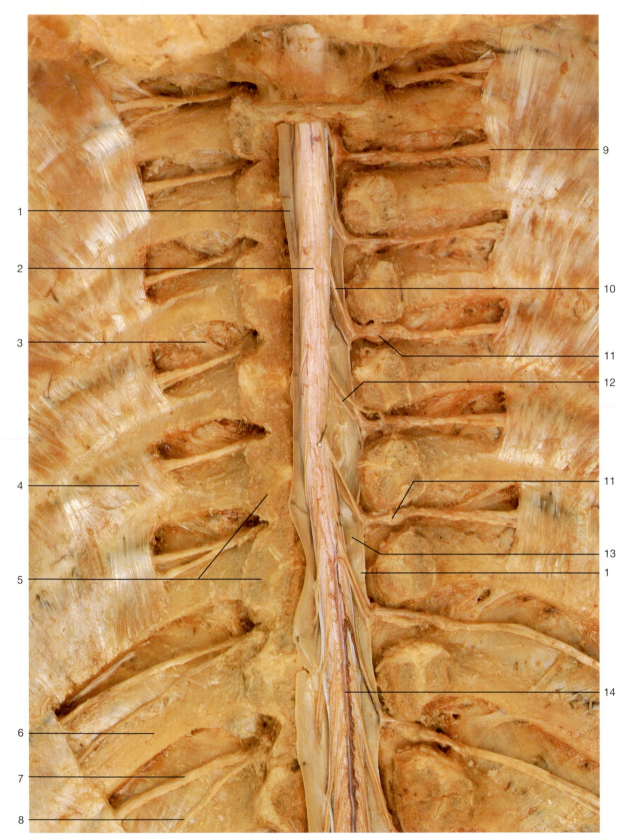

Spinal cord with intercostal nerves. Inferior thoracic region (anterior aspect). Ventral portion of thoracic vertebrae removed, dural sheath opened and spinal cord slightly reflected to the right to display the dorsal and ventral roots.

1	Dura mater	6	Eleventh rib	10	Anterior root filaments
2	**Spinal cord**	7	**Intercostal nerve**	11	Spinal ganglion
3	Costotransverse ligament	8	Collateral branch of intercostal nerve	12	Posterior root filaments
4	Innermost intercostal muscle	9	Intercostal nerve, entering the	13	Arachnoid mater
5	Vertebral arches (cut surfaces)		intermuscular interval	14	Anterior spinal artery

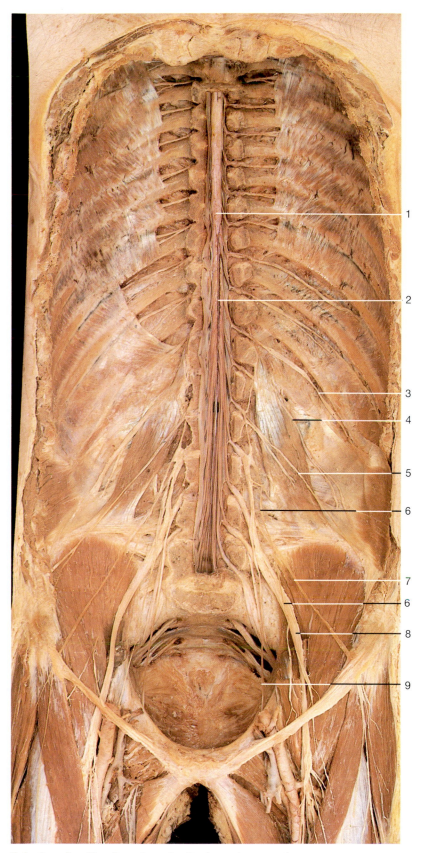

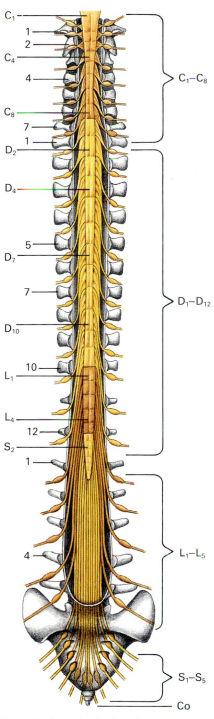

Organization of spinal cord segments
in relation to the vertebral column
(anterior aspect).

Spinal cord and lumbar plexus in situ (anterior aspect).

1	Conus medullaris	4	Iliohypogastric nerve	7	Lateral femoral cutaneous nerve
2	Filum terminale	5	Ilioinguinal nerve	8	Femoral nerve
3	Subcostal nerve	6	Genitofemoral nerve	9	Obturator nerve

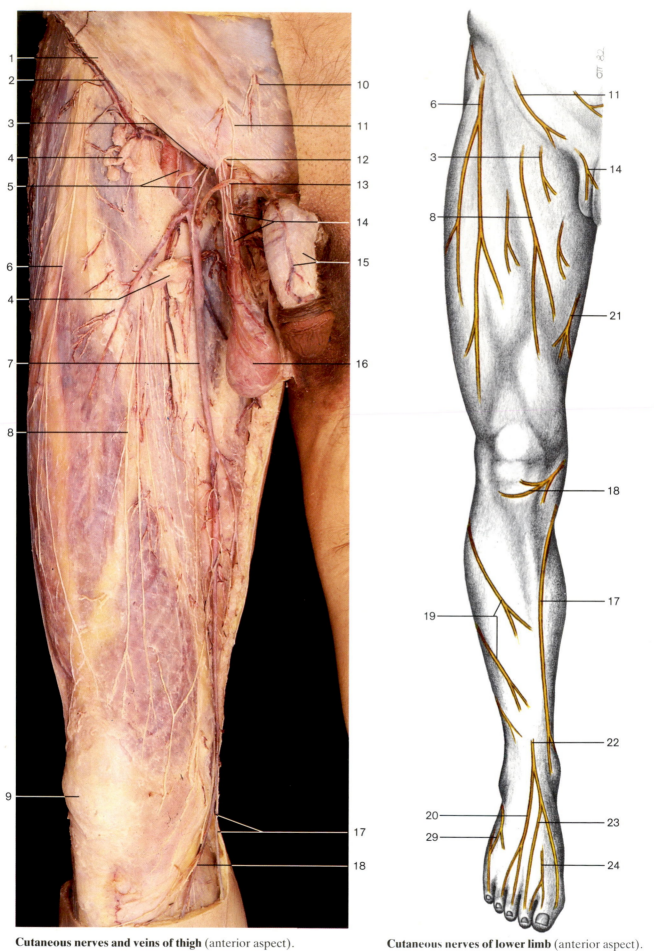

Cutaneous nerves and veins of thigh (anterior aspect).

Cutaneous nerves of lower limb (anterior aspect).
(Schematic drawing) (O.).

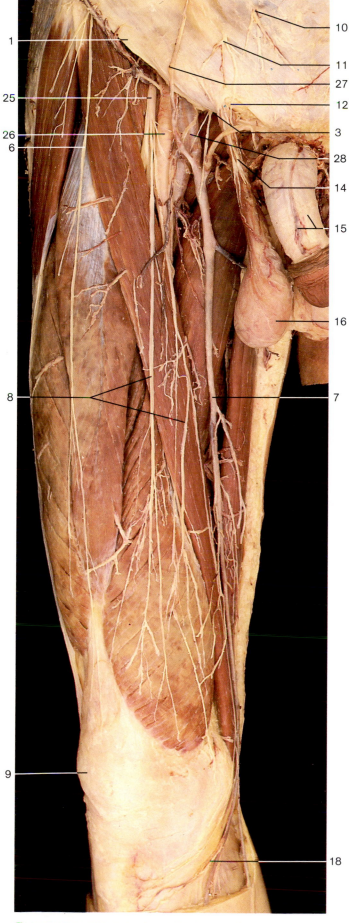

1 Inguinal ligament
2 Superficial circumflex iliac vein
3 Femoral branch of genitofemoral nerve
4 Superficial inguinal lymph nodes
5 Saphenous opening with femoral artery and vein
6 Lateral femoral cutaneous nerve
7 Great saphenous vein
8 Anterior cutaneous branches of femoral nerve
9 Patella
10 Terminal branches of subcostal nerve
11 Terminal branches of iliohypogastric nerve
12 Superficial inguinal ring
13 External pudendal vein
14 Spermatic cord with genital branch of genitofemoral nerve
15 Penis with superficial dorsal vein of penis
16 Testis and its coverings
17 Saphenous nerve
18 Infrapatellar branch of saphenous nerve
19 Lateral sural cutaneous nerves
20 Intermediate dorsal cutaneous branch of superficial peroneal nerve
21 Cutaneous branch of obturator nerve
22 Superficial peroneal nerve
23 Medial dorsal cutaneous branch of superficial peroneal nerve
24 Deep peroneal nerve
25 **Femoral nerve**
26 **Femoral artery**
27 Superficial epigastric vein
28 **Femoral vein**
29 Lateral dorsal cutaneous branch of sural nerve
30 **Inguinal nodes** (enlarged)
31 Lympathic vessels
32 Sartorius muscle

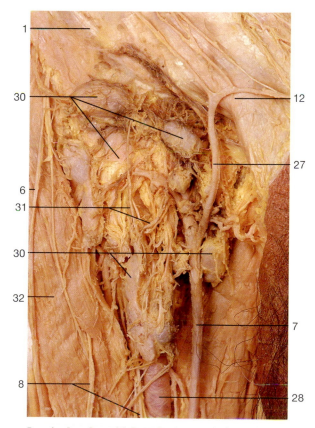

Cutaneous nerves and veins of thigh (anterior aspect).
The fascia lata and fasciae of the thigh muscles have been removed.

Inguinal nodes with lymphatic vessels (anterior aspect).

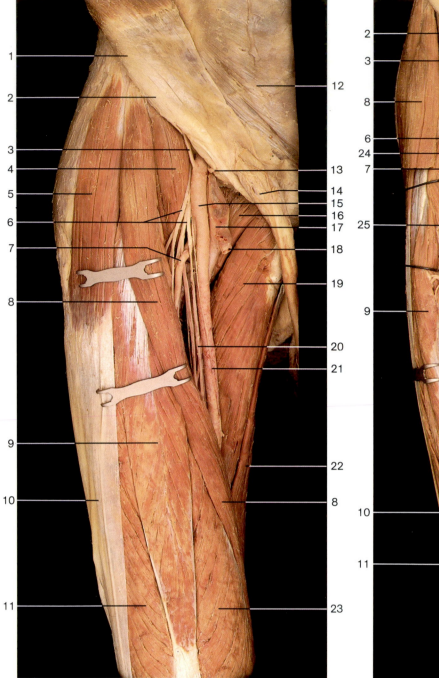

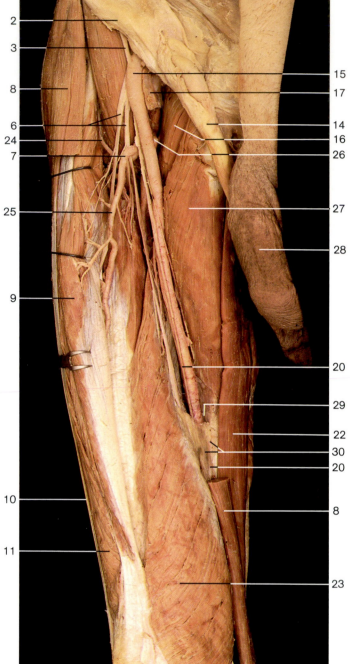

Anterior region of right thigh (ventral aspect).
The fascia lata has been removed, and the sartorius has been slightly reflected.

Anterior region of right thigh (ventral aspect).
The fascia lata has been removed, and the sartorius has been divided.

1 Anterior superior iliac spine
2 Inguinal ligament
3 Deep circumflex iliac artery
4 Iliopsoas
5 Tensor fasciae latae
6 Femoral nerve
7 Lateral circumflex femoral artery
8 Sartorius
9 Rectus femoris
10 Iliotibial tract
11 Vastus lateralis
12 Anterior sheath of rectus abdominis
13 Inferior epigastric artery
14 Spermatic cord
15 Femoral artery

16 Pectineus
17 Femoral vein
18 Great saphenous vein (divided)
19 Adductor longus
20 Saphenous nerve
21 Muscular branch of femoral nerve
22 Gracilis
23 Vastus medialis
24 Ascending branch of lateral circumflex femoral artery
25 Descending branch of lateral circumflex femoral artery
26 Medial circumflex femoral artery
27 Adductor longus
28 Penis
29 Entrance to adductor canal
30 Vastoadductory lamina of fascia beneath sartorius

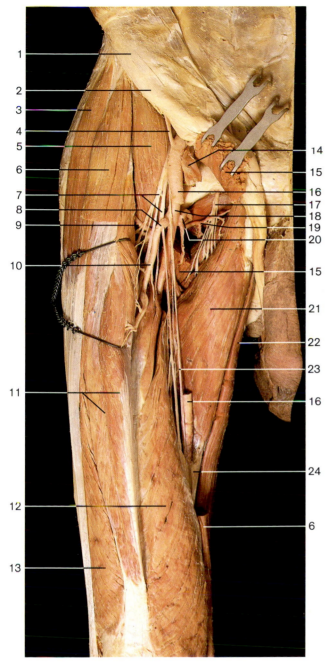

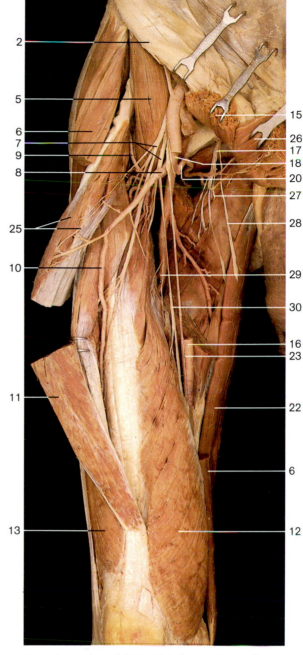

Anterior region of right thigh (ventral aspect).
The fascia lata has been removed. Sartorius, pectineus and femoral artery have been divided, to display the deep femoral artery with its branches. The rectus femoris has been slightly reflected.

Anterior region of right thigh (ventral aspect).
The sartorius, pectineus, adductor longus and rectus femoris have been divided and reflected. The greater part of the femoral artery has been removed.

1 Anterior superior iliac spine
2 Inguinal ligament
3 Tensor fasciae latae
4 Deep circumflex iliac artery
5 Iliopsoas
6 Sartorius (divided)
7 **Femoral nerve**
8 **Lateral circumflex femoral artery**
9 Ascending branch of lateral circumflex femoral artery
10 Descending branch of lateral circumflex femoral artery
11 Rectus femoris
12 Vastus medialis
13 Vastus lateralis
14 Femoral vein
15 Pectineus (divided)
16 Femoral artery (divided)

17 **Obturator nerve**
18 **Profunda femoris artery**
19 Ascending branch of medial circumflex femoral artery
20 **Medial circumflex femoral artery**
21 Adductor longus
22 Gracilis
23 Saphenous nerve
24 Distal part of vastoadductory lamina
25 Rectus femoris with muscular branch of femoral nerve
26 Adductor longus (divided)
27 Posterior branch of obturator nerve
28 Anterior branch of obturator nerve
29 Point at which perforating artery branches off from profunda femoris artery
30 Muscular branch to vastus medialis

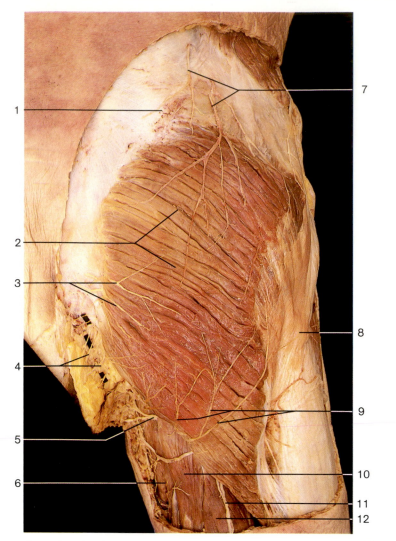

1 Iliac crest
2 Gluteus maximus
3 **Middle clunial nerves**
4 Anococcygeal nerves
5 Perineal branch of posterior femoral cutaneous nerve
6 Adductor magnus
7 **Superior clunial nerves**
8 Position of greater trochanter
9 **Inferior clunial nerves**
10 Semitendinosus
11 Posterior femoral cutaneous nerve
12 Long head of biceps femoris
13 Sacrotuberous ligament
14 **Sciatic nerve**
15 Quadratus femoris
16 Gluteus maximus (divided)
17 Tensor fasciae latae
18 Inferior gluteal nerve
19 Gluteus medius
20 **Piriformis**
21 Superior gemellus
22 Tendon of obturator internus
23 Inferior gemellus

Gluteal region (right side, dorsal aspect).

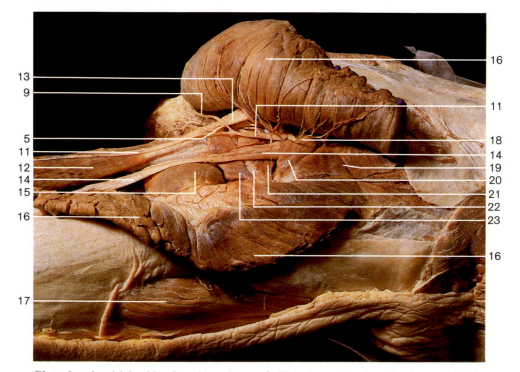

Gluteal region (right side, dorsolateral aspect). The gluteus maximus has been divided and reflected.

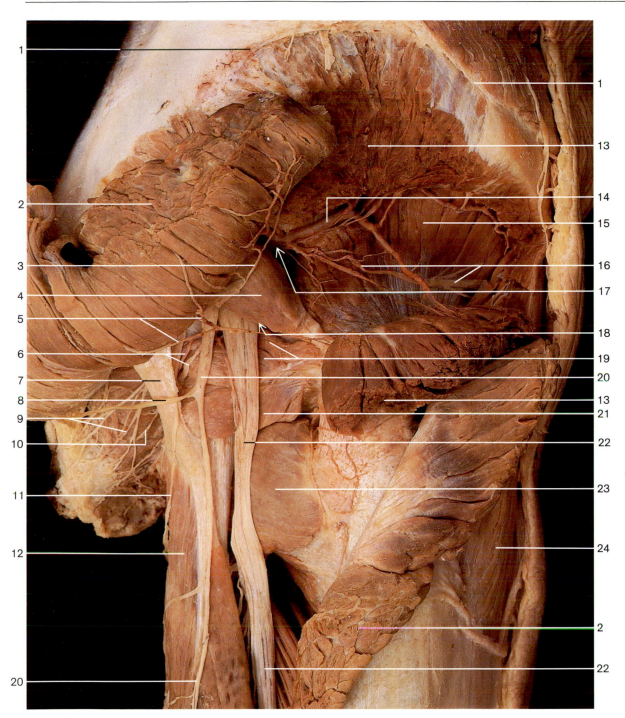

Gluteal region (right side, dorsal aspect). The gluteus maximus and gluteus medius have been divided and reflected. Notice the position of the foramina above and below piriformis and the lesser sciatic foramen.

1 Iliac crest
2 Gluteus maximus (divided)
3 Inferior gluteal nerve
4 Piriformis
5 Muscular branches
6 Pudendal nerve and internal pudendal artery within the
   lesser sciatic foramen (entrance to the pudendal canal)
7 Sacrotuberous ligament
8 Inferior clunial nerve
9 Inferior rectal nerves
10 Inferior rectal arteries
11 Perforating cutaneous nerve
12 Long head of biceps femoris

13 Gluteus medius (divided)
14 Deep branch of superior gluteal artery
15 Gluteus minimus
16 Superior gluteal nerve
17 **Suprapiriform foramen** } greater sciatic foramen
18 **Infrapiriform foramen** }
19 Tendon of obturator internus and superior gemellus
20 Posterior femoral cutaneous nerve
21 Inferior gemellus
22 **Sciatic nerve**
23 Quadratus femoris
24 Tensor fasciae latae

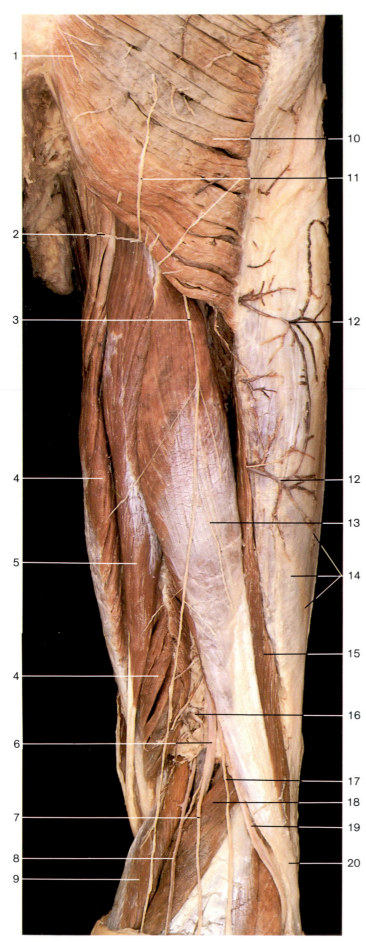

1   Middle clunial nerves
2   Perineal branch of posterior femoral cutaneous nerve
3   Posterior femoral cutaneous nerve
4   Semimembranosus
5   Semitendinosus
6   Tibial nerve
7   Medial sural cutaneous nerve
8   Small saphenous vein
9   Medial head of gastrocnemius
10 Gluteus maximus
11 Inferior clunial nerve
12 Cutaneous veins
13 Long head of biceps femoris
14 Iliotibial tract
15 Short head of biceps femoris
16 Popliteal fossa
17 Lateral sural cutaneous nerve
18 Lateral head of gastrocnemius
19 Common peroneal nerve
20 Tendon of biceps femoris
21 Inferior gluteal nerve
22 Sacrotuberous ligament
23 Inferior rectal branches of pudendal nerve
24 Anus
25 Gluteus medius
26 Piriformis
27 Sciatic nerve
28 Inferior gluteal artery
29 Gluteus maximus (divided)
30 Quadratus femoris
31 Sciatic nerve dividing into its two branches; the common peroneal nerve and the tibial nerve
32 Muscular branches of sciatic nerve to hamstring muscles
33 Popliteal artery
34 Popliteal vein
35 Small saphenous vein (divided)
36 Long head of biceps femoris (divided)
37 Superficial peroneal nerve

Cutaneous nerves of thigh (posterior aspect).
The fascia lata and the fasciae of muscles have been removed.

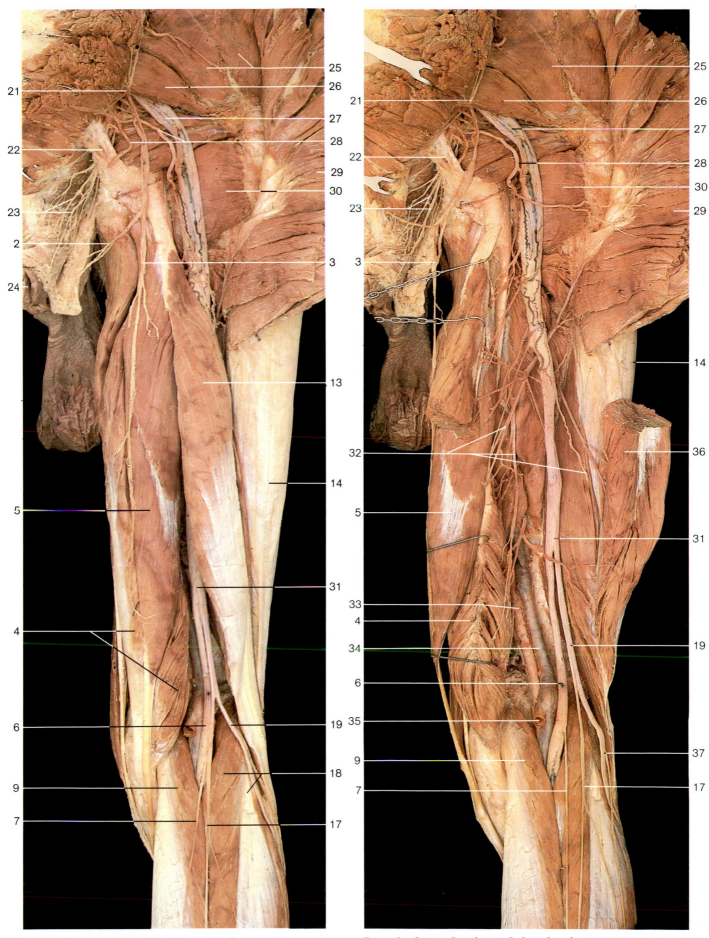

Posterior femoral region and gluteal region
(right side, dorsal aspect). The gluteus maximus has been divided and reflected.

Posterior femoral region and gluteal region
(right side, dorsal aspect). The gluteus maximus and the long head of biceps femoris have been divided and reflected.

443

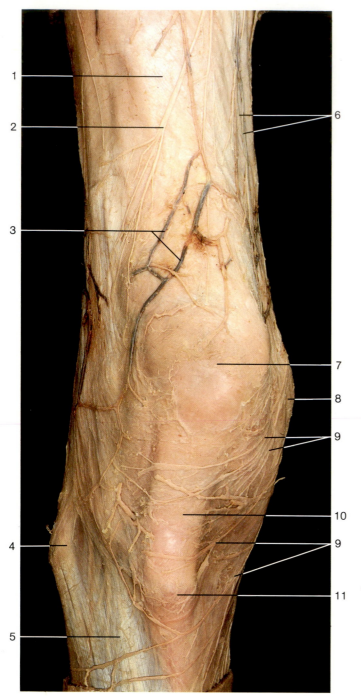

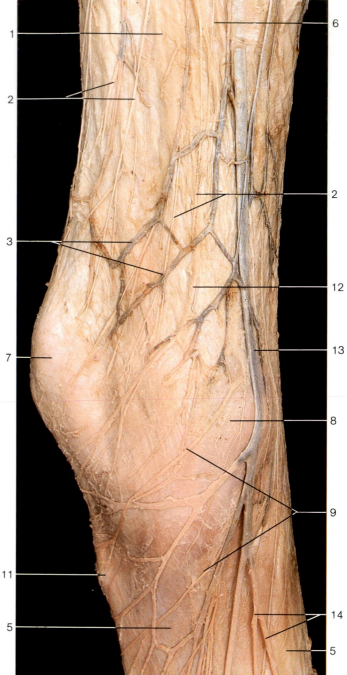

Anterior region of right knee; cutaneous nerves and veins (ventral aspect).

Right knee; cutaneous nerves and veins (medial aspect).

1 Fascia lata
2 Terminal branches of anterior cutaneous branches of femoral nerve
3 Venous network around knee
4 Position of head of fibula
5 Fascia cruris
6 Cutaneous branch of obturator nerve
7 Patella

8 Position of medial epicondyle of femur
9 Infrapatellar branches of saphenous nerve
10 Patellar ligament
11 Position of tuberosity of tibia
12 Terminal branch of anterior cutaneous branch of femoral nerve
13 Great saphenous vein
14 Tributaries of great saphenous vein from leg

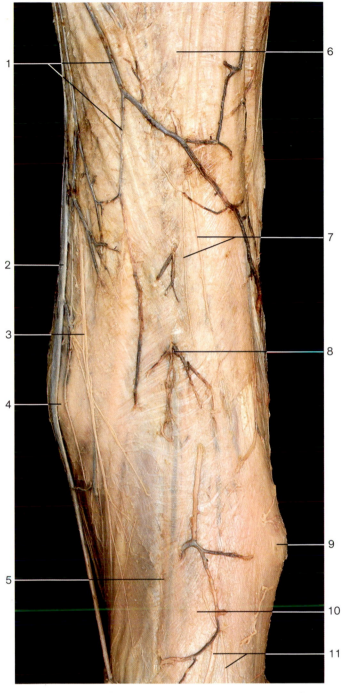

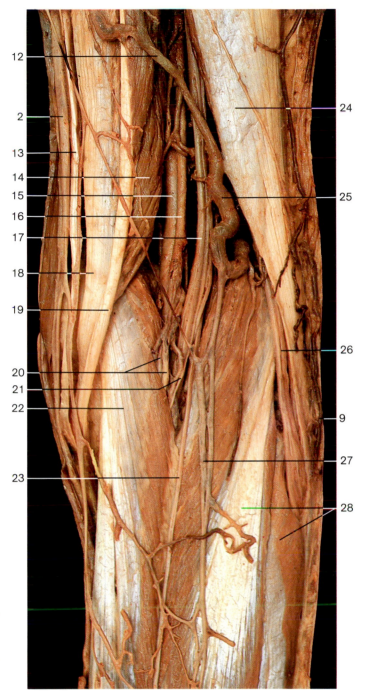

Posterior region of right knee; cutaneous nerves and veins (dorsal aspect).

Right popliteal fossa (dorsal aspect). The fasciae have been removed.

1 Cutaneous veins (tributaries of great saphenous vein)	15 **Popliteal artery**
2 Great saphenous vein	16 **Popliteal vein**
3 Cutaneous branch of femoral nerve	17 **Tibial nerve**
4 Position of medial epicondyle of femur	18 Tendon of semimembranosus
5 Position of small saphenous vein	19 Tendon of semitendinosus
6 Fascia lata	20 Sural artery and vein
7 Terminal branches of posterior femoral cutaneous nerve	21 Muscular branch of tibial nerve
8 Cutaneous veins of popliteal fossa	22 Medial head of gastrocnemius
9 Position of head of fibula	23 Medial sural cutaneous nerve
10 Superficial layer of fascia cruris	24 Biceps femoris
11 Lateral sural cutaneous nerve	25 Varicosity of vein
12 Superficial vein	26 Common peroneal nerve
13 Tendon of gracilis	27 Small saphenous vein
14 Semimembranosus	28 Lateral head of gastrocnemius

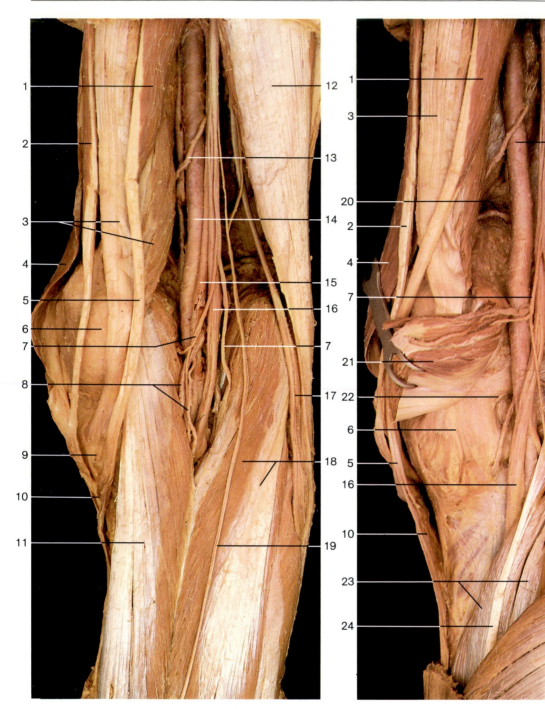

Right leg, posterior crural region (dorsal aspect).
The gastrocnemius has been divided and reflected.

Right leg, posterior crural region (deep layer, dorsal aspect). The
gastrocnemius and the soleus have been divided and reflected.

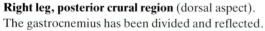

1 Semitendinosus	15 **Popliteal vein**
2 Gracilis	16 **Tibial nerve**
3 Semimembranosus	17 **Common peroneal nerve**
4 Sartorius	18 Lateral head of gastrocnemius
5 Tendon of semitendinosus	19 Medial sural cutaneous nerve
6 Position of medial condyle of femur	20 Medial superior genicular artery
7 Muscular branches of tibial nerve	21 Medial head of gastrocnemius (divided and reflected)
8 Sural arteries and veins	22 Medial inferior genicular artery
9 Tendon of semimembranosus	23 Soleus
10 Common tendon of gracilis, semitendinosus and sartorius	24 Tendon of plantaris
11 Medial head of gastrocnemius	25 Lateral superior genicular artery
12 Biceps femoris	26 Lateral inferior genicular artery
13 Muscular branch of popliteal artery	27 Plantaris
14 **Popliteal artery**	

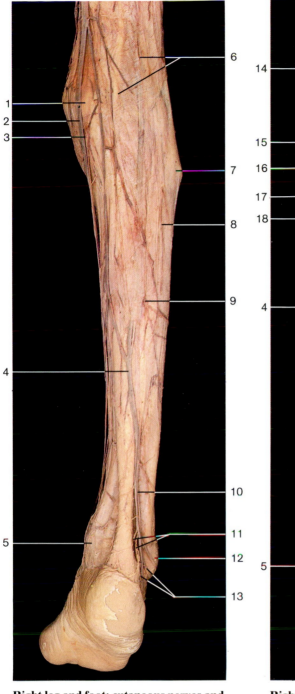
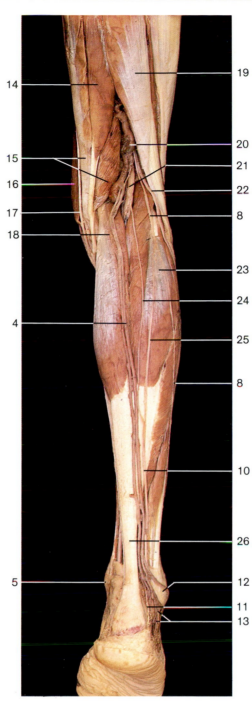

Right leg and foot; cutaneous nerves and veins (dorsal aspect).

Right leg and foot; cutaneous nerves and veins (dorsal aspect). The crural fascia and fasciae of the muscles have been removed.

1 Position of medial condyle of femur	14 Semitendinosus
2 Great saphenous vein	15 Semimembranosus
3 Saphenous nerve	16 Sartorius
4 Small saphenous vein	17 Tendon of gracilis
5 Medial malleolus	18 Medial head of gastrocnemius
6 Terminal branches of posterior femoral cutaneous nerve	19 Biceps femoris
7 Position of head of fibula	20 Varicosity of vein (pathological)
8 Lateral sural cutaneous nerve	21 **Tibial nerve**
9 Perforating vein (anastomosis between superficial and deep veins)	22 **Common peroneal nerve**
10 **Sural nerve**	23 Lateral head of gastrocnemius
11 Lateral calcaneal branches of sural nerve	24 Medial sural cutaneous nerve
12 Lateral malleolus	25 Communicating branch of peroneal nerve
13 Venous network	26 Tendo calcaneus

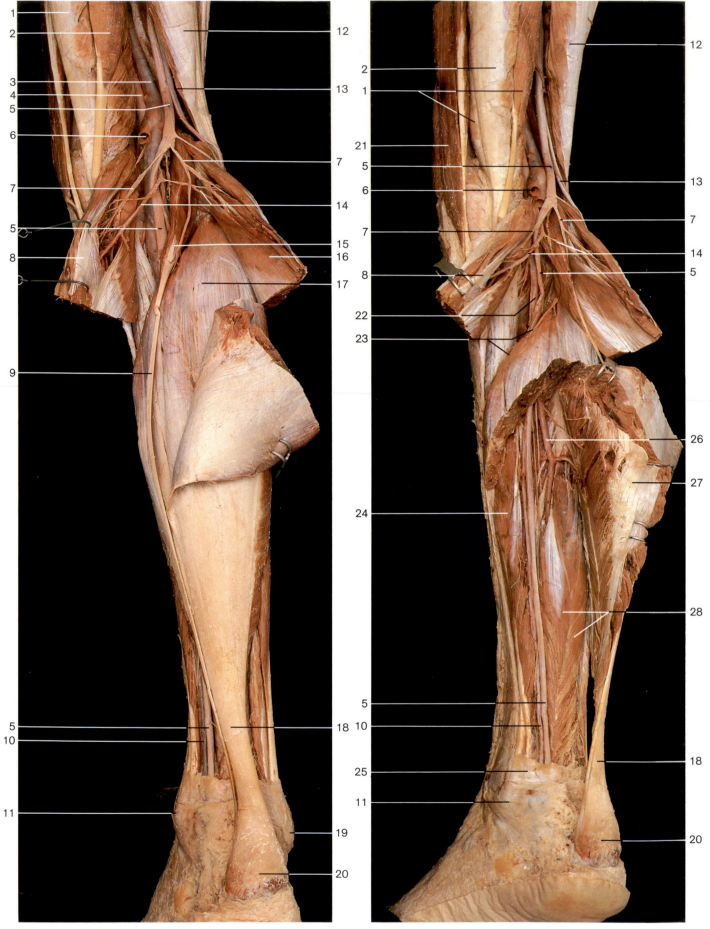

Right popliteal fossa, middle layer (dorsal aspect).
The cutaneous veins and nerves have been removed.

Right popliteal fossa, deep layer (dorsal aspect).
The medial head of gastrocnemius has been divided and
reflected.

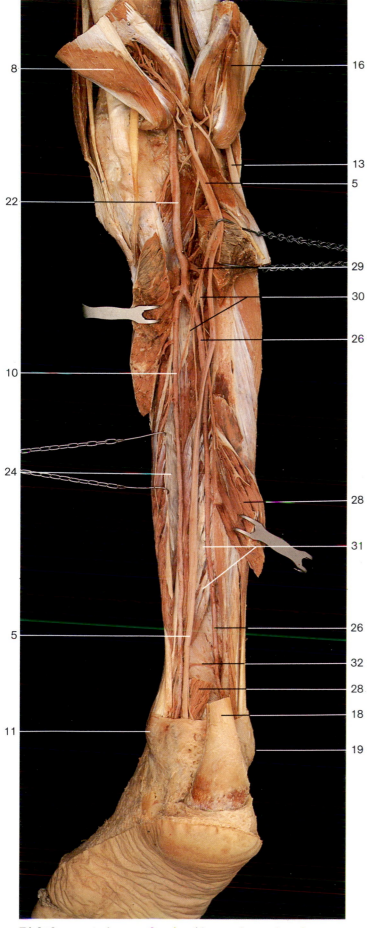

1 Semimembranosus
2 Semitendinosus
3 Popliteal vein
4 Popliteal artery
5 Tibial nerve
6 Small saphenous vein (divided)
7 Muscular branch of tibial nerve
8 Medial head of gastrocnemius
9 Tendon of plantaris
10 Posterior tibial artery
11 Medial malleolus
12 Biceps femoris
13 Common peroneal nerve
14 Sural arteries
15 Plantaris
16 Lateral head of gastrocnemius
17 Soleus
18 Achilles or calcaneal tendon
19 Lateral malleolus
20 Calcaneal tuberosity
21 Sartorius
22 Popliteal artery
23 Tendinous arch of soleus
24 Flexor digitorum longus
25 Flexor retinaculum
26 Peroneal artery
27 Triceps surae (divided)
28 Flexor hallucis longus
29 Anterior tibial artery
30 Muscular branches of tibial nerve
31 Tibialis posterior
32 Communicating branch of peroneal artery

Right leg, posterior crural region (deepest layer, dorsal aspect). The triceps surae and the long flexor hallucis have been divided and reflected.

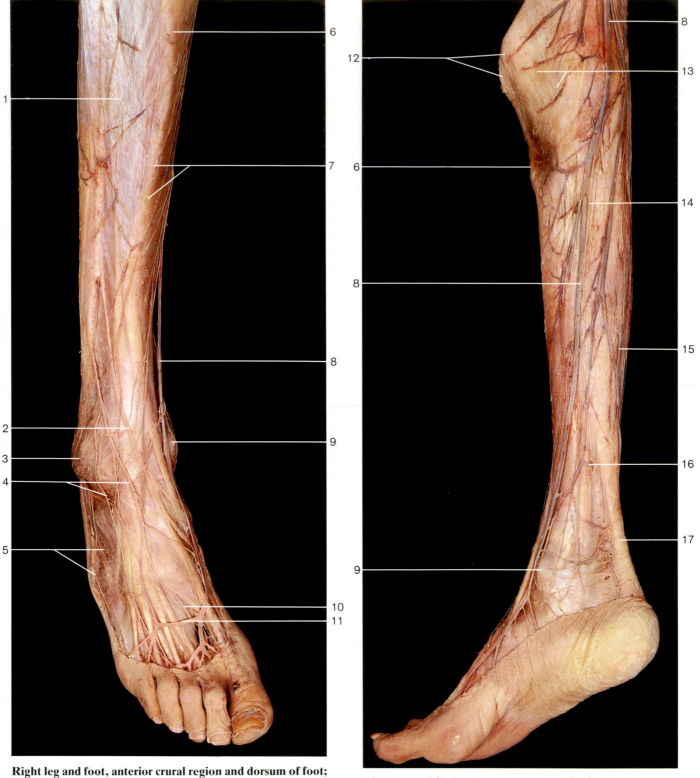

Right leg and foot, anterior crural region and dorsum of foot; cutaneous nerves and veins (ventral aspect).

Right leg and foot; cutaneous nerves and veins (medial aspect).

1   Fascia cruris
2   Medial cutaneous branch of superficial peroneal nerve
3   Lateral malleolus
4   Lateral cutaneous branch of superficial peroneal nerve
5   Cutaneous branch of sural nerve
6   Position of tuberosity of tibia
7   Anterior margin of tibia
8   Great saphenous vein
9   Medial malleolus

10   Deep peroneal nerve
11   Venous arch of dorsum of foot
12   Position of patella
13   Infrapatellar branches of saphenous nerve
14   Saphenous nerve
15   Small saphenous vein
16   Perforating vein
17   Tendo calcaneus

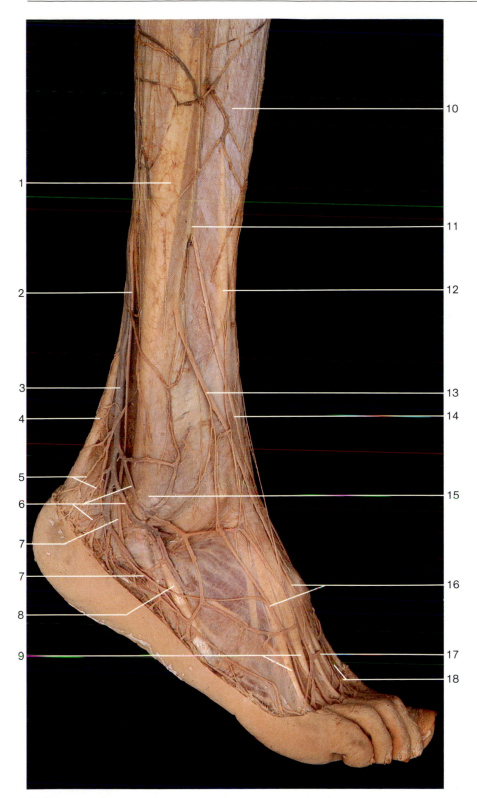

Right leg and dorsum of foot; cutaneous nerves and veins (lateral aspect).

1	Position of fibula	10	Fascia cruris
2	Sural nerve	11	Superficial peroneal nerve
3	Small saphenous vein	12	Position of tibia
4	Tendo calcaneus	13	Lateral cutaneous branch
5	Lateral calcaneal branches of sural nerve	14	Medial cutaneous branch ⎫ of superficial peroneal nerve
6	Venous network at lateral malleolus	15	Lateral malleolus
7	Cutaneous branch of sural nerve	16	Dorsal digital nerves
8	Tendon of peroneus brevis	17	Dorsal venous arch
9	Tendons of extensor digitorum longus	18	Deep peroneal nerve

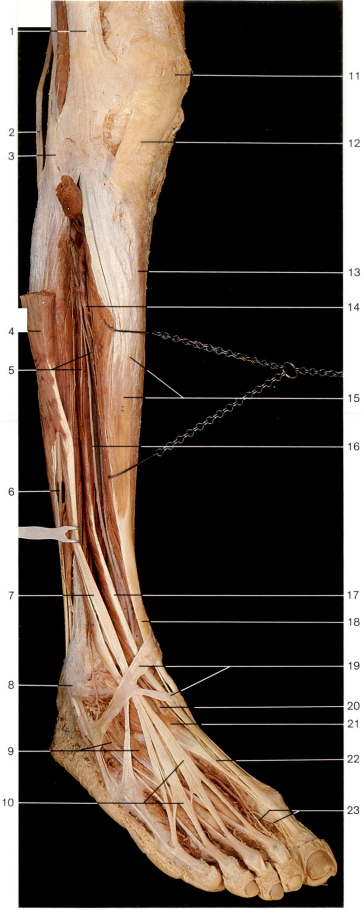

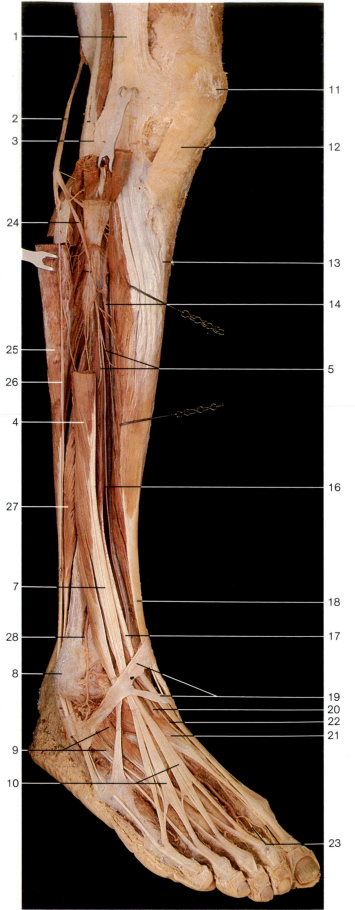

Right leg and dorsum of foot, middle layer (oblique anterior aspect). The extensor digitorum longus has been divided and reflected laterally.

Right leg, deep layer (oblique anterior aspect). The extensor digitorum longus and the peroneus longus have been divided or removed. The common peroneal nerve has been elevated to show its course around the head of fibula.

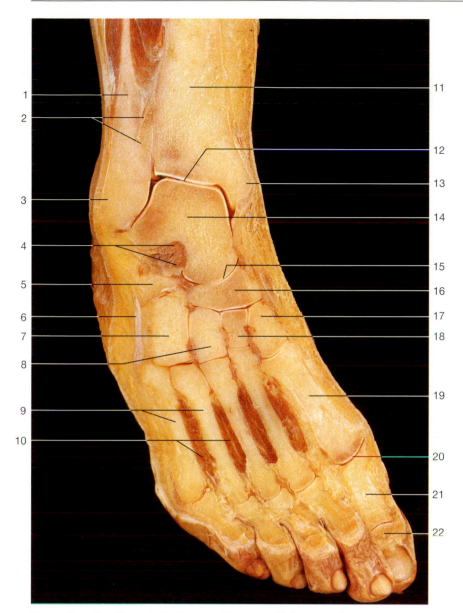

1 Fibula
2 Distal tibiofibular joint (syndesmosis)
3 Lateral malleolus
4 Interosseous talocalcaneal ligament
5 Calcaneus
6 Tendon of peroneus brevis
7 Cuboid bone
8 Lateral cuneiform bone
9 Metatarsal bones
10 Dorsal interosseous muscles
11 Tibia
12 **Talocrural joint**
13 Medial malleolus
14 Talus
15 **Talocalcaneonavicular joint**
16 Navicular bone
17 Medial cuneiform bone
18 Intermediate cuneiform bone
19 First metatarsal bone
20 Metatarsophalangeal joint of great toe
21 Proximal phalanx of great toe
22 Distal phalanx of great toe

Coronal section through the foot, and talocrural joint (anterior aspect).

◁

To page 452:

1 Iliotibial tract
2 **Common peroneal nerve**
3 Position of head of fibula
4 Extensor digitorum longus
5 Muscular branches of deep peroneal nerve
6 **Superficial peroneal nerve**
7 Tendon of extensor digitorum longus
8 Lateral malleolus
9 Extensor digitorum brevis
10 Tendons of extensor digitorum longus
11 Patella
12 Patellar ligament
13 Anterior margin of tibia
14 **Anterior tibial artery**
15 Tibialis anterior

16 Deep peroneal nerve
17 Extensor hallucis longus
18 Tendon of tibialis anterior
19 Extensor retinaculum
20 Dorsalis pedis artery
21 Extensor hallucis brevis
22 Deep peroneal nerve (on dorsum of foot)
23 Dorsal digital nerves (terminal branches of deep peroneal nerve)
24 **Deep peroneal nerve**
25 Peroneus longus (divided)
26 Superficial peroneal nerve (with peroneal muscles laterally reflected)
27 Peroneus brevis
28 Lateral anterior malleolar artery

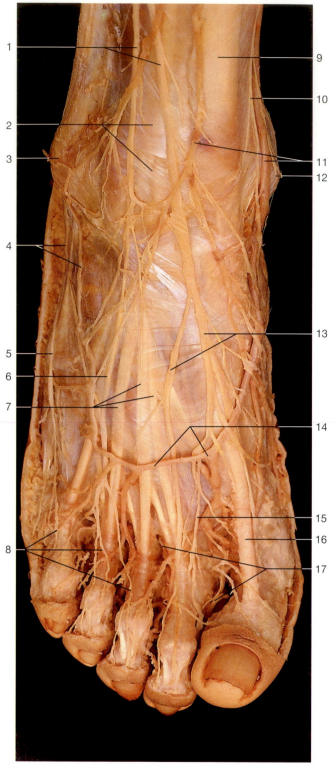

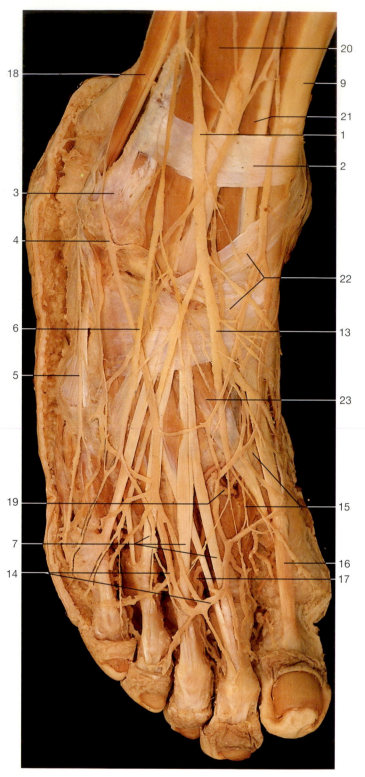

Dorsum of the right foot, superficial layer (anterior aspect).

Dorsum of the right foot, superficial layer. The fascia of the dorsum has been removed.

1 **Superficial peroneal nerve**
2 Superior extensor retinaculum
3 Lateral malleolus
4 Venous network of lateral malleolus, tributaries of small saphenous vein
5 Lateral dorsal cutaneous nerve (branch of sural nerve)
6 Intermediate dorsal cutaneous nerve
7 Tendons of extensor digitorum longus
8 Dorsal digital nerves

9 Tendon of tibialis anterior
10 **Saphenous nerve**
11 Venous network of medial malleolus, tributaries of great saphenous vein
12 Medial malleolus
13 Medial dorsal cutaneous nerves
14 **Dorsal venous arch**
15 Dorsal digital nerve (of deep peroneal nerve)

16 Tendon of extensor hallucis longus
17 Dorsal digital arteries
18 Peroneal muscles
19 Deep plantar branch of dorsalis pedis artery anastomosing with plantar arch
20 Extensor digitorum longus
21 Extensor hallucis longus
22 Inferior extensor retinaculum
23 Extensor hallucis brevis

1 Extensor retinaculum
2 Lateral malleolus
3 Lateral anterior malleolar artery
4 Tendons of peroneal muscles
5 Tendon of peroneus tertius
6 Extensor digitorum brevis
7 Tendons of extensor digitorum longus
8 Dorsal metatarsal arteries
9 Medial malleolus
10 Tendon of tibialis anterior
11 **Dorsalis pedis artery**
12 Deep peroneal nerve (on dorsum of foot)
13 Extensor hallucis brevis
14 Tendon of extensor hallucis longus
15 Dorsalis pedis artery with deep plantar branch to the plantar arch
16 Dorsal digital nerves (terminal branches of deep peroneal nerve)
17 Lateral tarsal artery
18 Extensor digitorum brevis (divided)
19 Arcuate artery
20 Dorsal interosseous muscles
21 **Deep peroneal nerve**

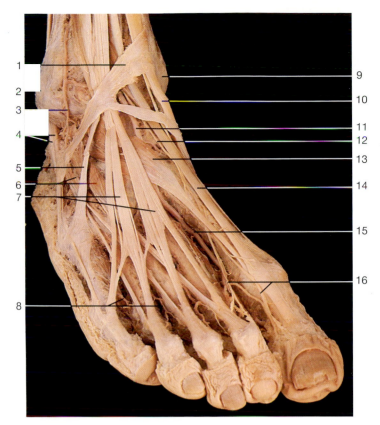

Dorsum of right foot, middle layer (anterior aspect).
The cutaneous nerves have been removed.

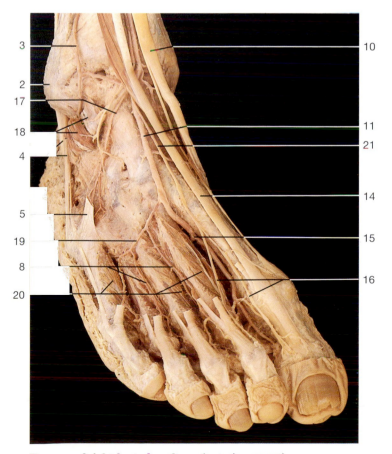

Dorsum of right foot, deep layer (anterior aspect).
The extensor digitorum and hallucis breves have been removed.

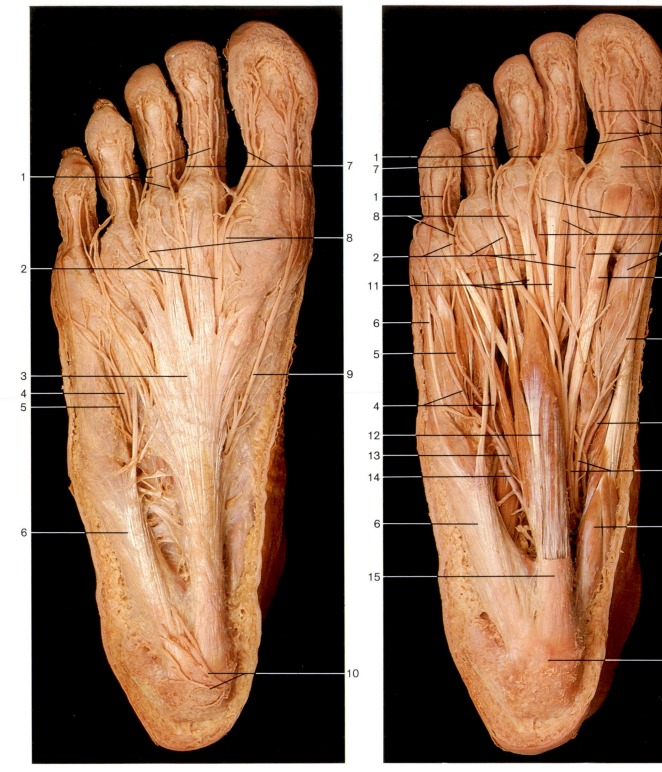

Sole of the right foot (superficial layer) (from below); dissection of cutaneous nerves and vessels.

Sole of the right foot (middle layer) (from below). The plantar aponeurosis has been removed.

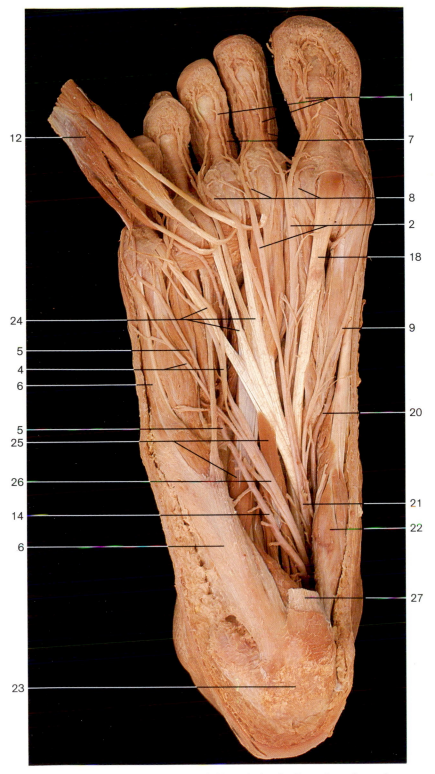

1 Proper plantar digital nerves
2 Common plantar digital nerves
3 Plantar aponeurosis
4 Superficial branch of lateral plantar nerve
5 Superficial branch of lateral plantar artery
6 Abductor digiti minimi
7 Proper plantar digital arteries
8 Common plantar digital arteries
9 Digital branch of medial plantar nerve to great toe
10 Medial calcaneal branches
11 Tendons of flexor digitorum brevis
12 Flexor digitorum brevis
13 **Superficial branch of lateral plantar nerve**
14 **Lateral plantar artery**
15 Plantar aponeurosis (remnant)
16 Digital synovial sheath
17 Lumbrical muscles
18 Tendon of flexor hallucis longus
19 Flexor hallucis brevis
20 **Medial plantar artery**
21 **Medial plantar nerve**
22 Abductor hallucis
23 Tuber calcanei
24 Tendons of flexor digitorum longus
25 Quadratus plantae
26 **Lateral plantar nerve**
27 Flexor digitorum brevis (divided)

Sole of the right foot (middle layer) (from below); dissection of vessels and nerves. The flexor digitorum brevis has been divided and anteriorly reflected.

457

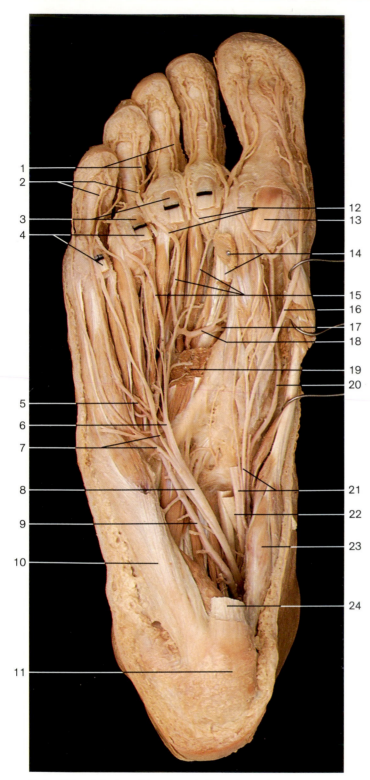

1 Proper plantar digital arteries
2 Proper plantar digital nerves
3 Tendons of flexor digitorum brevis
4 Tendons of flexor digitorum longus
5 Superficial branch of lateral plantar artery
6 Deep branch of lateral plantar nerve
7 Superficial branch of lateral plantar nerve
8 **Lateral plantar nerve**
9 **Lateral plantar artery**
10 Abductor digiti minimi
11 Tuber calcanei
12 Common plantar digital arteries
13 Tendon of flexor hallucis longus
14 Insertion of both heads of adductor hallucis
15 Plantar metatarsal arteries
16 Medial plantar nerve of great toe
17 Deep plantar branch of dorsalis pedis artery
   (perforating branch)
18 **Plantar arch**
19 Oblique head of adductor hallucis (divided)
20 **Medial plantar artery**
21 **Medial plantar nerve**
22 Crossing of tendons in sole of foot
23 Abductor hallucis
24 Origin of flexor digitorum brevis

Sole of the right foot (deep layer) (from below); dissection of
vessels and nerves. The flexor digitorum brevis, the
quadratus plantae with the tendons of the flexor digitorum
longus and some branches of the medial plantar nerve have
been removed. The flexor hallucis brevis has been
fenestrated to show the somewhat atypical course of the
medial plantar artery.

Index

461

superior 159, 220, 228–230, 235, 237, 243–247, 254, 256, 258, 259, 370
Vena vorticosa 124, 130
Venous sinuses 85
Ventricles of brain, fourth 91, 97, 108, 114
    lateral 102, 110, 112, 113
    third 91, 102, 108–110, 113
  of heart 228, 299
    left 235, 236, 242–244, 247, 259, 261
    right 235, 236, 242–244, 247, 256, 261
Vermis of cerebellum 98, 110, 217
    folium of 98
    uvula of 98
Vertebra(e) 5, 176
  arch of 177
  body of 177
  cervical 142, 147, 176, 178
  joints of 184
  lumbar 174, 176
  thoracic 176, 178, 181
    ligaments of 181

Vesicle, seminal 310–314, 316–318, 321
Vessel(s); *see* Artery, Vein, Lymph vessels
Vestibular apparatus 116
Vestibule 120
  aqueduct of 121
  bulb of 335, 336
  of oral cavity 53
  of vagina 326, 328, 334
Villi, intestinal 267
Vinculum breve, of tendon of finger 364
  longum 364
Visual pathway 128
Vomer 43–46
  ala of 46

W

Wall, abdominal, anterior 192–196
    structures on 278
    posterior 291, 293

    structures on 306, 307
  thoracic and abdominal 187, 191
    anterior 188, 238, 239
    posterior, structures on 306
Walls of tympanic cavity 119
Window, round 119
Wing, greater, of sphenoid bone 29, 38
  lesser 29, 38
Wrist, skeleton of 348
  ligaments of 352

Z

Zygomatic arch 24, 49, 55, 61
Zonula fibers 124